AF182557

J.G. Grudzinskas, M.G. Chapman, T. Chard
and O. Djahanbakhch (Eds.)

# The Fallopian Tube

## Clinical and Surgical Aspects

With 87 Figures

Springer-Verlag
London Berlin Heidelberg New York
Paris Tokyo Hong Kong
Barcelona Budapest

Jurgis G. Grudzinskas, MB BS, BSc, MD, FRCOG, FRACOG
Professor, Academic Unit of Obstetrics and Gynaecology, 4th Floor, Holland Wing, The Royal London Hospital, Whitechapel, London E1 1BB, UK

Michael G. Chapman, MB BS, MRCOG
Professor, Department of Obstetrics and Gynaecology, Guy's Hospital, New Guy's House (2nd Floor), London Bridge, London SE1 9RT, UK

Timothy Chard, MD, FRCOG
Professor, Department of Reproductive Physiology, St Bartholomew's Hospital, Medical College, West Smithfield, London EC1A 7BE, UK

Ovrang Djahanbakhch
Senior Lecturer, Department of Obstetrics and Gynaecology, Newham General Hospital, London E13 8SL and Academic Unit of Obstetrics and Gynaecology, The Royal London Hospital, Whitechapel, London E1 1BB, UK

*Front cover illustration:* Montage of Fig.3.1, Schematised secretory, ciliary, peg and indifferent cells *[see p. 38]* and Fig.7.3, LEC-falloposcope system (with kind permission from Imagyn Medical, Inc) *[see p. 101]*.

ISBN-13: 978-1-4471-1989-0 e-ISBN-13: 978-1-4471-1987-6
DOI: 10.1007/978-1-4471-1987-6

British Library Cataloguing in Publication Data
Fallopian Tube: Clinical and Surgical Aspects
I. Grudzinskas, J. G.
618.1
ISBN-13: 978-1-4471-1989-0

Library of Congress Cataloging-in-Publication Data
The Fallopian tube: clinical and surgical aspects / J.G. Grudzinskas . . . [et al.] eds.
p. cm.
Includes bibliographical references and index.
ISBN-13: 978-1-4471-1989-0 (alk. paper)
1. Fallopian tubes—Congresses. 2. Fallopian tubes—Diseases—Congresses. 3. Fallopian tubes—Surgery—Congresses. 4. Tubal pregnancy—Congresses. I. Grudzinskas, J.G. (Jurgis Gediminas)
[DNLM: 1. Fallopian Tube Diseases—congresses. 2. Fallopian Tubes—pathology—congresses. 3. Fallopian Tubes—pathology—congresses. WP 300 F1964 1993]
RG421.F36 1993
618.1—dc20
DNLM/DLC
for Library of Congress 93-34147

Apart from any fair dealing for the purposes of research or private study, or criticism or review, as permitted under the Copyright, Designs and Patents Act 1988, this publication may only be reproduced, stored or transmitted, in any form or by any means, with the prior permission in writing of the publishers, or in the case of reprographic reproduction in accordance with the terms of licences issued by the Copyright Licensing Agency. Enquiries concerning reproduction outside those terms should be sent to the publishers.

© Springer-Verlag London Limited 1994
Softcover reprint of the hardcover 1st edition 1994

The publisher makes no representation, express or implied, with regard to the accuracy of the information contained in this book and cannot accept any legal responsibility or liability for any errors or omissions that may be made.

Typeset by Asco Trade Typesetting Ltd., Hong Kong
69/3830-543210 Printed on acid-free paper

# Preface

The examination of the human fallopian tubes was, until recently, restricted to observations on gross anatomical disposition and tubal patency. These studies, for decades, were the domain of doctors and physiologists whose primary interest was population control and family planning, funded largely by organisations and agencies seeking alternatives to steroidal contraceptives. For a "worrying" but short period after the birth of Louise Brown in 1978 as the consequence of successful in-vitro fertilisation and embryo transfer, the fallopian tube was considered to be "dispensable" given that the metabolic milieu in which human fertilisation takes place could be effortlessly reproduced in a Petri dish, in in-vitro fertilisation procedures.

However, a number of factors have acted together to renew interest in the fallopian tube, namely new techniques in cell biology, microinstrument developments (in particular in imaging), an interdisciplinary transfer of skills from interventional radiology and cardiology to gynaecology, the surgeon's wish to improve surgical techniques, and better techniques to monitor early pregnancy. These factors have led surgeons to develop the new diagnostic and therapeutic strategies and techniques listed here. This volume contains contributions from the majority of keynote speakers at a conference held in London in April 1992 from which its title is derived. Better diagnostic procedures should lead to the implementation of rational effective treatments. This is the recurring theme throughout this volume, the principal change in therapeutic strategies being the diminished extent of ablative surgery used either in tubal disease or tubal ectopic pregnancy. The case for medical treatment of ectopic pregnancy, as well as expectant management, is also discussed here.

Since the birth of Louise Brown, the fallopian tube can no longer be claimed to have been traversed by each and every one of us, but the new information makes it no less interesting or important an organ. The majority of the contributions to this volume argue this case strongly.

# Contents

# Contributors

J.C. Anderson
Sydney IVF, 187 Macquarie Street, Sydney 2000, Australia

C.L.R. Barratt
University Department of Obstetrics and Gynaecology, Jessop Hospital for Women, Sheffield S3 7RE, UK

S. de Blok
Onze Lieve Vrounwe Gasthuis, le Oosterparkstraat 179, 1091 HA Amsterdam, The Netherlands

A. Bongso
Department of Obstetrics and Gynaecology, National University of Singapore, Kent Ridge, Singapore 0511

I.A. Brewis
Department of Molecular Biology and Biotechnology, University of Sheffield, Sheffield, S10 2UH, UK

I.A. Brosens
Department of Obstetrics and Gynaecology, University Hospital Gasthuisberg, B-3000 Leuven, Belgium

B. Cacciatore
Departments I and II, Obstetrics and Gynaecology, Helsinki University Hospital, Helsinki, Finland

O. Djahanbakhch
Department of Obstetrics And Gynaecology, Newham General Hospital, London E13 8SL, UK

L.J. Edwards
Department of Biology, University of York, Heslington, York YO1 5DD, UK

M.H. Emanuel
Spaarne Hospital, Department of Obstetrics and Gynaecology, Van Heythuijzenweg 1, PO Box 1644, 2003 BR Haarlem, The Netherlands

G.M. Filshie
Department of Obstetrics and Gynaecology, University Hospital, Queen's Medical Centre, Nottingham NG7 2UH, UK

C.-Y. Fong
Department of Obstetrics and Gynaecology, National University of Singapore, Kent Ridge, Singapore 0511

R. Forman
Guy's Hospital, London SE1 9RT, UK

N. Gleicher
Department of Obstetrics and Gynaecology, Immunology/ Microbiology, University of Health Sciences, The Chicago Medical School, North Chicago, Illinois, USA

V. Gomel
Department of Obstetrics and Gynaecology, University of British Columbia, Vancouver, BC, Canada

S.M. Gray
The Hull IVF Unit, The Princess Royal Hospital, Salthouse Road, Hull HU8 9HE, UK

J.G. Grudzinskas
Joint Academic Unit of Obstetrics, Gynaecology and Reproductive Physiology, The London Hospital Medical College, The Royal London Hospital, Whitechapel Road, London E1 1BB, UK

R.P.S. Jansen
Sydney IVF, 187 Macquarie Street, Sydney 2000, Australia

J.F. Kerin
Department of Obstetrics and Gynaecology, Flinders Medical Centre, Bedford Park, South Australia 5042, Australia

E. Kervancioglu
Department of Obstetrics and Gynaecology, Newham General Hospital, London E13 8SL, UK

H.J. Leese
Department of Biology, University of York, Heslington, York YO1 5DD, UK

B. Lindblom
Department of Obstetrics and Gynaecology, Karolinska Institute, Huddinge University Hospital, S-141 86 Huddinge, Sweden

S.D. Maguiness
Department of Obstetrics and Gynaecology, Newham General Hospital, London E13 8SL, UK

J.E. Martin
Department of Morbid Anatomy, London Hospital Medical College, Whitechapel, London E1 1BB, UK

S.-C. Ng
Department of Obstetrics and Gynaecology, National University of Singapore, Kent Ridge, Singapore 0511

J.M. Pearce
Department of Obstetrics and Gynaecology, St George's Hospital, Blackshaw Road, London SW17 0QT, UK

S. Ratnam
Department of Obstetrics and Gynaecology, National University of Singapore, Kent Ridge, Singapore 0511

F. Risquez
Centro Medico La Trinidad, Caracas, Venezuela

G. Robinson
Department of Histopathology, University Hospital, Queen's Medical Centre, Nottingham NG7 2UH, UK

M. Seppälä
Departments I and II, Obstetrics and Gynaecology, Helsinki University Hospital, Helsinki, Finland

K. Shrimanker
Joint Academic Unit of Obstetrics, Gynaecology and Reproductive Physiology, The London Hospital Medical College, The Royal London Hospital, Whitechapel Road, London E1 1BB, UK

L.S. Skiera
Department of Biology, University of York, Heslington, York YO1 5DD, UK

C.G.W.A. Stappers-de Kuijer
Spaarne Hospital, Department of Obstetrics and Gynaecology, Van Heythuijzenweg 1, PO Box 1644, 2003 BR Haarlem, The Netherlands

C. Sutton
Department of Obstetrics and Gynaecology, Royal Surrey County Hospital, Egerton Road, Guildford, Surrey GU2 5XX, UK

A.S. Thurmond
Oregon Health Sciences University, 3181 SW Sam Jackson Park Road, Portland, Oregon 97201, USA

C.J. Verco
Department of Obstetrics and Gynaecology, Modbury Hospital, Modbury, South Australia 5092, Australia

K. Wamsteker
Spaarne Hospital, Department of Obstetrics and Gynaecology, Van Heythuijzenweg 1, PO Box 1644, 2003 BR Haarlem, The Netherlands

M.A. Warren
Department of Biomedical Science, University of Sheffield, Sheffield S10 2TN, UK

M. Williams
University Department of Obstetrics and Gynaecology, Jessop Hospital for Women, Sheffield S3 7RE, UK

R.M.L. Winston
Institute of Obstetrics and Gynaecology, Royal Postgraduate Medical School, Hammersmith Hospital, DuCane Road, London W12 ONN, UK

P. Ylöstalo
Departments I and II, Obstetrics and Gynaecology, Helsinki University Hospital, Helsinki, Finland

J. Yovich
PIVET Medical Centre, 166-168 Cambridge Street, Leederville, Perth, Western Australia 6007, Australia

J.-R. Zorn
Clinique Universitaire Baudelocque, Paris, France

Section I

# Microanatomy, Physiology and Metabolism of the Fallopian Tube

Chapter 1

# Fallopian Tube Anatomy, Microanatomy, Microcirculation and Counter-current Exchange

C.J. Verco

## Introduction

Anatomists before Falloppius had observed and described the uterine tubes, now known as oviducts or fallopian tubes. The definitive description, however, was written by Gabriel Falloppius, in Observationes Anatomicae (1561), ensuring eponymous remembrance. This translation of his description is characteristic. "This seminal duct originates from the cornua uteri; it is thin, very narrow, of white colour and looks like a nerve. After a short distance, it begins to broaden and to coil like a tendril, winding in folds almost up to the end. There, having become very broad, it shows an extremitas of nature of skin and colour of flesh, the utmost end being very ragged and crushed, like the fringe of worn out clothes. Further, it has a great hole which is held closed by the fimbriae which lap over each other. However, if they spread out and dilate, they create a kind of opening which looks like the flaring bell of a brazen tube. Because the course of the seminal duct, from its origin up to its end, resembles the shape of this classical instrument – anyhow, whether the curves are existing or not – I named it tuba uteri. These uterine tubes are alike not only in men, but also in the cadavers of sheep and cows, and all the other animals which I dissected." (Herrlinger and Feiner 1964).

This chapter will outline tubal anatomy and embryology and examine tubal microanatomy, vascular anatomy, microcirculation and relevant aspects of circulatory physiology.

# Embryology

The Müllerian (paramesonephric) ducts appear in the human between the fifth and sixth week after fertilisation. They form as bands of coelomic epithelium at the cranial end of the urogenital ridge. Each grows caudally, lateral to its ipsilateral Wolffian duct, turning inwards and crossing anterior to the Wolffian duct; they then join at the back of the urogenital sinus. The lower ends fuse to form the uterus and upper part of the vagina; the upper parts separate to form the fallopian tubes. The Müllerian ducts fuse from below upwards beginning at 7 and ending at 12 weeks (Williams 1989). Congenital abnormalities of the fallopian tubes are rare; unilateral or bilateral tubal agenesis, a missing segment or tubal narrowing, which may extend as far as tubal obstruction, are all possible (Golan et al. 1989).

# Tubal Morphology

The human fallopian tubes are paired, tubular, seromuscular organs attached laterally to the ovary and medially to the lateral aspect of the uterine fundus with which they are continuous. Situated in the upper margins of the broad ligaments of the uterus, each tube is about 10 cm long, the medial end opens into the superior angle of the cavity of the uterus and the lateral into the peritoneal cavity close to the ipsilateral ovary. The abdominal ostium is situated at the base of a funnel-shaped expansion of the tube, the infundibulum, the circumference of which is enhanced by irregular processes called fimbriae. The ovarian fimbria is longer and more deeply grooved than the others and is closely applied to the tubal pole of the ovary. Passing medially the infundibulum opens into the thin-walled ampulla forming more than half the length of the tube; it is succeeded by the isthmus, a round and cord-like structure constituting the medial one-third. The intramural part of the tube continues from the isthmus through the uterine wall, about 1 cm in length, into the uterine cavity (Williams 1989).

# Microanatomy

The tube consists of an external serosal layer, an intermediate stratum of muscle and an internal mucosal layer. The tubal lumen, a potential space (Blandau 1978, Verco et al. 1983), progressively diminishes in size from the fimbrial ostium to the uterus, the most significant luminal diameter change being at the ampullary isthmic junction (AIJ) (Halbert et al. 1988). The serosal layer has subjacent areolar tissue, being continuous with the peritoneum of the broad ligament, the upper margins of which are the mesosalpinges.

## Tubal Mucosa

The mucosa consists of an epithelium with an underlying stratum of connective tissue, the lamina propria, which contains nerves, blood and lymphatic vessels (Williams 1989). The mucosa is invaginated to form folds or plicae and is more extensively folded in the ampulla, there being six to eight major plicae, than in the isthmus, where there are four (Williams 1989). The epithelium consists of columnar and ciliated cells, at least three kinds being identified – ciliated cells, columnar cells and intercalated or peg cells; the basement membrane is considered to be incomplete (Williams 1989). A fourth epithelial cell, a basal or indifferent cell, has also been reported (Pauerstein and Woodruff 1967). Ciliated cells are most frequently found on the apices of the mucosal folds; the proportion of ciliated cells decreases from about 70% at the fimbria to 50% in the ampulla near the AIJ (Fredericks 1986).

During the proliferative phase of the menstrual cycle, human tubal epithelium contains numerous ciliated cells in the ampulla and infundibulum, which are particularly plentiful at the apices of the plicae (Patek et al. 1972a). Non-ciliated cells are more plentiful at the plical base. Ciliated cells in the isthmus, limited in number, appear mainly in strands demarcated by the protruding surfaces of non-ciliated cells. During the late secretory phase, secretory cells bulge into the tubal lumen, there being no evidence of cilial degeneration (Patek et al. 1972a). Tubal epithelial height may decrease after ovulation (Kim-Bjorklund et al. 1991) and Patek et al. (1972a) concluded that oestrogen dependent cyclical changes are mainly observed in the secretory cells. But fimbrial deciliation after ovulation is also seen (Verhage et al. 1979).

The tubal mucosa is slow growing and independent of cyclical changes (Patek 1977). Ciliogenesis has been described (Cornier et al. 1980) and deciliation may be delayed 20 years after the menopause (Patek et al. 1972b). The epithelium maintains its ciliation and secretory cell appearance if oestrogen is administered in post-menopausal women (Gaddum-Rosse et al. 1975).

Ciliary beat in the isthmus and ampulla is directed towards the uterus in women (Blandau 1978). Increased frequency of human female cilial beat of 18% in the isthmus and 16% in the ampulla has been observed at the time of ovulation (Critoph and Denis 1977). Verdugo et al. (1980) found that ciliary activity (measured by laser scattering spectroscopy) was stimulated by prostaglandins (PG) $PGF_{2\alpha}$, $PGE_1$ and $PGE_2$ in epithelial cell cultures. Brosens and Vasquez (1976) performed fimbrial microbiopsies, and observed that 54%–70% of fimbrial epithelial cells were ciliated in fertile women. Although their findings suggest an important role for cilia in tubal transport, absent cilial dynein arms seen in a fertile woman with the immotile or dyskinetic cilia syndrome (Sturgess et al. 1980) raises interesting doubts about the relative significance of cilial activity in tubal function.

Notwithstanding contrasting observations of cyclic changes in ciliated cells, there seems general agreement that secretory cell changes are pronounced and consistent (Fredericks 1986). Cell heights increase during the follicular phase and achieve maximal height near the time of ovulation. At this time, secretory and ciliated cells reach equal heights, secretory cell microvilli being swollen and adhering to each other (Fredericks 1986). Secretory cells enlarge and bulge into the tubal lumen, their microvilli distributed less evenly, and "peg" cells, which may represent exhausted secretory cells, are seen (Fredericks 1986). During the ovarian cycle, the secretory cells undergo ultrastructural change with variations in Golgi apparatus compactness and endoplasmic reticulum prominence (Fredericks 1986).

## Tubal Musculature

The myosalpinx is made up of external longitudinal or spiral and internal circular strata of non-striated muscle, thickest in the proximal isthmus and intramural portions where there is also an inner stratum of longitudinal muscle (Lindblom and Norstrom 1986). The extramural portion of the uterotubal junction exhibits outer longitudinal muscle bundles which originate from the outer longitudinal layer of the myometrium and extend towards the ampulla as a well-defined continuous layer. Subjacent is a vascular plexus and deep to this plexus the myosalpinx is comprised of bundles which pass in an uneven circular pattern, bifurcating, from the outer muscle layer towards the bases of the mucosal folds. Some of the outer longitudinal muscle bundles of the isthmic myosalpinx pass abruptly sideways as they approach the ampulla enveloping the subjacent muscle (Muglia et al. 1991). The architecture of the outer, longitudinally arranged muscle bundles in the ampulla is plexiform. The muscle arrangements described suggest that the myosalpinx is more likely to generate random contraction waves capable of stirring rather than contractions which are primarily constrictive or propulsive (Muglia et al. 1991).

Although there is close apposition between myosalpingeal muscle fibres, cell to cell contacts fulfilling the criteria of "gap junctions" have not been demonstrated. The mesosalpinx, ovarian ligaments and uterus all have muscle fibres which may affect tubal function (Lindblom and Norstrom 1986).

Localised peristaltic contractions originate in isolated segments or loops to travel a short distance; segmental contractions and worm-like writhing involve the entire oviduct. Contractions directed away from the ovary are more common than those directed towards it. In general, the ampulla is less active than the isthmus (Hafez 1979). Before ovulation, contractions are gentle with some individual variations in rate and pattern. At ovulation, contractions become vigorous, the mesosalpinx and mesotubarium superior contract independently and intermittently, to draw the tube into a crescent, sliding the fimbria over the surface of the ovary and causing continuous change in the tubal contour. The fimbria contract rhythmically and "massage" the ovarian surface (Hafez 1979). Endogenous oestrogen stimulates and endogenous progesterone depresses tubal activity (Lindblom et al. 1980), the effect being seen within 3 days.

## Neuroanatomy

The automatic innervation of the human tube is both sympathetic and parasympathetic. The afferent innervation, carrying pain sensation, accompanies the sympathetic nerves and is derived from T10 to L2. Parasympathetic innervation is uncommon and is derived from segments S234 (Paton et al. 1978). The tubal nerves originate not only from the pre- and para-vertebral ganglia but also from adrenergic ganglia adjacent to the utero-vaginal junction (Owman et al. 1967; Helm et al. 1982).

The ampullary muscle layer contains few nerves, the majority being vasomotor fibres in contrast with the isthmus (Helm et al. 1982), there being more nerve fibres, the majority supplying circular muscle. The number of nerves observed decreases towards the intramural part, the innervation being denser than that found in the adjacent uterine smooth muscle. Excitatory and inhibitory adrenoreceptors exist in the tube (Paton et al. 1978). In addition, peptidergic nerve fibres have been observed in the human isthmus and ampulla (Bishop et al. 1979).

The pharmacological response of the tube varies during the menstrual cycle (Marshall 1981). During menstruation and throughout the proliferative phase, the human tube is very sensitive to alpha adrenergic compounds (Korenga and Kadota 1981; Helm et al. 1982; Sjoberg et al. 1983) and oxytocin (Maia and Coutinho 1976; Hafez 1979). After ovulation and during the luteal phase, the response to norepinephrine (Korenga and Kadota 1981; Helm et al. 1982; Sjöberg et al. 1983) and oxytocin is decreased and the inhibitory effects of beta adrenergic compounds is more pronounced (Maia and Coutinho 1976; Hafez 1979; Strom et al. 1981, 1983). The frequency of spontaneous human isthmic and ampullary contractions increases progressively during the proliferative phase of the menstrual cycle, to a maximum at the time of ovulation (Helm et al. 1982). Alpha receptor activity is low near the beginning and the end of the ovulatory cycle (Moawad et al. 1976) but is enhanced during the period when oestrogen levels rise and before progesterone levels become significantly high. The beta receptor activity is enhanced by raised progesterone levels (Strom et al. 1981, 1983; Fredericks et al. 1982), suggesting that the tubal adrenergic innervation is associated with relaxation of the circular muscle. This increase in isthmic luminal diameter could enable trans-isthmic passage of the fertilised ovum.

The implication is that progesterone may cause isthmic myosalpingeal quiescence (Korenga and Kadota 1981; Fredericks et al. 1982; Blair and Beck 1976; Strom et al. 1981, 1983) and that isthmic ovum transport is facilitated. Oestrogens may enhance "tube locking," with delay in ovum transport at the AIJ, and progesterone may accelerate isthmic ovum transport (Pauerstein et al. 1974; Blair and Beck 1976; Korenga and Kadota 1981; Strom et al. 1981, 1983; Helm et al. 1981, 1982).

Peptidergic nerve fibres are seen in the human isthmic and ampullary subepithelial layer, there being very few fibres in the surrounding muscle (Bishop et al. 1979). These fibres are more abundant in the isthmus (Helm et al. 1981). Vasoactive polypeptide (VIP) inhibits spontaneous smooth muscle activity in human tubal strips (Helm et al. 1981) and is responsible for the neurogenic inhibition of motor activity in the human isthmus (Helm et al. 1982; Owman et al. 1983). This may be the mechanism by which the isthmus opens and allows the embryo to pass into the uterus (Owman et al. 1983).

## Tubal Vasculature

Branches of the uterine artery, to the human oviduct, supply the isthmus and branches of the ovarian artery the remaining parts of the tube. Either artery alone, however, may supply the whole tube (Eddy and Pauerstein 1980).

The venous drainage follows that of the arterial supply (Eddy and Pauerstein 1980). Tubal venous drainage in the ovarian vein is particularly significant as the ovarian vein and artery are closely related in the human ovarian pedicle (Bendz 1977; Bendz and Hansson 1982). Areas of contact between the ovarian artery (Bendz et al. 1982a) and vein are characterised by thinning of the ovarian vein wall (Bendz 1977; Bendz et al. 1982a). This anatomical arrangement is consistent with the hypothesis that there is a countercurrent transfer of factors from ovarian veins to artery (Bendz 1977; Bendz and Hansson 1982; Bendz et al. 1982a; Hunter et al. 1983).

Lymphatic channels follow the course of ovarian and uterine veins and drain to the aortic or lumbar nodes (Eddy and Pauerstein 1980). Three separate lymphatic networks drain the mucosa, muscle and serosa respectively; these combine, emerging from the oviduct and entering the mesosalpinx (Andersen 1927, 1928; Eddy and Pauerstein 1980).

### Tubal Microvasculature

The human tubal subserosa is supplied by arterioles which arise from juxtatubal arterial arcades, the myosalpinx being supplied by tortuous arteries which pass through it to give rise to the mucosal arterioles (Koritke and Gillet 1967; Koritke et al. 1968a,b). Mucosal arterioles are coiled and terminate in a dense submucosal capillary network draining into irregular calibre venules which pass, parallel to each other and at right angles to the long axis of a mucosal fold (Koritke and Gillet 1967; Gillet and Leissner 1967; Muller et al. 1968), to join deeper venules. Fimbrial microvascular architecture (MVA) differs from that of the isthmic or ampullary mucosa in that arteries are more numerous (Koritke et al. 1968a) and are located peripherally around a centrally located fimbrial core venule (Koritke and Gillet 1967; Gillet and Koritke 1967; Koritke et al. 1968a; Muller et al. 1968). During the proliferative phase, mucosal arterioles become increasingly coiled and this coiling progresses, during the secretory phase, to a maximum at the time of menstruation (Gillet and Leissner 1967; Gillet and Koritke 1967; Koritke et al. 1968a,b). These vascular changes are most marked in the fimbria (Koritke et al. 1968a,b). Mucosal venules are markedly dilated at the time of ovulation and maximally dilated at the time of menstruation (Gillet and Leissner 1967; Koritke et al. 1968a,b). Mucosal venule diameters range from 75 μm in the proliferative phase to 175 μm premenstrually and 120 μm at the time of menstruation (Koritke et al. 1968a). Mucosal arteriolar coils progressively tighten during pregnancy (Gillet and Koritke 1967; Koritke et al. 1968b). After the menopause, mucosal arterioles and venules are dilated and the mucosal arterioles are less tightly coiled (Gillet and Koritke 1967; Koritke et al. 1968b). Mucosal capillaries are normally 10 μm in diameter; premenstrually capillary diameters increase to 20–25 μm (Koritke et al. 1968a).

Rabbit oviduct MVA varies characteristically along the length of the tube; the major differences are in the subserosal and submucosal microvasculature. There is an extensive interlocking venous plexus in the isthmic subserosa; ampullary subserosal vasculature, in contrast, is comprised of parallel branching arteries and veins. Isthmic plicae are well supplied with arterioles which branch little before terminal ramification, into capillaries which drain either down the fold or directly to centrally located plical core venules. Ampullary plical arterioles are less frequently observed and either branch low in a mucosal fold or pass to the top of a fold, along which they run before terminal ramification into capillaries. Ampullary plical capillaries drain to large venules that originate high in the plical core. Fimbrial arterioles and venules exhibit parallel branching; near the edge of a fimbrial fold the arterioles branch terminally into capillaries which drain to the large, accompanying and frequently observed core venules (Verco et al. 1983). It is suggested firstly, that isthmic subserosal venous plexus dilatation (caused by either a rise in venous pressure or a fall in venous wall smooth-muscle tone) could, within the limiting perimeter of the serosal connective tissue, occlude the isthmic lumen to ovum or embryo transport. Secondly, the observed differences in the MVA imply a greater blood delivery to the submucosal capillary network of the isthmus and a greater venous drainage capacity in the ampulla. This suggests that there may be a net movement of intravascular fluid to the interstitium and possibly thence to the tubal lumen in the isthmus, and a net movement of tubal fluid from the tubal lumen to the mucosal interstitium and thence to the subepithelial capillaries in the ampulla (Verco et al. 1983). A pattern of tubal luminal fluid movement may thus be initiated or a pre-existing pattern of fluid flow along the tube modified.

Observation of variations in rabbit oviduct MVA after oophorectomy, during pregnancy and during ovum transport suggests a sensitivity and perhaps even the dependence of the tubal vasculature on local or circulating ovarian, embryonic or placental hormones (Verco et al. 1983, 1984).

Isthmic subserosal venous plexus dilatation 36 h after ovulatum is less than that at 12 h and is similar to the observed in controls; this is consistent with the proposition that dilatation of the isthmic subserosal venous plexus limits isthmic wall distensibility and thus contributes to the known pre-isthmic delay in ovum transport.

Experimental rabbit hydrosalpinges exhibit isthmic and ampullary luminal dilatation, reduction in the extent of projection of the primary mucosal fold MVA into the lumen, and loss of secondary mucosal fold MVA (Verco et al. 1982; Verco and Gannon 1984). Plical MVA is preserved; in contrast, interplical subepithelial capillaries are not perfused. Isthmic and ampullary subserosal venous distension is greater in the hydrosalpinx than in controls or in adjacent tubal segments (Verco et al. 1982; Verco and Gannon 1984). Subepithelial capillary perfusability and permeability to native rabbit and bovine serum albumin are reduced in the hydrosalpinx, particularly between plicae (Verco and Gannon 1984, 1985). Poor interplical subepithelial capillary perfusion is probably the underlying mechanism of interplical deciliation, previously reported in this model (Vasquez et al. 1981; Kleinstein et al. 1982). Preservation of the plical MVA, the absence of interplical subepithelial capillary perfusion, and reduced interplical subepithelial capillary perfusion indicate, since all mucosal subepithelial capillaries are exposed to the same increased tubal intraluminal hydrostatic pressure, that the microvascular changes are primarily due to stretching of the tubal wall (Verco et al. 1982; Verco and Gannon 1984, 1985). The larger and more extensive mucosal arterioles of the hydrosalpinx suggest increased blood pressure in the hydrosalpinx; in addition, the subserosal venous dilatation observed in the hydrosalpinx implies superregulation of blood flow and thus increased blood flow in the hydrosalpinx. A net increase in capillary fluid outflow and a net decrease in capillary fluid absorption would therefore be predicted. Interstitial fluid in the hydrosalpinx could pass between the epithelial cells through "leaky" tight intercellular junctions which are rendered more "leaky" by stretching of the epithelium (Verco and Gannon 1984, 1985). The reduction in subepithelial capillary permeability to albumin, in the hydrosalpinx model, would decrease osmotically driven absorption of luminal fiuid. Taken together, increased hydrosalpinx blood pressure and blood flow, reduced subepithelial capillary perfusion and macromolecular permeability would result in an increase in mucosal interstitial fluid, an increase in epithelial transudation, a reduction in osmotically driven transepithelial luminal fluid absorption and reduced subepithelial capillary fluid absorption (Zweifach 1977). These mechanisms would explain the maintenance of the hydrosalpinx in this model. Reduced human fertility after salpingoneostomy for hydrosalpinges may be due to persistence of vascular changes similar to those described above.

## Patterns of Oviduct Blood Flow

Verco and Gannon (1984, 1985) demonstrated that the tube is well perfused and, in addition, the MVA is readily permeable to macromolecules (Verco et al. 1983, 1984). Current measurements of human endometrial blood flow by laser doppler flowmetry (which measures red cell flux) reveal considerable minute-to-minute variations in blood flow ranging from 0.05–1.2 ml/min/g (Verco et al. 1991). A small number of fimbrial blood flow estimations at the time of laparoscopy reveal flow rates ranging from 0.60–1.2 ml/min/g. The study of transvaginal colour flow velocity wave forms may lead to a better understanding of tubal and ovarian arterial and venous systems (Deutinger et al. 1989; Steer et al. 1990; Bourne et al. 1990; Kurjak et al. 1991). These techniques, however, are not considered to provide an accurate assessment of events in the arteriovenous systems of these organs. In addition, blood flow in the larger blood vessels does not necessarily indicate the haemodynamics of the capillaries, the exchange vessels (Zweifach 1977). Oviduct blood flow studies, in future, should be directed at an understanding of sub-epithelial capillary blood flow and hydraulic conductivity (or coefficient of filtration). It is relevant to know if the sub-epithelial capillaries are absorbing or filtering out electrolytes, fluid, protein, etc; the net fluid flux, when documented, will enhance knowledge of the pathways used by ova/embryo-derived factors to communicate, probably by cascade initiation (Yi-Qian et al. 1991), appropriate "messages" influencing tubal, ovarian and uterine function.

### Ovarian Venous to Ovarian Artery Counter-current Exchange

The proximity of the utero-ovarian vein and the ovarian artery, in sheep, resulted in the demonstration of the counter-current transfer of prostaglandin $F_{2\alpha}$, from the utero-ovarian vein to the ovarian artery and hence to the ovary (Barrett et al. 1971; Goding et al. 1972; McCracken et al. 1972). The human ovarian artery and vein are in close contact and where the ovarian artery is in contact with ovarian veins thinning of the vein wall has been reported (Bendz 1977; Bendz et al. 1982a) and the potential for counter-current exchange suggested.

A counter-current transfer of progesterone and antipyrine between the human ovarian veins and the ovarian artery in the ovarian pedicle has been demonstrated (Bendz et al. 1982b). Albumin is not exchanged, which suggests that macromolecules do not pass freely across these vessel walls.

## Conclusion

The many observations relating to fallopian tube anatomy and physiology reported in this chapter, to which one must add the vast extant tubal literature, reflect the long-standing interest in tubal function. Nonetheless, many opportunities exist to examine further this fascinating and enigmatic organ. The biological importance of normal tubal function in the preservation and maintenance of mammalian species continues to encourage such endeavours.

It is necessary to determine the leakiness of tubal epithelial intercellular (gap) junctions. The freeze factor technique used by Murphy et al. (1981) is a suitable method for obtaining such observations. As it is likely that gap junction leakiness is focal in relation to intra-tubal ova or embryo(s), careful tissue preparation will be necessary. In addition, sub-epithelial oedema warrants some examination; the transient accumulation of tissue fluid may well contribute to tubal occlusion.

Tubal vasculature, at its simplest, supplies "nutrients" and removes "waste"; at increasing levels of complexity, the microvasculature may play an important role in gamete and embryo transport and, furthermore, provide a mechanism for biochemical communication between the oviduct, ovary and uterus. For example it is possible that the direction of tubal venous drainage changes from the ovarian vein, with counter-current exchange to ovarian artery and thence "marker" transport to tube and ovary, to the uterine vein with counter-current exchange to the uterine artery and thereby "communication" from the ovary and tube to the uterine vein and thence to the uterine artery and uterus. There is, therefore, considerable opportunity for speculation on the precise role of the tube vasculature, microvasculature and blood flow in oviduct function. Definitive experiments are, clearly, possible but will be technically difficult; the reward, however, will be a substantial increase in our understanding of the complex interactions resulting in normal tubal function.

## References


Andersen DH (1927) Lymphatics of the fallopian tube of the sow. Contrib Embryo Carneg Instn 19:136–147

Andersen DH (1928) Comparative anatomy of the tubo-uterine junction. Histology and physiology in the sow. Am J Anat 42:255–305

Barrett S, Blockley MA de B, Brown JM, Cumming SA, Goding JR, Mole MJ, Obst JM (1971) Initiation of the estrus cycle in the ewe by infusions of $PGF_{2\alpha}$ into the auto transplanted ovary. J Reprod Fertil 24:136–137

Bendz A (1977) The anatomical basis for a possible counter current exchange mechanism in the human adnexa. Prostaglandins 13:355–362

Bendz A, Hansson HA (1982) Structure of veins and arteries in the human ovarian pedicle. Unpublished monograph, pp 1–4

Bendz A, Hansson HA, Svendsen P, Wiquist N (1982a) On the extensive contact between veins and arteries in the human ovarian pedicle. Acta Physiol Scand 115:179–182

Bendz A, Lundgren O, Hamberger L (1982b) Countercurrent exchange of progesterone and antipyrine between human utero-ovarian vessels, and of antipyrine between the femoral vessels in the cat. Acta Physiol Scand 114:611–616

Bishop AE, Polak JM, Bloom SR (1979) Vasoactive intestinal polypeptide innervation of the genital tract of women. J Endocrinol 81:141P–142P

Blair WD, Beck LR (1976) Demonstration of postovulatory sphincter action by the isthmus of the rabbit oviduct. Fertil Steril 27:431–441

Blandau RJ (1978) Mechanism of tubal transport – comparative aspects. In: Brosens I, Winston R (eds) Reversibility of female sterilization. Academic Press, London: Grune and Stratton, New York, pp 1–20

Bourne TH, Campbell S, Whitehead MI, Royston P, Steer CV, Collins WP (1990) Detection of endometrial cancer in post-menopausal women by transvaginal ultrasonography and colour flow imaging. Br Med J 301:369

Brosens IA, Vasquez G (1976) Fimbrial microbiopsy. J Reprod Med 16:171–178

Cornier E, Chatelet F, Grenier J, Valade S, Salat-Baroux J, Roland J (1980) Ciliated epithelium of the fallopian tube in women. An ultrastructural study (author's translation). Journal De Gynaecologie, Obstetrique Biologie De La Reproduction (Paris) 9:505–511

Critoph RN, Denis KJ (1977) Ciliary activity in the human oviduct. Br J Obstet Gynaecol 84:216–218

Deutinger J, Reinthaller A, Bernaschek G (1989) Transvaginal pulsed doppler measurement of blood flow velocity in the ovarian arteries during cycle stimulation and after follicle puncture. Fertil Steril 51:466–470

Eddy CA, Pauerstein CJ (1980) Anatomy and physiology of the fallopian tube. Clin Obstet Gynaecol 23:1177–1193
Fredericks CM (1986) Morphological and functional aspects of the oviductal epithelium. In: Siegler AM (ed) The fallopian tube: basic studies and clinical contributions. Futura Publishing Company Inc., New York, pp 67–80
Fredericks CM, Anderson WR, Smith CE, Mathur RS (1982) Patterns of periovulatory oviductal motility and progesterone in the unanaesthetized rabbit. Biol Reprod 27:340–350
Gaddum-Rosse P, Rumery RE, Blandau RJ, Thiersch JB (1975) Studies on the mucosa of postmenopausal oviducts: surface appearance, ciliary activity and the effect of oestrogen treatment. Fertil Steril 26:951–969
Gillet JY, Koritke JG (1967) Spiral arterioles of the human oviduct mucosa. Acta Anat 68:609
Gillet JY, Leissner P (1967) Variations of microvascularisation of oviduct during the ovarian cycle in women. Acta Anat 68:608–609
Goding JR, Baird DT, Cumming SA, McCracken JA (1972) The functional assessment of autotransplanted endocrine glands. Acta Endocrinol Suppl (Copenh) 158:169–199
Golan A, Langer R, Bukovsky I, Csapi E (1989) Congenital anomalies of the Müllerian system. Fertil Steril 51:747–755
Hafez ESE (1979) Function of the fallopian tube in human reproduction. Clin Obstet Gynaecol 22:61–79
Halbert SA, Szal SE, Broderson SH (1988) Anatomical basis of a passive mechanism for ovum retention at the ampullo-isthmic junction. Anat Rec 221:841–845
Helm GH, Ottesen B, Fahrenkrug J, Larsen JJ, Owman C, Sjöberg NO, Stolberg B, Sundler F, Walles B (1981) Vasoactive intestinal polypeptide (VIP) in the human female reproductive tract: distribution and motor effects. Biol Reprod 25:227–234
Helm GH, Hoakanson R, Leander S, Owman C, Sjöberg NO, Sporrong B (1982) Neurogenic relaxation mediated by vasoactive intestinal polypeptide (VIP) in the isthmus of the human fallopian tube. Regul Pept 3:145–153
Herrlinger R, Feiner E (1964) Why did Versalius not discover the fallopian tubes? Med Hist 8:335–341
Hunter RHF, Cook B, Poyser NL (1983) Regulation of oviduct function in pigs by local transfer of ovarian steroids and prostaglandins: a mechanism to influence sperm transport. Eur J Obstet Gynaecol Reprod Biol 14:225–232
Kim-Bjorklund T, Landgren B-M, Hamberger LD, Johannisson E (1991) Comparative morphometric study of the endometrium, the fallopian tube, and the corpus luteum during the postovulatory phase in normally menstruating women. Fertil Steril 56:842–850
Kleinstein J, Neubuser D, Mussmann J (1982) Mechanically induced tube damage in aritifical hydrosalpinx. Gynaecol Obstet Invest 14:292–299
Korenga M, Kadota T (1981) Changes in mechanical properties of the circular muscle of the isthmus of the human fallopian tube in relation to hormonal domination and postovulatory time. Fertil Steril 36:343–350
Koritke JG, Gillet JY (1967) Microvascularisation of oviduct in women. Acta Anat 68:612–613
Koritke JG, Gillet JY, Leissner P (1968a) La microvascularisation de la muqueuse tubaire et ses variations au cours du cycle ovarien chez la femme. Mikroscopisch-Anatomische Forschung 88:48–56
Koritke JG, Muller P, Gillet JY (1968b) Vascularisation of the oviduct in the woman. Bulletin of the Federal Societies of Gynaecol Obstet 20:405–406
Kurjak A, Kupesic-Urek S, Schulman H, Zalud I (1991) Transvaginal colour flow doppler in the assessment of ovarian and uterine blood flow in infertile women. Fertil Steril 56:870–873
Lindblom B, Norstrom A (1986) The smooth-muscle architecture of the human fallopian tube. In: Siegler AM (ed) The fallopian tube: basic studies and clinical contributions. Futura Publishing Company, New York, pp 13–20
Lindblom B, Hamberger L, Ljung B (1980) Contractile patterns of isolated oviductal smooth muscle under different hormonal conditions. Fertil Steril 33:283–287
Maia H, Coutinho EM (1976) Motility of the human oviduct in vivo. In: Harper MJK, Pauerstein CJ, Adams CE, Coutinho EM, Croxatto HB, Paton DM (eds) Ovum transport and fertility regulation. Scriptor, Copenhagen, pp 221–227
Marshall JM (1981) Effects of ovarian steroids and pregnancy on adrenergic nerves of uterus and oviduct. Am J Physiol 240:165–174
McCracken JA, Carlson JC, Giew ME, Goding JR, Baird DT, Green K, Samuelsson B (1972) Prostaglandin $F_{2\alpha}$ identified as a luteolytic hormone in sheep. Nature 238:129–134

Moawad AH, Hedqvist P, Kim MH (1976) Correlation of plasma oestrogens and progesterone levels with the in vitro adrenergic responses in the isthmus of the human oviduct. In: Harper MJK, Pauerstein CJ, Adams CE, Coutinho EM, Croxatto HB, Paton DM (eds) Ovum transport and fertility regulation. Scriptor, Copenhagen, pp 276–292
Muglia U, Vizza E, Correr S, Germana G, Motta PM (1991) The three-dimensional architecture of the myosalpinx in the rabbit as revealed by scanning electron microscopy. J Submicros Cytol Pathol 23:525–532
Muller M, Koritke JC, Gillet JY (1968) Vascular architecture of the fallopian tube in the woman. Bulletin of the Federal Societies of Gynaecology and Obstetrics 20:407–409
Murphy CR, Swift JG, Mukherjee TM, Rogers A (1981) Effects of ovarian hormones on cell membranes in the rat uterus. Cell Biophys 3:57–69
Owman CH, Rosengren E, Sjöberg NO (1967) Adrenergic innervation of the human female reproductive organs: a histochemical and chemical investigation. Obstet Gynaecol 30:763–773
Owman CH, Helm G, Sjöberg NO (1983) Non-adrenergic, non-cholinergic neurogenic relaxation mediated by vasoactive intestinal polypeptide (VIP) in the isthmus of the human fallopian tube. Int J Fertil 28:12
Patek E (1977) The proliferative behaviour of the human fallopian tube epithelium. Acta Cytol 21:777–780
Patek E, Nilsson L, Johannisson E (1972a) Scanning electron microscope study of the human fallopian tube. Report I. The proliferative and secretory stages. Fertil Steril 23:459–465
Patek E, Nilsson L, Johannisson E (1972b) Scanning electron microscopic study of the human fallopian tube. Report II. Foetal life, reproductive life and post-menopause. Fertil Steril 23:719–733
Paton DM, Widdicombe JH, Rheaume DE, Johns A (1978) The role of the adrenergic innervation of the oviduct in the regulation of mammalian ovum transport. Pharmacol Rev 29:67–102
Pauerstein CJ, Woodruff JD (1967) The role of the "indifferent" cell of the tubal epithelium. Am J Obstet Gynecol 98:121–125
Pauerstein CJ, Anderson V, Chatkoff M, Hodgson GJ (1974) Effect of estrogen and progesterone on the time-course of tubal ovum transport in rabbits. Am J Obstet Gynecol 120:299–308
Sjöberg NO, Helm G, Owman CH, Sporrong B, Walles B (1983) Electron microscopic, biochemical and pharmacological evidence for functional adrenergic innervation of the smooth musculature in the humam fallopian tube. Int J Fertil 28:4
Steer CV, Campbell S, Pampiglione EJS, Kingsland CR, Mason BA, Collins WP (1990) Transvaginal colour flow imaging of the uterine arteries during the ovarian and menstrual cycles. Hum Reprod 5:391–395
Strom C, Edin R, Dahlstrom A, Ahlman H (1981) In vivo studies of the motility of the isthmic segment in the perfused rabbit oviduct. Acta Physiol Scand 13:491–498
Strom C, Dahlstrom A, Lindblom B, Ahlman H (1983) In vivo studies on motility of the isthmic portion of the perfused rabbit oviduct. Int J Fertil 28:4
Sturgess JM, Chao J, Peter-Turner JA (1980) Transposition of ciliary microtubules. Another cause of impaired ciliary motility. N Engl J Med 303:318–322
Verco CJ, Gannon BJ (1984) Microvascular architecture, vascular perfusability and capillary macromolecular permeability in the mechanically induced rabbit hydrosalpinx. In: Courtice FC, Garlick DG, Perry MA (eds) Progress in microcirculation research II. Committee on Postgraduate Medical Eduction, University of South Wales, Sydney, pp 232–238
Verco CJ, Gannon BJ (1985) Vascular perfusability and capillary macromolecular permeability in the mechanically induced rabbit hydrosalpinx. Acta Anat 122:126–132
Verco CJ, Jones WR (1981) Monamniotic twin pregnancy complicated by massive fetal-maternal haemorrhage. Aust New Z J Obstet Gynaecol 21: 186–187
Verco CJ, Hawkins DF (1982) Pregnancy after renal transplantation J Obstet Gynaecol 3:29–33
Verco CJ, Gannon BJ, Jones WR (1983) Fallopian tube microvasculature in the rabbit. Aust J Exp Biol Med Sci 61:127–138
Verco CJ, Gannon BJ, Jones WR (1984) Variations in rabbit oviduct microvascular architecture following gonadotrophin induced ovulation. J Reprod Fertil 71:15–19
Verco CJ, Carati CJ, Gannon BJ (1991) Human endometrial microvascular perfusion. 47th Meeting, Am Fertil Society, Program Supplement 52–53
Verdugo P, Rumery RE, Tam PY (1980) Hormonal control of oviductal ciliary activity: effect of prostaglandins. Fertil Steril 33:193–196

Verhage HG, Bareither ML, Jaffe RC, Akbar M (1979) Cyclic changes in ciliation, secretion and cell height of the oviductal epithelium in women. Am J Anat 156:505–521
Williams PL (1989) Gray's Anatomy. 37th Edn. Churchill Livingstone, UK, pp 1438–1439
Yi-Qian Y, Kudolo GB, Harper MJK (1991) Platelet activating factor (PAF) binding sites in the rabbit oviduct. In: Croxatto HB, Villalon M (eds) Biology of the mammalian oviduct. Archivos de Biologica y Medicina Experimentales 24:275–281
Zweifach BW (1977) Perspectives in microcirculation. In: Kaley G, Altura BM (eds) Microcirculation. Vol 1. University Park Press, Baltimore, pp 1–19

Chapter 2

# In Vivo and In Vitro Behaviour of Human Tubal Epithelial Cells: Their Relevance to Assisted Reproduction

A. Bongso, C.-Y. Fong, S.-C. Ng and S. Ratnam

## Introduction

The fallopian tube in the human and other mammals is a highly specialised structure which assures one of the most fundamental roles in the reproductive process – the meeting of spermatozoa and the oocyte under optimal conditions to encourage fertilisation, early cleavage and safe transport of the cleaving embryo down to the uterus for implantation. The fallopian tube is not simply an inert pipe, but it has immense functional significance in the development of early human life. It is derived from the cranial region of the primitive Müllerian ducts and histologically follows the basic plan of the entire reproductive tract viz., a muscular coat on which lies a submucosa and an epithelial lining. In recent years, the human fallopian tube has attracted great interest in the field of assisted reproduction. Man's intervention in the reproductive process has raised many fundamental questions on the cell biology of the fallopian tube. This chapter attempts to address some of these questions by examining the in vivo and in vitro behaviour of tubal epithelial cells and assessing their relevance to assisted reproduction.

## Functional Microanatomy of the Fallopian Tube In Vivo

The human fallopian tube has four distinct regions: the infundibulum, ampulla, isthmus and uterotubal junction. Each displays characteristic histological features and physiological functions. In the human female, the length of the tube is 11 cm with a range of 8 to 15 cm (Pauerstein and Eddy 1979). These values are for Caucasian women. Asian women have slightly shorter tubes with a mean length of 9.4 cm; the isthmus, ampullary and infundibular regions measure 6.9, 1.5 and 1.0 cm respectively (Bongso et al. 1991b). Interactions occur between the gametes, embryo and tubal epithelium. An oviductal cycle is now recognised; both the ciliated and secretory cells are influenced by changes in hormones during the menstrual cycle.

### Musculature of the Fallopian Tube

The musculature comprises circular and longitudinal layers, with the circular muscle layer increasing in thickness from the infundibulum to the uterotubal junction. The arrangement of the two muscle layers varies between species. In the human, the circular muscle layer is sandwiched between inner and outer longitudinal layers (Nilsson and Reinius 1969). Peristaltic contraction of the muscle layers allows the gametes to be brought together for fertilisation and transport of the cleaving embryo from the ampulla to the uterus. The circular muscle layers of the isthmus are richly innervated, the ampullary-isthmic junction rather less so, while the ampulla and infundibulum have very poor innervation (Brundin 1965; Owman et al. 1967).

### Cell Form and Function of the Tubal Mucosa

The longitudinal folds of the mucosa are most accentuated in the ampulla, the site where fertilisation occurs. The entire tubal mucosa has a columnar epithelial lining resting on connective tissue. The epithelium has two distinct cell types, ciliated and secretory cells. Although the ratio of ciliated to secretory cells is largely determined by hormonal influences, ciliated cells are most prominent in the fimbriated infundibulum. They bear upright cilia; their primary role is to propel the gametes and embryo within the tube. Ultrastructurally, the cilia carry the 9+2 axoneme made up of microtubules. The beat rate of the cilia is dictated by the levels of oestrogen and progesterone, with activity being greatest at the time of ovulation.

The secretory cells are most abundant in the ampullary region. In the follicular phase, these cells have several varieties of microvilli and contain abundant amounts of endoplasmic reticulum. Secretory material is accumulated in these cells and then released into the lumen for nourishment of the oocyte and embryo, and perhaps also to play a role in the fertilisation process. The exact role of the secretions in the preparation of sperm prior to fertilisation, such as capacitation and the acrosome reaction, is not known.

## The Oviductal Cycle

The first description of a distinct oviductal cycle in women was by Novak and Everett in 1928. The ciliated and secretory cells undergo cyclical changes under the influence of oestrogen–progesterone during the menstrual cycle. The most comprehensive work on the human oviductal cycle is that by Verhage et al. (1979) and Donnez et al. (1985). Cytomorphometric studies showed that the epithelial cells attained their maximum height and degree of ciliation during the late follicular phase in the ampulla and fimbriae. In the late luteal phase, atrophy and deciliation occurred, especially in the fimbrial region. Hypertrophy and reciliation commenced in the early follicular phase. During pregnancy and throughout the post-partum period further atrophy and deciliation occurred (Verhage et al. 1979).

Atrophy and deciliation were shown to be associated with elevated serum progesterone levels while hypertrophy and reciliation were related to low levels of progesterone. Oestrogen stimulated epithelial cell hypertrophy, secretion and ciliogenesis. This ciliation–deciliation cycle was confirmed by Donnez et al. (1985). It was also shown that, at ovulation, the isthmic secretion became more viscous than those of the ampulla and the volume of this material was greatest at mid-cycle. Progesterone suppressed the secretion. The isthmic mucous secretions were claimed to play an important role in the transport of sperm (Jansen 1984).

The secretory cells also undergo changes throughout the menstrual cycle. Their height and activity reach a maximum close to the time of ovulation, and during the follicular phase they are well developed and possess evenly distributed microvilli. Once the contents are discharged the cell height diminishes, usually during ovulation (Patek 1974).

## Fallopian Tube Fluid

There is fluid in the normal fallopian tube throughout reproductive life. It is most abundant when gametes or embryos are present (Hunter 1988) and may play an important role during fertilisation and early cleavage. Fluid in the tubes is believed to be formed by (a) selective transudation from the blood and (b) active secretion from the epithelial lining. Hamner (1973) suggested rates of 1.3 ml per 24 h for fluid accumulation; Mastroianni and Go (1979) reported that the rate of fluid production increased significantly during the late proliferative phase of the cycle. Lippes et al. (1981), however, claimed that the largest volumes of fluid were obtained around the time of ovulation. Studies on the proteins in human tubal fluid with gel electrophoresis revealed patterns similar to serum, together with a unique $\beta$-glycoprotein (Moghissi 1970). Lippes et al. (1981) demonstrated specific proteins in the tubal fluid at the time of ovulation, which disappeared in 3 to 5 days. These proteins migrated in the albumin and $\beta$-globulin regions. Fazleabas and Verhage (1986) reported a human follicular phase protein similar to the 130 000 Mr protein observed in baboon tubal fluid. More recently, two oviduct-specific secretory glycoproteins of 15 and 25 kd were described in the human fallopian tube (Shrimanker et al. 1991; Maguiness et al. 1992). A wide range of energy substrates is found in tubal fluid, the most important being pyruvate, lactate, glucose and glycogen. These compounds play important roles in the metabolism of the gametes and preimplantation embryo (Biggers and Borland 1976; Hardy et al. 1989).

# Fertilisation and Early Cleavage

In the human fertilisation occurs in the ampulla of the fallopian tube. The sperm undergoes three important changes: capacitation, the acrosome reaction and hyperactivated motility (Yanagimachi 1988). These changes occur while the sperm swims from the cervix to the ampulla of the fallopian tube. The final steps involved in the sperm acrosome reaction and hyperactivation take place at the zona pellucida of the oocyte before the single sperm gains entry. The oocyte undergoes the cortical reaction in which cortical granules migrate to the periphery of the ooplasm, allowing the entry of only a single sperm and blocking polyspermy. The sperm nucleus decondenses in the ooplasm to form the male pronucleus. The male and female pronuclei are seen at about 16–20 h after the sperm has encountered the oocyte. The fusion of the two pronuclei (syngamy) takes place in the ampullary-isthmus region at 22–25 h after sperm–egg interaction followed by the first cleavage division at 26–28 h. The embryo divides to form the 4-cell stage while in the isthmic region; this occurs at 44–48 h. Cleavage to 8–12 cells (72 h), morula (96 h) and early cavitation to form a blastocyst (120 h) occurs in the isthmic region of the fallopian tube.

# In Vitro Behaviour of Tubal Epithelial Cells

Long before it was possible to fertilise mammalian oocytes in vitro in liquid media, the rabbit oviduct was used as an incubator for the air transport of sheep embryos in the livestock industry (Hunter et al. 1962). It was also shown that fertilised oocytes of farm animals could cleave regularly within the rabbit oviduct (Boland 1984). Live offspring were obtained when cattle embryos were grown in rabbit oviducts in vivo and then transferred to the uterus of infertile cows (Stubbings 1988).

In vitro culture methods offer a tool for direct study of the human fallopian tube. Maintaining an intact human fallopian tube in organ culture for several days has not so far been possible; it would require a very intricate perfusion system. The growth of single cells in tissue culture, however, is feasible. Before attempts at growing fallopian tubal cells in culture were carried out, separated stromal and gland cells from the rabbit, guinea-pig and human endometrium were characterised in primary monolayer culture (Ricketts et al. 1983; Chaminadas et al. 1986; Bongso et al. 1988). Modification of these methods for fallopian tubal epithelial cells permitted the growth and maintenance of cell lines which could be used for the study of hormone-related cell differentiation as well as gamete–embryo–cell interactions in assisted reproduction.

## Setting-up and Maintaining Tubal Epithelial Cells

A simple method for the establishment and maintenance of human tubal ampullary epithelial cell cultures was reported by Bongso et al. (1989c). The same procedure could be used for other parts of the fallopian tube. Healthy fallopian tubes were collected from premenopausal women undergoing hysterectomy. The tubes were collected aseptically in Hank's balanced salt solution (HBSS, Grand Island Biol Co (GIBCO), New York, USA), supplemented with 100 iu/ml penicillin (GIBCO) and 100 μg/ml streptomycin (GIBCO). The cultures could be set up immediately or stored at 4 °C to be set up the following day. The tubes are first washed in HBSS in large sterile Petri dishes and the ampulla dissected away from the rest of the tube. The ampulla is transferred to clean HBSS in another Petri dish and carefully slit open to expose the inner epithelial surface. Small 1-mm square pieces of the epithelial surface are then cut and transferred to clean HBSS with a pair of pointed fine curved scissors and watch-makers' forceps. The epithelial cells are separated from connective tissue or muscle cells by gently teasing each piece with two sets of watch-makers' forceps under a stereomicroscope. Single and clusters of epithelial cells are then collected into centrifuge tubes and centrifuged at 300 g for 5 min. The supernatant is decanted and the cell button resuspended in clean HBSS and spun down again at 300 g for 5 min. The final cell pellet is resuspended in Chang's A + B medium (Irvine Sc, USA). A small aliquot is examined under inverted optics to confirm that the cells are epithelial by observing the beating motion of the cilia of ciliated cells. The cells are seeded into 25 $cm^2$ plastic screw-cap tissue-culture flasks (Nunclon, Roskilde, Denmark) containing 3 ml of Chang's A + B medium. Chang's medium is supplemented with 2 mM L-glutamine (GIBCO) and double the recommended dosage of an antibiotic–antimycotic mixture of penicillin, streptomycin and amphotericin B (GIBCO). The flasks are incubated at 37 °C in an atmosphere of 5% $CO_2$ in air and left undisturbed for 3 days. The flasks are examined on the 4th day and once islands or patches of cells attached to the plastic base are observed, the medium is changed with fresh Chang's A + B medium. Once several islands are formed, by around the 7th to 10th day, the cells are passaged into new flasks. For passaging, the cells are dislodged by using 0.5% trypsin:0.53 mM EDTA (GIBCO) for 5 min at 37 °C in 5% $CO_2$ in air. The cells are washed with medium to remove traces of trypsin and seeded into new flasks. Several passages could be maintained until senescence and cell death.

## Primary Cultures

Primary cultures of human ampullary epithelial cells were usually observed at around 6 to 10 days (Table 2.1). Using phase-contrast inverted optics the beating motion of cilia could be observed in primary culture. The cells were tightly packed, with prominent nucleoli and an epithelioid pattern. Several circular cells undergoing mitosis were found in the periphery of each island of cells. There was no significant relationship between cell growth and in vitro behaviour with respect to the age of the patient and stage of menstrual cycle. Cells collected in the follicular, ovulatory and luteal phases all showed epithelial characteristics in primary culture (Fig. 2.1). Scanning electron micrographs of primary cultures revealed the presence of the two cell types, ciliated and secretory cells. However, there were fewer ciliated cells than secretory cells and many of the ciliated cells were shedding their cilia and transforming to the non-ciliated secretory type. The secretory cells had

**Table 2.1.** In vitro characteristics of human tubal ampullary cells

| Culture | Approximate time to form monolayer (days) | Type of growth (LM) | Cell type | Surface structures (SEM) | Modal chromosome number |
|---|---|---|---|---|---|
| Primary | 6 to 10 | Epithelioid | C + S | Cilia, microvilli | 46 |
| 1st Passage | 4 to 5 | Epithelioid | S | Microvilli | 46 |
| 2nd Passage | 3 to 4 | Epithelioid + Fibroblast-like | S | Microvilli | 46 |
| 3rd to 8th Passage | 3 to 4 | Fibroblast-like | S | Microvilli | 46 |
| 9th to 15 Passage | 3 to 4 | Wide, band-like, prominent cytoskeleton | S | Few microvilli | 461 |

LM, light microscopy; SEM, scanning electron microscopy; C, ciliated; S, secretory.

**Table 2.2.** Embryo quality in human ampullary coculture

| Experiment | In vitro system | Number of patients | Number of embryos (2PN) | 2 to 6 cells (%) Absent/slight fragments | Morula (%) | Cavitating blastocysts (%) |
|---|---|---|---|---|---|---|
| 1 | Human ampulla + $T_6$ + 15% HS | 12 | 23 | 91[a] | 78[d] | 69[g] |
| | $T_6$ + 15% HS (control) | | 18 | 72[a] | 50[d] | 33[g] |
| 2 | Human ampulla + Medicult + 10% HS | 36 | 74 | 89[b] | 76[e] | 68[h] |
| | Medicult + 10% HS (control) | | 70 | 70[b] | 39[e] | 31[h] |
| 3 | 48 h conditioned medium (Medicult) | 18 | 67 | 88[c] | 58[f] | 47[i] |
| | Medicult (control) | | 61 | 68[c] | 37[f] | 29[i] |

2PN, 2-pronuclear stage; a:$p<0.01$; b:$p<0.01$; c:$p<0.01$; d:$p<0.01$; e:$p<0.01$; f:$p<0.05$; g:$p<0.01$; h:$p<0.01$; i:$p<0.05$.

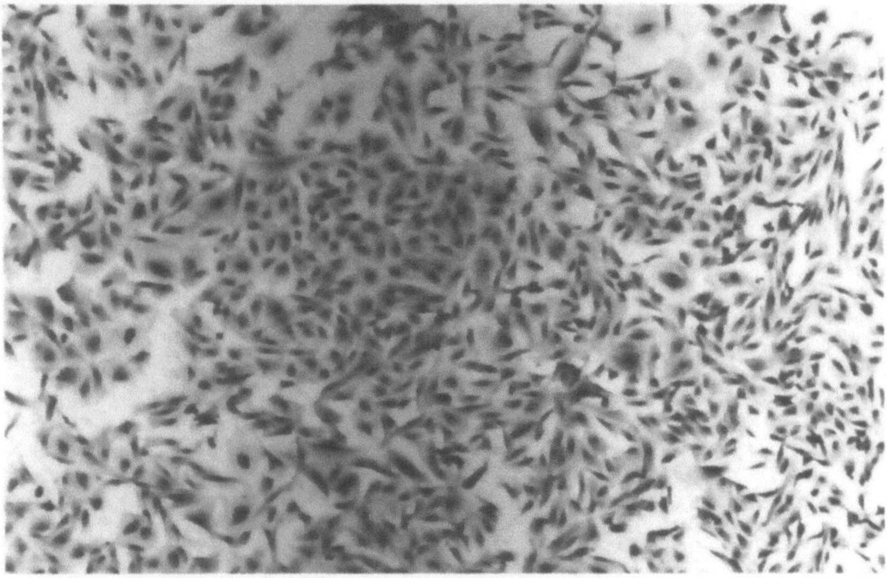

**Fig. 2.1.** Epithelioid cell pattern in ampullary epithelial cells in vitro. Primary culture (×200).

numerous varieties and numbers of microvilli on their surfaces and both cell types showed large areas of cytoplasm, ruffled plasma membranes and several cytoplasmic processes or filopodia. Transmission electron micrographs also confirmed that most of the cells became the secretory type as the length of time in culture increased. The secretory cells were basically of two types – Type I and II (Bongso et al. 1989c). The majority of cells were Type I which had reticulate nucleoli, abundant rough endoplasmic reticulum (RER), well-developed Golgi complexes and dense elongate mitochondria of varied shapes. Secretory vesicles were predominantly clear but occasionally had dark contents. Lipid globules were also present in these cells. Rounded protrusions were observed on the free surfaces of these cells which contained RER and vesicular inclusions. Type II secretory cells were less frequent and had oval translucent mitochondria, less prominent nucleoli and less RER. The secretory vesicles were electron-dense and associated with Golgi complexes. The fact that most of the non-secretory cells transform in culture to the secretory type suggests that the ampullary epithelium is fundamentally secretory in nature.

## Ampullary Epithelial Cell Lines

Human ampullary cells could be maintained alive through at least 15 passages. The time taken between passages to form confluent monolayers was usually around 3–4 days (Table 2.1). Cell morphology changed with continuous passaging. The first passage was usually epithelioid (Fig. 2.2) while the second and third passages became fibroblast-like (Fig. 2.3). The fibroblast-like cells were long, spindle-shaped cells with several long drawn-

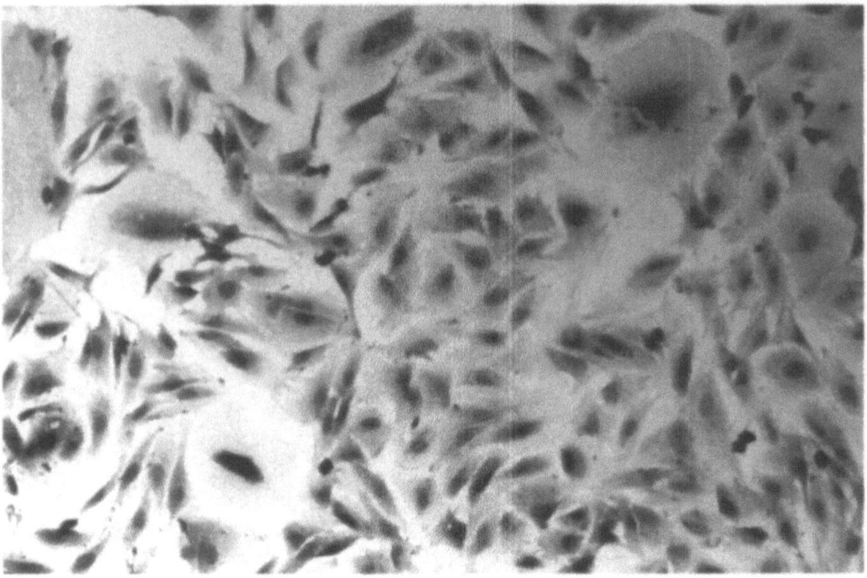

**Fig. 2.2.** Epithelioid cell pattern in ampullary epithelial cells in vitro. 1st passage (×500).

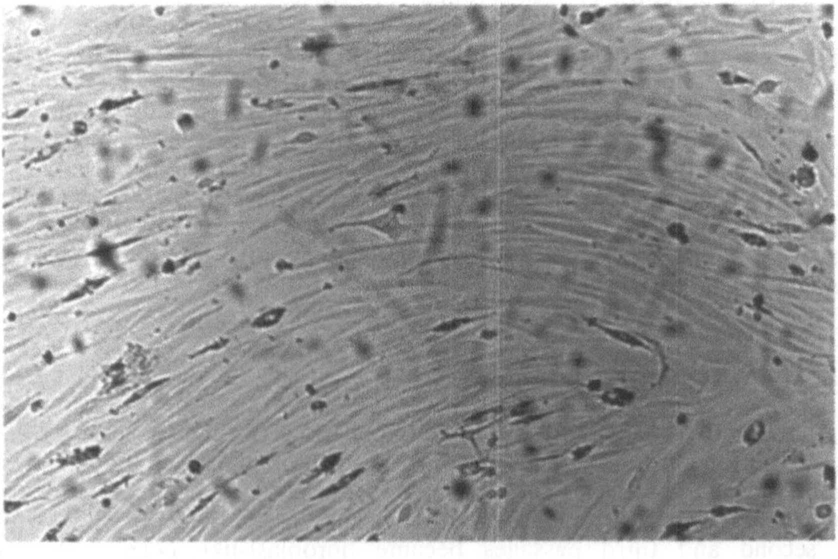

**Fig. 2.3.** Fibroblast-like cell pattern in ampullary epithelial cells in vitro. 5rd passage (×200).

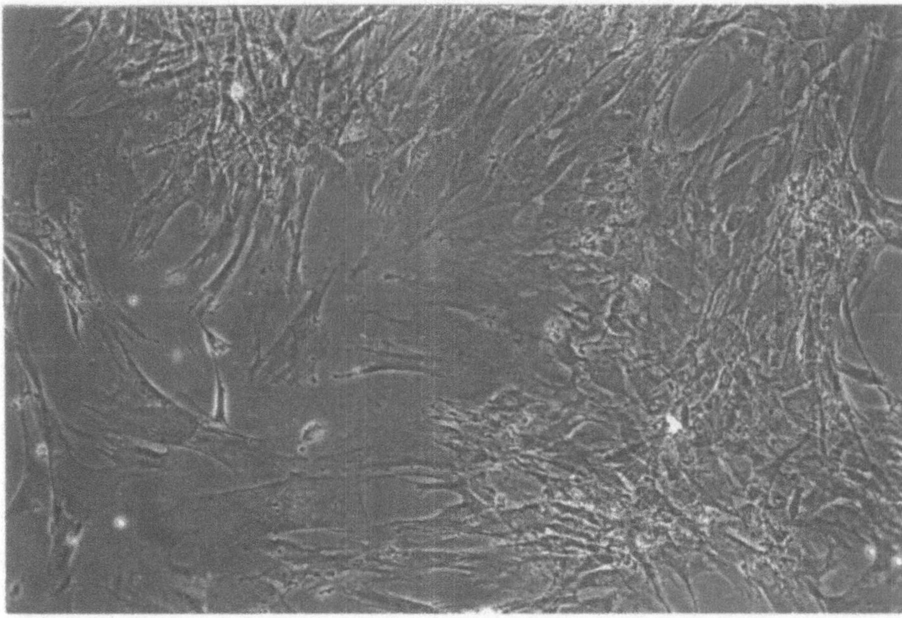

**Fig. 2.4.** Broad band-like cell pattern in ampullary epithelial cells in vitro. 10th passage (×200).

out cytoplasmic processes. In passages thereafter, the spindle-shaped cells became flat, wider band-like cells with prominent cytoskeleton-like structures (Fig. 2.4). Scanning electron micrographs of passaged cultures revealed the complete absence of ciliated cells, and all secretory cells had abundant numbers and varieties of microvilli on their cell surfaces. Transmission electron micrographs of these cells continued to reveal secretory vesicles with electron-dense material. Karyological studies on cells from the various passages showed that the normal diploid chromosome number of 46 was retained all the way to the 15th passage (Fig. 2.5). Many cells also had polyploid sets of chromosomes (Fig. 2.6) (Bongso et al., unpublished data). It will be interesting to investigate the relationship of such cells with a normal genetic make-up but change in morphology to cell function.

Chang's A + B medium was the most suitable for the growth of primary and first passage cultures, while RPMI 1640 or Ham's F10 supplemented with serum was adequate to maintain the growth of further passages. A source of serum was also necessary to allow attachment of cells to the plastic bases and spreading of cells via mitosis. In the absence of a protein source, primary cultures and early passages did not form confluent monolayers but the cells piled up and underwent degeneration. Chang's A + B, RPMI 1640 and Ham's F10 were used in open systems, where the screw-caps of the flasks were kept loose to allow exposure of the cells to a free flow of 5% $CO_2$ in air, and also to maintain the pH of the medium. The risk of microbial contamination is always present in an open system. To overcome this Chang's C medium was successfully used in a closed system which limited

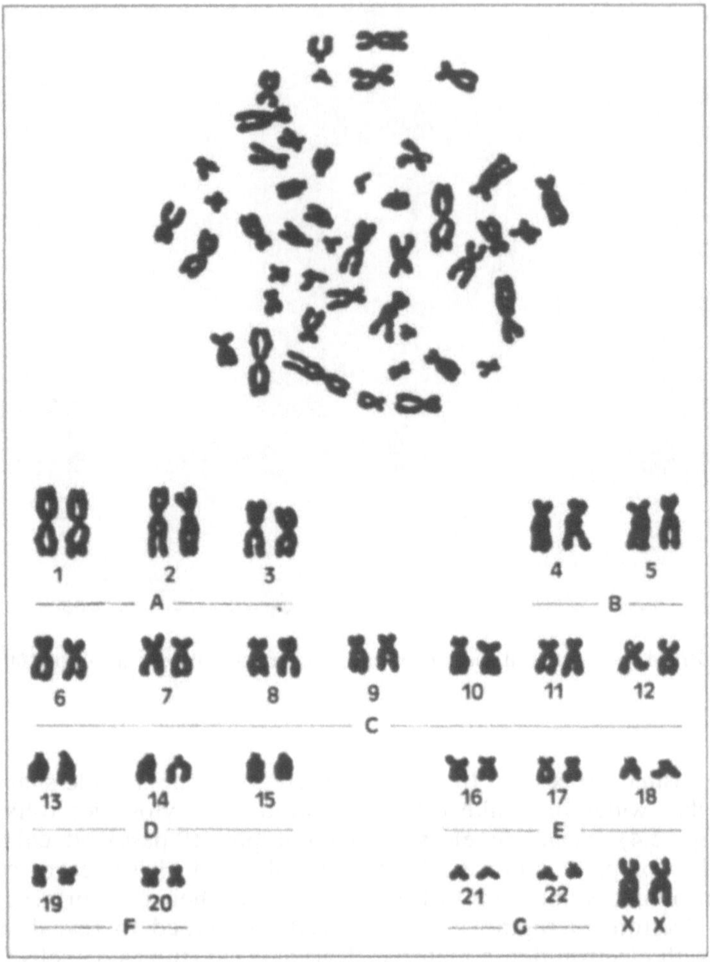


**Fig. 2.5.** Karyotype of ampullary epithelial cells in culture. 10th passage. Note modal chromosome number of 46, and morphology of chromosomes similar to normal human karyotype.

the risk of contamination. However, the medium rapidly became acidic and frequent changing of medium was necessary.

## Ampullary Cell Lines as Cocultures for Assisted Reproduction

Tubal transfer techniques such as gamete intrafallopian technique (GIFT) and tubal embryo transfer (TET) are associated with higher pregnancy rates than uterine transfers of the in-vitro fertilisation and embryo replacement

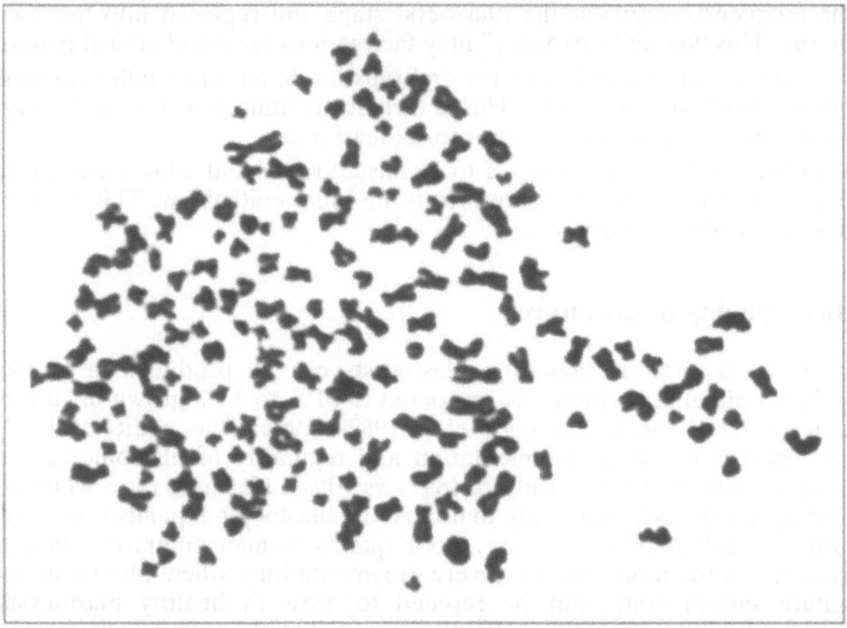

**Fig. 2.6.** Metaphase plate showing polyploid set of chromosomes in ampullary epithelial cells in culture. 10th passage.

method (IVF–ER). There are three possible reasons for this: (i) the tubal environment is most appropriate and superior for embryonic development, (ii) discrete, but as yet unidentified, tubal factors improve embryo quality and (iii) the post-ovulatory uterine environment is hostile (Yovich et al. 1988). Further, although embryos produced in IVF laboratories appear to be of good quality morphologically, many such embryos once replaced into the uterus fail to implant or sustain implantation. It thus appears that currently practised in vitro conditions for IVF–ER are suboptimal as the embryos produced may be of reduced viability; this could be a major cause of low implantation and rates of successful pregnancy outcome. It is also interesting to note that only 15% to 20% of IVF–ER embryos cleave to the blastocyst stage (Bolton et al. 1989). When blastocysts grown in culture medium alone were replaced, the pregnancy rates were the same as with transfer at the 2–6-cell stage (Bolton et al. 1991). In farm animals oocytes are fertilised in vivo in the tubal environment. Blastocysts are flushed from the uterus of donor animals and transferred to recipients, yielding pregnancy rates of over 60% (Iritani 1988).

All this suggests that the viability of human embryos might be improved if fertilisation and growth occurs in a replicated part of the human fallopian tube in vitro. Three approaches to providing a tubal environment are possible:

1. To transfer the patient's two-pronuclear stage embryos into the fallopian tube of another woman. The patient's embryos will then be flushed from

the recipient's uterus at the blastocyst stage and replaced into her own uterus. This type of "surrogacy" may face serious legal and ethical issues.
2. To fertilise oocytes and grow the embryos inside an intact fallopian tube maintained in organ culture. This is technically difficult as the method requires intricate perfusion systems for at least 5 days.
3. Another promising approach is to fertilise oocytes and allow cleavage to occur on feeder layers prepared from the tubal epithelium. This concept has been called "coculture".

## Embryo Quality in Coculture

Some 68% to 69% of cavitating blastocysts can be produced in human ampullary epithelial coculture as compared to 31% to 33% grown in culture medium alone (Table 2.2) (Bongso et al. 1989b, 1992). The quality of the 2–6-cell embryos based on fragmentation and regularity of blastomeres was also significantly better in coculture (89% vs 70%). Hatching rates were not significantly different, suggesting that once the blastocyst expands it may not require an endometrial coculture. Poor quality human embryos (unequal blastomeres with moderate to severe fragmentation) when placed in the coculture system could not be rescued to grow to healthy blastocysts, although Menezo and Ouhibi (1990) claimed that they observed a rescue effect when human embryos were grown in Vero cell coculture. These workers, however, did not describe the exact morphology of their poor quality embryos. We believe that severe fragmentation of embryos in some patients may be an intrinsic embryo problem not related to external deleterious culture factors; such patients will consistently produce fragmented embryos in every assisted reproduction cycle. It is doubtful whether even coculture could improve embryo quality.

## Fertilisation Rates in Coculture

Fertilisation occurs in the ampulla of the fallopian tube in the human and most animals. It is therefore presumed that the secretions from the ampullary epithelium may play a role in the fertilisation process through the induction of capacitation and the acrosome reaction and the initiation of hyperactivated motility. Fertilisation rates have been studied in the human ampullary coculture system (Bongso et al. 1991c). The confluent monolayer interfered with the sperm–egg encounter because the sperm heads became bound to the monolayer or the sperm buried their heads into gaps within the monolayer. If the monolayer was dislodged into single circular cells using trypsin–EDTA and $1 \times 10^5$ cells were added to insemination dishes containing sperm and eggs, 85% of oocytes were fertilised, compared to 67% in culture medium alone ($p < 0.01$). These results were observed for patients with normal and subnormal sperm parameters. The ensuing embryos in coculture were of significantly better quality than the controls (79% vs 67%; $p < 0.05$). Sperm survival at 48 h after insemination was also greater in coculture compared to controls. The sperm acrosome reaction in coculture did not appear to be dramatically increased but motility increased significantly as assessed by computer-automated sperm motion analysis (Cellsoft, Cryoresources, USA) (Bongso et al., unpublished data). The increased motility may have been responsible for the increase in fertilisation rates since it has been shown that sperm motility is the single most important criterion influencing human fertilisation rates (Bongso et al. 1989a). Also, rabbit oviductal coculture did not appear to increase the acrosome reaction of rabbit sperm (Boice et al. 1990).

## Specificity of Cocultures

Cells from different reproductive and non-reproductive sources such as cumulus, ovary, uterus, kidney, spleen and chick embryo, when used for coculture, showed improved viability for a number of mammalian preimplantation embryos (Bongso et al. 1991b). Positive coculture effects were also observed when mouse embryos were grown on feeder layers of human ampulla, human cumulus, mouse ampulla, mouse cumulus and mouse muscle (Bongso et al. 1991a). These results suggest that a specific cell type may not be needed. Further, the species of the cell source used for coculture does not seem to be important since positive effects have been observed when embryos of one species are placed on cell monolayers of other species (Bongso et al. 1991b). Comparative studies of coculture effects between embryos and cells of the same species (homologous effects) with those involving different species (heterologous effects) have not yet been adequately tested.

## Mechanism of Action of Human Tubal Coculture System

The mechanism of the beneficial effects of the ampullary epithelial cells is unknown. Two mechanisms are possible. The cells might condition the culture medium by removing undesirable factors and/or secreting embryotrophic factors. A greater number of cavitating blastocysts can be produced in conditioned medium compared to conventional culture medium for routine IVF–ER (47% vs 29%, $p < 0.05$). The number of good-quality embryos, with slight to no fragments and regular blastomeres, was significantly greater in conditioned medium (88% vs 68%, $p < 0.01$) (Fong et al., unpublished data). Positive coculture effects were also observed with conditioned medium used to grow Vero (monkey kidney) cells (Follett et al. 1991). However, in this report the human embryos studied were polyspermic. Polyploid embryos usually do not fragment and produce regular blastomeres when grown in conventional culture medium. Thus, the positive coculture effects observed with Vero cell-conditioned medium may not be accurate. On polyacrylamide gel electrophoresis, several bands can be observed in ampullary cell-conditioned medium, which are not present in the Vero cell-conditioned medium lanes. It is therefore possible that the effects of human ampullary cells may be due not only to conditioning effect but also to specific proteins secreted by the cells. Glycoproteins specific to the epithelium of the oviduct have been observed in the human (Moghissi 1970; Lippes et al. 1981; Julkunen et al. 1986; Shrimanker et al. 1991), the mouse (Kapur and Johnson 1985), cattle (Gerena and Killian 1990), sheep (Gandolfi et al. 1989) and baboon (Fazleabas and Verhage 1986). The molecular weights ranged from 36 to 215 kd. Gandolfi et al. (1989) showed that two glycoproteins (SOP 46 and SOP 92) secreted from the sheep oviduct were responsible for bypassing the embryonic block in sheep embryos grown on sheep oviductal epithelial monolayers.

## Screening of Ampullary Cell Lines for Microbes

Human ampullary cell lines require screening for microbes before they can be used as feeder layers in assisted reproduction. This is important to prevent the risk of disease transmission directly to the embryo or to the patient. Cell lines can be screened by conventional direct or indirect fluorescent antibody techniques, immunoelectron microscopy and microbiological plating tests.

Of most concern is the transmission of the human immunodeficiency virus (HIV). Several methods for screening tubal cell lines for this organism can been used (Fig. 2.7).

1. The patient providing the tubes for coculture is subjected to two HIV antibody tests: the first at the time of hysterectomy and the second 6 months later. The cultured cells could be frozen, thawed and used only when both tests are negative.
2. By an immunoenzymatic method, we have shown that human ampullary epithelial cells do not possess CD4 receptor sites on their cell membranes. Glycoproteins on the HIV virus coat have to attach to CD4 before they can infect the cell.
3. The DNA of tubal epithelial cells could be tested for the viral genome by extraction and use of an HIV gene probe. We recently observed that ampullary epithelial cells from female transexual patients undergoing reassignment surgery grew very well in culture despite the large doses of testosterone given to these patients. The in vitro behaviour of the epithelial cells was very similar to the cells of women undergoing hysterectomy for sterilisation. Since it is mandatory that transexual patients should be HIV negative before surgery, their tubal epithelial cells would be ideal material to develop HIV-free cell lines as cocultures for assisted reproduction.

## Pregnancy and Implantation Rates Following Human Ampullary Cell Coculture

Human tubal cell lines were developed for coculture with the primary objective of mimicking the environment of the fallopian tube in vivo. In the first trial, 50 patients gave their consent to replace cocultured embryos. The majority of these patients had had at least two previously failed attempts at assisted reproduction and were over the age of 35 years. Such patients were entitled to the replacement of 4 embryos according to Ministry of Health

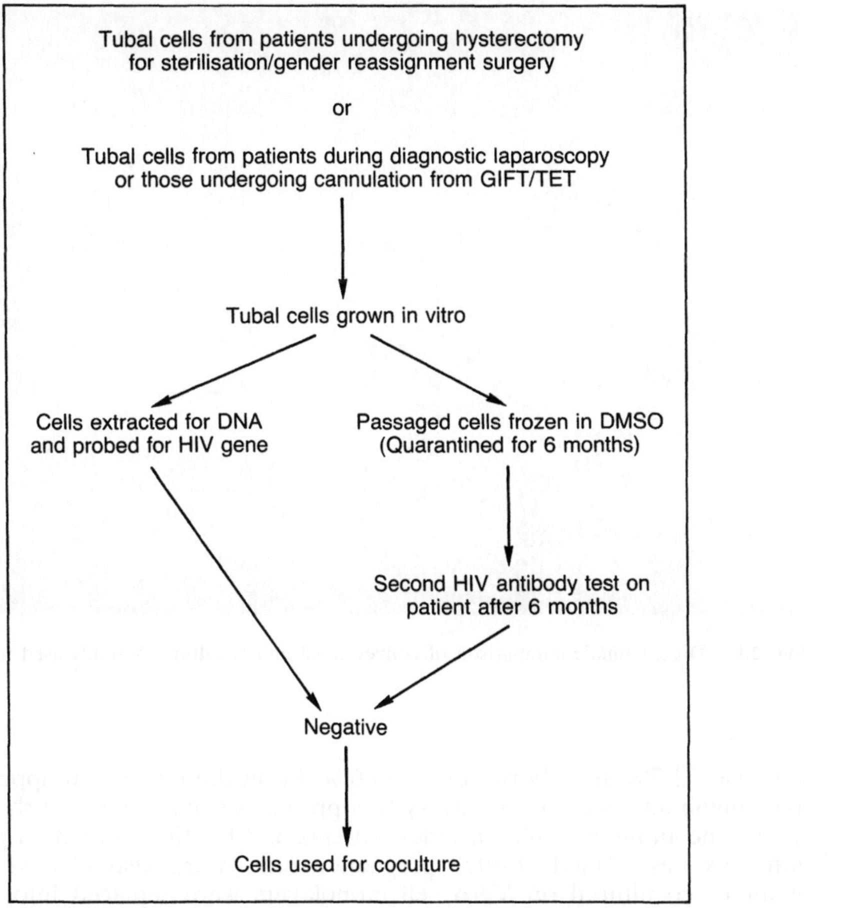


**Fig. 2.7.** Methods of obtaining an HIV-free coculture.

ethical guidelines. When up to 4 embryos were available on Day 2 at the 2–6-cell stage, all four were replaced either into the tubes or into the uterus at this particular stage. If 5 or more embryos were available on Day 2, a sequential transfer was performed (Fig. 2.8). For sequential transfer, 3 embryos were replaced on Day 2 post-insemination (2–6-cell stage) into the tubes or uterus and the remaining embryos grown up to the blastocyst stage. One blastocyst was then replaced into the uterus on Day 5. The steps involved in the preparation of the coculture system for the patients are shown in Fig. 2.9. The overall clinical pregnancy and implantation rates of the 50 patients (30 IVF; 20 TET) in this preliminary trial were 44% and 31.8% respectively (Table 2.3) (Bongso et al. 1991d, 1992). The pregnancy and implantation rates of the 30 IVF and 20 TET patients, when examined separately, were 37% and 31.0% and 55% and 32.6%. Sixty eight per cent of all pregnant patients were over 35 years of age and 68% of the pregnant patients had had at least 2 previously failed cycles. The multiple pregnancy

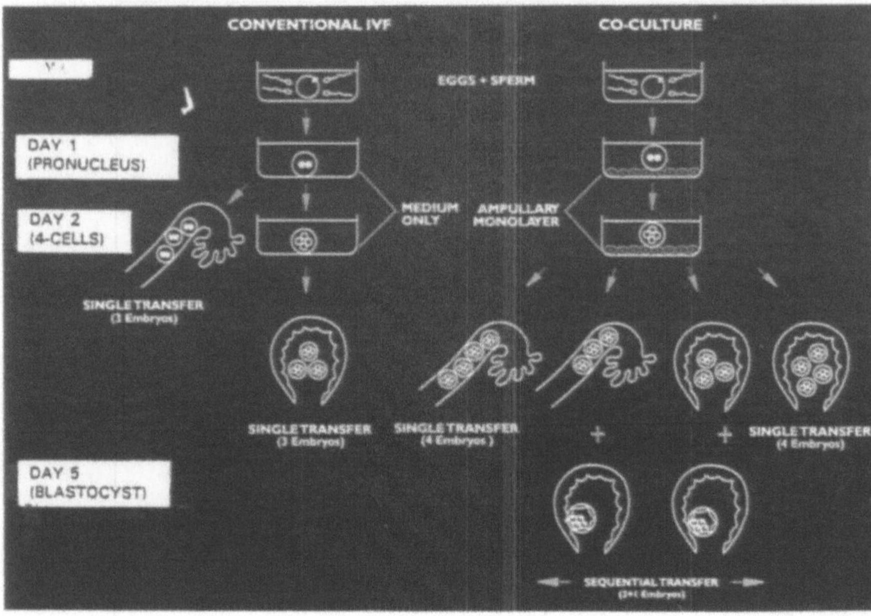


**Fig. 2.8.** Diagrammatic comparison of conventional and coculture methods used for clinical trial.

rate was 22.7% and abortion rate 13.6%. From these results it appears that the human ampullary coculture system produces viable embryos; the system yields encouraging results in older patients and for those in whom previous attempts have failed. Better pregnancy rates were also observed when embryos cocultured on Vero cell monolayers were replaced into patients who had at least 4 previously failed cycles (Menezo et al. 1991). Weimer et al. (1989) reported a 35% implantation rate when human embryos were cocultured on bovine uterine epithelial cells (Table 2.3). It is thus fairly conclusive that the presence of a feeder layer of cells is beneficial to the human embryo in vitro, as reflected in improved pregnancy rates. Whether the

**Table 2.3.** Implantation rates after coculture

| Cell type | Number of patients | Patient category | Embryo stage at transfer | Implantation rate (%) | Author |
|---|---|---|---|---|---|
| Bovine uterine epithelium | 40 | IVF | 2 to 6 cell | 35 | Wiemer et al. (1989) |
| Vero | – | IVF[a] | 2 to 6 cell | 40[b] | Menezo et al. (1992) |
| | 51 | IVF[a] | Blastocyst | 53[b] | |
| Human tubal epithelium | 30 | IVF | 2 to 6 cell | 31[c] | Bongso et al. (1992) |
| | 20 | TET | 2PN/2 to 6 cell | 33[c] | |

[a] All patients had at least four previously failed cycles.
[b] $p < 0.05$.
[c] 68% of pregnant patients were >35 yr and had at least two previously failed cycles.

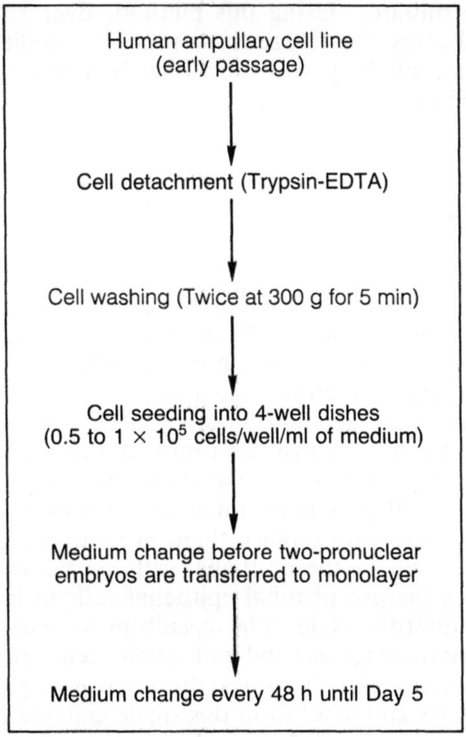


**Fig. 2.9.** Setting up of coculture system for embryonic growth. Note cocultures are set up 24 h before oocyte recovery.

beneficial effects will be greater in a more physiological system such as the human tubal epithelial monolayer needs to be investigated.

## Cryopreservation of Tubal Epithelial Cells

The maintenance of tubal epithelial cell lines requires frequent monitoring, passaging and the changing of culture media. This is labour-intensive and costly. To avoid this, cells could be frozen in liquid nitrogen and maintained as a cell bank. When required for coculture, the cells could be rapidly thawed, washed, seeded into flasks and confluent monolayers established once again. Human tubal epithelial cells have been successfully frozen using a slow stepwise method with a programmable freezing machine (Bongso et al. 1990). Thaw-survival rates were best when 10% dimethylsulphoxide (DMSO) was used as a cryoprotectant, followed by controlled freezing in the machine from room temperature down to −30 °C at 1 °C.min. When the temperature reached −30 °C, the cryotubes were rapidly plunged into liquid nitrogen. Thawing was achieved by warming the frozen cells in a water-bath at 37 °C for a few minutes. Using this method, over 80% of viable cells could be generated after the freeze-thaw process. Studies are in progress to investigate the morphology and functional behaviour of frozen-thawed human tubal epithelial cells.

## Future Aspects

Recent work on the in vitro behaviour of tubal epithelial cells has given much insight on the roles of these cells in fertilisation and early conception. By maintaining such cells in vitro it is now possible to study the interaction between these cells, their secretions, the gametes and the early preimplantation embryo. The ability to generate blastocysts on such feeder layers opens a new area of investigation in assisted reproduction. It has still to be confirmed whether the replacement of cocultured blastocysts alone will yield better pregnancy rates. If pregnancy rates are improved, it might be logical to freeze such blastocysts and replace them in natural cycles. The effect of specific proteins released by the epithelial cells on the embryo needs more investigation as does the use of tubal epithelial cells to improve the quality of sperm in the subfertile male. The coculture system may be useful in preimplantation genetic diagnosis and embryonic stem cell production.

Recently, blastomeres were removed by micromanipulation from 8-cell human embryos; DNA amplified from this single cell was used to provide diagnosis of sex and single gene defects in that embryo. The detection of chromosomal defects is not possible because only a single cell is available. Blastocyst biopsy will provide more cells without harm to the remainder and the coculture system may contribute to providing the required number of blastocysts for such a diagnosis. Embryonic cells from hatched embryos usually require a feeder layer of cells to grow on, spread and yield patches of stem cells. Tubal epithelial cells, which embryologically are of reproductive tract origin, may be ideal feeder layers for stem-cell production when compared to the non-reproductive sources of cell monolayers used for this purpose.

*Acknowledgements*. The authors wish to thank Ms Harjeet Kaur for her excellent secretarial skills in preparing this manuscript.

## References

Biggers JD, Borland RM (1976) Physiological aspects of growth and development of the preimplantation mammalian embryo. Ann Rev Physiol 38:95–119

Boice ML, Duby RT, Robl JM (1990) Rabbit sperm function after coculture with uterine epithelial cells. Theriogenology 34:113

Boland M (1984) Use of the rabbit oviduct as a screening tool for the viability of mammalian eggs. Theriogenology 21:126–137

Bolton V, Hawes SM, Taylor CT, Parsons JH (1989) Development of spare human pre-

implantation embryos in vitro: an analysis of the correlations among gross morphology, cleavage rates and development to blastocyst. J In Vitro Fertil Embryo Transfer 6:30–35
Bolton VN, Wren ME, Parsons JH (1991) Pregnancies after in vitro fertilization and transfer of human blastocysts. Fertil Steril 55:830–832
Bongso A, Gajra B, Ng PL, Wong PC, Ng SC, Ratnam SS (1988) Establishment of human endometrial cell cultures. Hum Reprod 3:705–713
Bongso A et al. (1989a) Effect of sperm motility on human in vitro fertilization. Archives Andrology 22:185–190
Bongso A, Ng SC, Sathananthan H, Ng PL, Rauff M, Ratnam SS (1989b) Improved quality of human embryos when cocultured with human ampullary cells. Hum Reprod 4:706–713
Bongso A, Ng SC, Sathananthan H, Ng PL, Rauff M, Ratnam SS (1989c) Establishment of human ampullary cell cultures. Hum Reprod 4:486–494
Bongso A, Ng SC, Ratnam SS (1990) Cocultures: their relevance to assisted reproduction. Hum Reprod 5:893–900
Bongso A, Ng SC, Fong CY, Mok H, Ng PL, Ratnam SS (1991a) Cocultures in human assisted reproduction: support of embryos in vitro and their specificity. In: Frontiers in human reproduction, Ann NY Acad Sci 620:438–444
Bongso A, Ng SC, Fong CY, Ratnam SS (1991b) Cocultures: a new lead in embryo quality improvement for assisted reproduction. Fertil Steril 56:179–191
Bongso A, Ng SC, Fong CY, Ratnam SS (1991c) Improved fertilization rates of human oocytes in coculture. J In Vitro Fertil Embryo Transfer 8:216–221
Bongso A, Ng SC, Ratnam SS, Chan C, Anandakumar C, Wong YC, Goh V, Devendra S, Soon SB, Fong CY, Vasuthevan S (1991d) Pregnancies after fertilization and cleavage in human coculture. J In Vitro Fertil Embryo Transfer 8:116–118
Bongso A, Ng SC, Fong CY, Anandakumar C, Marshall B, Edirisinghe R, Ratnam SS (1992) Improved pregnancy rate after transfer of embryos grown in human fallopian tubal cell coculture. Fertil Steril 58: 569–574.
Brundin J (1965) Distribution and function of adrenergic nerves in the rabbit fallopian tube. Acta Physiol Scand 66, Suppl 259:1–57
Chaminadas C, Chopper AY, Royez A, Prost O, Remy-Martin JP, Adessi GM (1986) Culture of endometrial and stromal cells of guinea-pig endometrium and the effect of oestradiol-17$\beta$ on the epithelial cells. J Reprod Fertil 77:547–558
Donnez J, Casanas-Roux F, Caprasse J, Ferin J, Thomas K (1985) Cyclic changes in ciliation, cell height and mitotic activity in human tubal epithelium during reproductive life. Fertil Steril 43:554–560
Fazleabas AT, Verhage HG (1986) The detection of oviduct specific proteins in the baboon (*Papio anubis*). Biol Reprod 35:455–460
Follett KL, Hammitt DG, Bennett MR, Syrop CH (1991) Enhanced development of human embryos cocultured with Vero cells. Proc Amer Fertil Soc, Oregon, USA, Abst p 184
Gandolfi F, Tiziana A, Brevini AL, Richardson L, Brown CR, Moor RM (1989) Characterization of proteins secreted by sheep oviduct epithelial cells and their function in embryonic development. Development 106:303–312
Gerena RL, Killian GJ (1990) Electrophoretic characterization of proteins in oviduct fluid of cows during the estrous cycle. J Exp Zool 256:113–120
Hamner CE (1973) Oviductal fluid – composition and physiology. In: Greep RO, Astwood EB (eds) Handbook of physiology, Section 7, Endocrinology II. American Physiology Society, Washington DC, pp 141–151
Hardy K, Hooper MAK, Handyside AH, Rutherford AJ, Winston RML, Leese JH (1989) Non-invasive measurement of glucose and pyruvate uptake by individual human oocytes and preimplantation embryos. Hum Reprod 4:188–191
Hunter GL, Bishop GP, Adams CE, Rowson LE (1962) Successful long distance aerial transport of fertilized sheep ova. J Reprod Fertil 3:33–40
Hunter RHF (ed) (1988) The fallopian tubes: their role in fertility and infertility. Springer-Verlag, London, pp 30–52
Iritani A (1988) Current status of biotechnological studies in mammalian reproduction. Fertil Steril 50:543–551
Jansen RPS (1984) Endocrine response in the fallopian tube. Endocrinol Rev 5:525–532
Julkunen M, Wahlstrom T, Seppala M (1986) Human fallopian tube contains placental protein 14. Am J Obstet Gynecol 154:1076–1079
Kapur RP, Johnson LV (1985) An oviductal fluid glycoprotein associated with ovulated mouse ova and early embryos. Developmental Biol 112:89–93

Lippes J, Krasner J, Alfonso LA, Dacalos ED, Lucero R (1981) Human oviductal fluid proteins. Fertil Steril 36:623–629
Maguiness SD, Shrimanker K, Djahanbakhch O, Grudzinskas JG (1992) Oviduct proteins. Contemp Rev Obstet Gynaecol 4:42–50
Mastroianni L Jr, Go KJ (1979) Tubal secretions. In: Beller FK, Schumacher GFB (eds) The biology of the fluids of the female genital tract. Elsevier, North Holland, 335–344
Menezo Y, Ouhibi N (1990) Embryo coculture. Assisted Reprod Tech, Androl 1, 29–308
Menezo Y, Dumont M, Montagut J, Hazout A, Nicollet B, Herbaut N (1991) Coculture and delayed transfer at the blastocyst stage for multiple failures of embryo transfer in IVF programmes. 7th World Congress on IVF and Assisted Procreations. Abstract p 122, 149
Menezo Y, Hazout A, Dumont M, Herbaut N, Nicollet B (1992) Coculture of embryos on Vero cells and transfer of blastocysts in humans. Hum Reprod 7:101–106
Moghissi KS (1970) Human fallopian tube fluid 1. Protein composition. Fertil Steril 21:821–829
Nilsson O, Reinius S (1969) Light and electron microscopic structure of the oviduct. In: Hafez ESE, Blandau RJ (eds) The mammalian oviduct. University of Chicago Press, Chicago, p 57–83
Novak E, Everett HS (1928) Cyclical and other variations in the tubal epithelium. Am J Obstet Gynecol 16:499–505
Owman CH, Rosengren E, Sjoberg NO (1967) Adrenergic innervation of the human female reproductive organs: a histochemical and chemical investigation. Obstet Gynecol 30:763–773
Patek E (1974) The epithelium of the human fallopian tube. Acta Obstet Gynecol Scand 53, Suppl 31:1–28
Pauerstein CJ, Eddy CA (1979) Morphology of the fallopian tube. In: Beller FK, Schumacher GFB (eds) The biology of the fluids of the female genital tract. Elsevier, North Holland, pp 299–317
Ricketts AP, Hagensee M, Bullock DW (1983) Characterization in primary monolayer culture of separated cell types from rabbit endometrium. J Reprod Fertil 67:151–160
Shrimanker K, Maguiness SD, Djahanbakhch, Grundzinskas JG (1991) Two tubal proteins (TEP-1 and TEP-2): identification and preliminary characterization. 7th World Congress on IVF and Assisted Procreations, Abstract p 119, 97
Stubbings B (1988) *Maturation of oocytes for cattle in vitro fertilization*. PhD dissertation. University of Guelph, Ontario, Canada
Verhage HG, Bareither ML, Jaffe RC, Akbar M (1979) Cyclic changes in ciliation, secretion and cell height of the oviductal epithelium in women. Am J Anat 156:505–510
Weimer KE, Cohen J, Amborski GF, Wright G, Wiker S, Munyakasi L, Godke RA (1989) In vitro development and implantation of human embryos following culture on fetal bovine uterine fibroblast cells. Hum Reprod 4:595–600
Yanagimachi R (1988) Mammalian fertilization. In: Knobil E, Neill JD (eds) The physiology of reproduction. Raven Press, New York, pp 135–186
Yovich JH, Yovich JM, Edirisinghe WR (1988) The relative chance of pregnancy following tubal or uterine transfer procedures. Fertil Steril 49:858–864

Chapter 3

# Fallopian Tube Epithelial Cell Culture

O. Djahanbakhch, E. Kervancioglu, S.D. Maguiness
and J.E. Martin

## Introduction

There is limited knowledge about the biological events which occur in the fallopian tube during the ovarian cycle and the early events of reproduction. The physiological mechanisms which control the timing of gamete interaction and fertilisation are not yet clearly understood. As the fallopian tube provides the environment in which early embryo development takes place these events may have a significant effect on all the subsequent events of the pregnancy. Physiological study of the fallopian tube has been hampered by its inaccessibility. The fluid in the tubal lumen has been studied using tubal cannulation, demonstrating that while the majority of the constituents of tubal fluid appear to originate from serum, there are proteins which may be specific to it (Lippes et al. 1981; Lippes and Wagh 1989; Wagh and Lippes 1989). The role of these proteins is unknown.

A problem with tubal cannulation is that the presence of the cannula may affect the constituents of the tubal fluid. Furthermore it is difficult to study fluid from different sections of the tube. To facilitate more detailed study and specifically to investigate the tubal mucosa which is in contact with the gametes and pre-embryo, many workers have established in vitro cultures of tubal epithelial cells (McComb et al. 1986; Bongso et al. 1989a; Ouhibi et al. 1989; Takeuchi et al. 1991; Kervancioglu et al. 1992). Most studies have had only limited success and use complex culture media. This chapter reviews these studies and describes a simple, inexpensive method by which we have been able to culture tubal epithelial cells successfully for up to 60 days.

# Histological Organisation of Fallopian Tube Mucosa

The mucosa of the fallopian tube is convoluted into folds longitudinally around the lumen. The size and complexity of these folds increases progressively along the lumen towards the fimbriated end where there are many secondary and tertiary folds superimposed on the primary fold. Each fold consists of a single epithelial cell layer on a basement membrane. This is surrounded by a connective tissue layer, the lamina propria, which separates the epithelial layer from the muscle layer, the tunica muscularis.

In the epithelial layer four types of cell have been identified. The commonest are ciliated and secretory cells. Less commonly seen are the smaller peg (intercalary) and basal (indifferent) cells. In the lamina propria plasma cells are present. The commonest of these, which are present throughout the length of the tube, secrete IgA (Kutteh et al. 1988). Plasma cells of the IgG or IgM class are present, but are less frequently seen.

The ciliated cells are cuboidal in shape and contain a fine granular cytoplasm. These cells are further characterised by their vesiculated endoplasmic reticulum, long mitochondria and cytoplasmic droplets. The nucleus is usually centrally located and is round or oval in shape. A perinuclear halo of clear cytoplasm is often seen. The cilia are attached to a refractile row of basal granules beneath the cell membrane (Fig. 3.1). They are approximately 7 $\mu$m long and consist of two central filaments surrounded by nine double lateral filaments.

Ciliated cells are most commonly seen on the apical aspect of the mucosal folds. Along the length of the mucosal folds some workers have reported a uniform distribution, while others suggest a progressive decrease in their

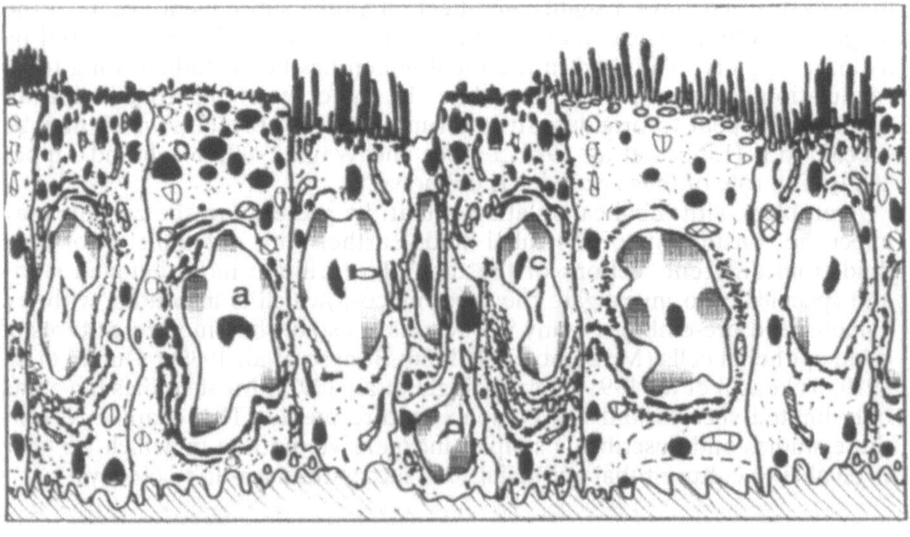


**Fig. 3.1.** Schematised secretory (a), ciliary (b), peg (c) and indifferent (d) cells.

occurrence from the fimbriated end to the isthmus (Ferenczy et al. 1972; Patek et al. 1972a,b; Critoph and Dennis 1977).

Secretory cells have a more granular cytoplasm (secretory granules), a well-developed endoplasmic reticulum and golgi bodies. The mitochondria are smaller than in ciliated cells and the nucleus is dark and oval with its longitudinal axis parallel to that of the cell (Fig. 3.1). As with the secretory epithelial cells of the endometrium the position of the nucleus varies throughout the ovarian cycle.

Secretory cells are distributed throughout the length of the fallopian tube, being most common in the ampulla where they constitute approximately 50% of epithelial cells.

Intercalary cells appear as small cells with little cytoplasm and a long dark nucleus, compressed between adjacent cells (Fig. 3.1). It is thought that they may be exhausted secretory cells as they are seen most often in the luteal phase of the ovarian cycle (Fredricks 1986). The basal cells are small, rounded and also have sparse cytoplasm surrounding a dark nucleus and are located adjacent to the basement membrane.

## Changes in the Oviduct Mucosa during the Ovarian Cycle

The appearance of cells in the epithelial layer of the fallopian tube varies during the ovarian cycle. This appears to be in direct response to changes in circulating levels of ovarian steroids since the concentration of both cytosol and nuclear receptors for oestradiol and progesterone vary with the stage of the ovarian cycle (Pollow et al. 1981). Evidence for binding to these receptors has been reported in tissue studies which have demonstrated high concentrations of oestradiol and progesterone in the fallopian tube compared with serum (Batra et al. 1980; Devoto et al. 1980).

Ciliated cells in the tubal epithelial layer become reduced in height during the menstrual phase (Patek et al. 1972a). The cells become progressively higher during the follicular phase achieving maximum height during the periovulatory phase. In the luteal phase the cells become broader and lower.

While there is no cyclic shedding and regeneration of cilia as observed in the infundibulum of the Rhesus monkey (Brenner 1969), Verhage et al. (1979) reported 12%–14% deciliation in the luteal phase, with regeneration in the early follicular phase of the next cycle. The cilia appear "droopy" during the menstrual phase. They become progressively more erect during the follicular phase and are regularly distributed on the surface of the cell. The cilia beat most vigorously at or just after ovulation. At this time the strokes of the cilia in the fimbria, ampulla and isthmus are synchronised and orientated towards the isthmic-ampullary junction (Borell et al. 1957; Blandau 1969; Blandau and Verdugo 1976).

There is disagreement about the occurrence of specific ultrastructural changes during the ovarian cycle. However, there may be an increase in the number and size of cytoplasmic granules, and mitochondria, as the cycle progresses. The majority of secretory cells of the tubal epithelium appear low during the menstrual phase. Some, which are spherical in shape, appear in clusters and bulge into the tubal lumen. These appearances are retained from the late luteal phase of the previous cycle. During the follicular phase the secretory cells increase in height and are covered with tall, well-shaped microvilli. In the periovulatory period the microvilli become swollen and adhere to each other, forming tuft-like formations. In the luteal phase the tall secretory cells bulge into the tubal lumen, creating an irregular epithelial border. The microvilli of these cells are less evenly distributed on their surface (Patek et al. 1972a,b).

These changes are associated with ultrastructural alterations which reflect changing secretory activity (Ludwig and Metzer 1976; Pauerstein 1975). At the onset of the proliferative phase the golgi apparatus is compact, the endoplasmic reticulum limited and mitochondria diminished. These structures become progressively more prominent during the follicular phase and at about Day 10 ribonucleic acid (Palade) granules become numerous. By the end of the follicular phase secretory granules appear beneath the cell membrane adjacent to the tubal lumen. In the luteal phase the endoplasmic reticulum dilates and secretory droplets and granules appear. At the same time the golgi apparatus expands and the mitochondria decrease in number. Some secretory cells rupture and release their contents during the midluteal phase. Overall, secretory activity during the menstrual cycle is more prominent in the isthmus than in the ampulla.

## Functional Aspects of Tubal Epithelium

The proteins which are secreted by tubal epithelium are reviewed in Chapter 5. Their roles in the events of early reproduction are unknown, though there is evidence of interaction between gametes, the pre-embryo and tubal fluid which contains the products of secretion by the epithelial cells.

In sheep, Gandolfi et al. (1989) demonstrated that the oviduct produced two polypeptides, referred to as sheep oviduct proteins 92 and 46 (SOP 92, SOP 46); these were detected within the first 4–5 days of oestrus. Labellng studies showed that these proteins were bound to the zona pellucida of oocytes collected from the oviduct, and were absent from oocytes which had no contact with the oviduct.

There is increased capacitation of bovine spermatozoa in oviductal fluid (Parrish et al. 1989). Human spermatozoa with poor mobility have been shown to have an increased ability to penetrate a zona-free hamster oocyte in the presence of a medium based on the composition of human tubal fluid compared with Ham F10 medium alone (Cai and Marik 1990). The value of using culture media with the characteristics of human tubal fluid is less clear, with some reporting improved pregnancy rates (Quinn et al. 1985) while others found no improvement (Cummins et al. 1986).

In current in vitro fertilisation programmes the pre-embryo is usually transferred to the uterine cavity 2 days after fertilisation when it has reached the 2–4-cell stage. The theoretical reason for this is that longer term culture might lead to a developmental block and fragmentation or loss of viability.

In natural reproduction the pre-embryo enters the uterine cavity about 6 days after fertilisation. Thus, in current assisted-conception practice a rather immature pre-embryo is transferred to the uterine cavity where the endometrium is not necessarily receptive for implantation. Coculture of the pre-embryo with epithelial cells from the fallopian tube and transfer to the endometrial cavity at a more physiological time may improve embryo quality and implantation rate.

## Oviduct Epithelial Cell Culture

Cell culture provides a useful means of studying various aspects of the function of epithelial cells of the fallopian tube such as metabolism, protein synthesis, and response to drugs and infection. The effect of different physicochemical conditions (pH, temperature, osmotic pressure, oxygen and carbon dioxide tension) and physiological agents such as hormones and other regulatory substances on the fallopian tube can be observed in cells obtained from the different sites at each stage of the ovarian cycle.

In cell culture the characterisation and homogeneity of the sample can be tightly controlled. Single cell types can be individually assessed or the interaction of two different cell types can be observed (Byres et al. 1986). The use of polarised cell cultures allows the direction of substrate uptake and protein secretion to be studied (Carson et al. 1988). The translocation of hormone receptor complexes, fluctuations in cellular metabolic pools and cell-to-cell interactions can be examined (Freshney 1987).

The disadvantages of cell culture systems are that the original histology is lost, together with any paracrine influences. Cells which are cultured on an uncoated plastic surface lose the polarisation normally present in intact tissue. Premature senescence and de-differentiation may occur in cells cultured on either glass or plastic surfaces (Gospodarowicz et al. 1980). Since it has been shown that extracellular matrices (ECM) stimulate proliferation and prevent de-differentiation (Hadley et al. 1985), and these is no reported study on human fallopian tube epithelial cell culture, we currently use a commercially available ECM on a permeable filter for culture of epithelial cells (Fig. 3.2).

## Methodology

### Isolation of Fallopian Tube Epithelial Cells

The method we have used to isolate epithelial cells of fallopian tube is to dissect off the tubal mucosa and cut it into small pieces approximately 1 $mm^3$ with fine scissors. The tissue pieces are washed to remove any traces of blood and placed in culture medium. After 7–10 days of this primary culture the tissue explants are removed to fresh medium.

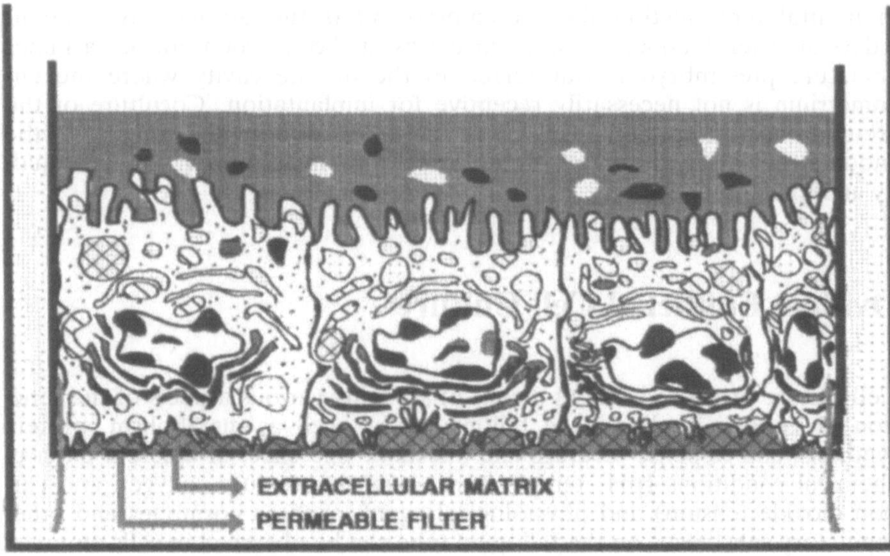


**Fig. 3.2.** Schematised epithelial cells in the dual environmental chamber.

Mechanical isolation (Bongso et al. 1989a) involves dislodging epithelial cells by using a needle and syringe to flush the lumen of the fallopian tube with Hank's Balanced Salt Solution (HBSS). If the cell numbers obtained using this method were inadequate the authors resorted to gently scraping the epithelial layer.

Enzymatic disaggregation of the epithelial layer can be achieved using trypsin (Ouhibi et al. 1989), collagenase (Takeuchi et al. 1991), or a combination of the two (Jung-Testas et al. 1986). Care needs to be taken with these enzymes as trypsin has been shown to have a deleterious effect on the cells if the reaction is performed at 37 °C (Freshney 1987). At lower temperatures (4 °C) a higher yield of viable cells can be obtained after 14 h. If serum-free medium is used the effect of trypsin has to be neutralised with an inhibitor, e.g., soyabean trypsin inhibitor.

## Media Requirements and Maintenance

Various media have been used for the culture of human fallopian tube epithelial cells: Chang, B2, MEM, Ml99, RPMI 1640. With the exception of Chang's medium (Bongso et al. 1989a) all these media require the addition of 7.5% to 20% serum. When cells become confluent they are detached from their substrate with trypsin/EDTA and transferred to fresh media in new culture dishes to allow further cell proliferation in subculture. Without serum supplementation, primary culture has been carried on for up to 56 days in the presence of albumin, insulin and transferrin (Henrikson et al. 1990). However, the cell number did not increase after Day 10 and subculture was not successful. Supplements used by others include lactalbumin hydrolysed epidermal growth factor and serotonin (Takeuchi et al. 1991).

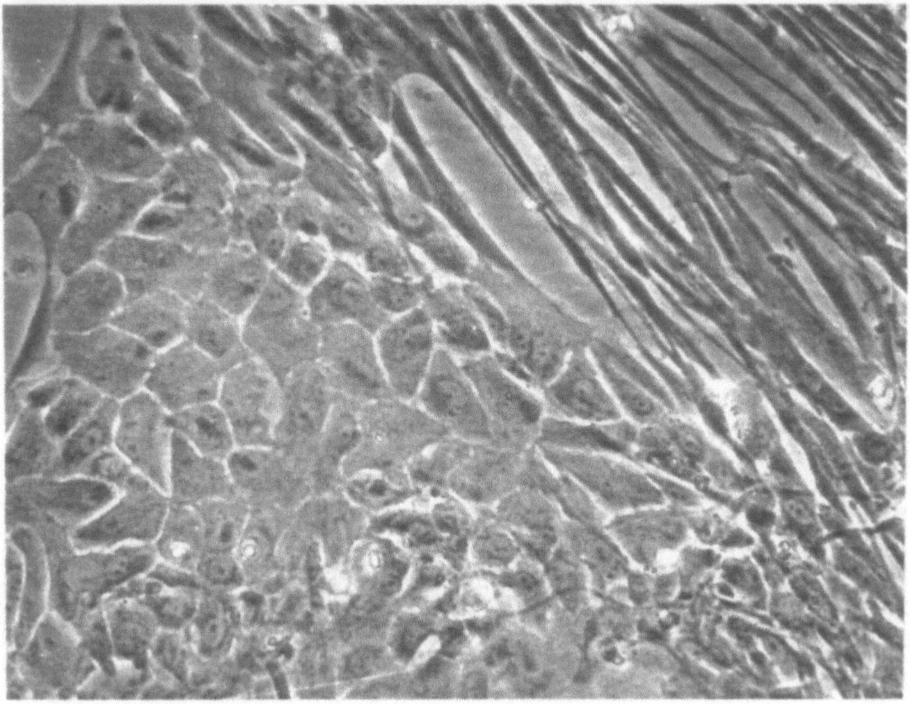

**Fig. 3.3.** Fibroblastic contamination seen in primary culture (×180).

We have successfully cultured and subcultured tubal epithelial cells for 60 days in MEM Earle's, a conventional medium used for assisted conception procedures, supplemented with fetal bovine serum.

## Selection of Epithelial Cells

A major problem encountered in epithelial cell culture is contamination by fibroblast overgrowth (Fig. 3.3). Different methods have been devised to select epithelial cells preferentially and prevent fibroblast proliferation.

1. Cloning. As with any normal tissue, cultured cells may only survive through a limited lifespan; thus when a clone is eventually produced the surviving cells may have only limited viability.
2. Selective media. L-valine and D-valine have been used to select epithelium from fetal lung and umbilical cord (Gilbert and Migeon 1975).
3. Selective detachment. If a heterogeneous monolayer is treated with trypsin, fibroblasts are preferentially removed. If EDTA is used, epithelial cells are readily removed.
4. Differential attachment. This method has been used to separate fibroblasts and epithelial cells in the chick oviduct (Jung-Testas et al. 1986).
5. The substrate. Different substrates favour the attachment of different cell types. Collagen in gel form has been used to promote the growth of epithe-

lial cells (Lillie et al. 1980). Some plastic surfaces, with different electrical charges, favour epithelial cell growth relative to that of fibroblasts.

## Confirmation of Cell Type

Phase contrast microscopy is widely used to identify cells as epithelial-like or fibroblast-like. A more accurate assessment of cell type can be made by demonstrating the staining characteristics of intermediate filament proteins: cytokeratin (epithelial cells), vimentin (mesodermal cells), and desmine (muscle cells). It is important to include positive and negative controls. Our control experiments included one in which the primary antibody was excluded. Anti-cytokeratin and anti-vimentin antibodies were used in parallel experiments on cells from the same culture well. After staining with the primary antibody, antibody-containing cells can be observed using different methods e.g. PAP or Biotin-Avitin (Fig. 3.4).

Electron microscopy can identify specific characteristics of epithelial cells e.g. microvilli (sometimes covered by glycocalyx), intercelluar junction complexes and polarised cytoplasmic structures (Fig. 3.5a,b,c). Polarised cells showed a columnar pattern and prominent epithelial patches where non-polarised cells were flat (Fig. 3.6).

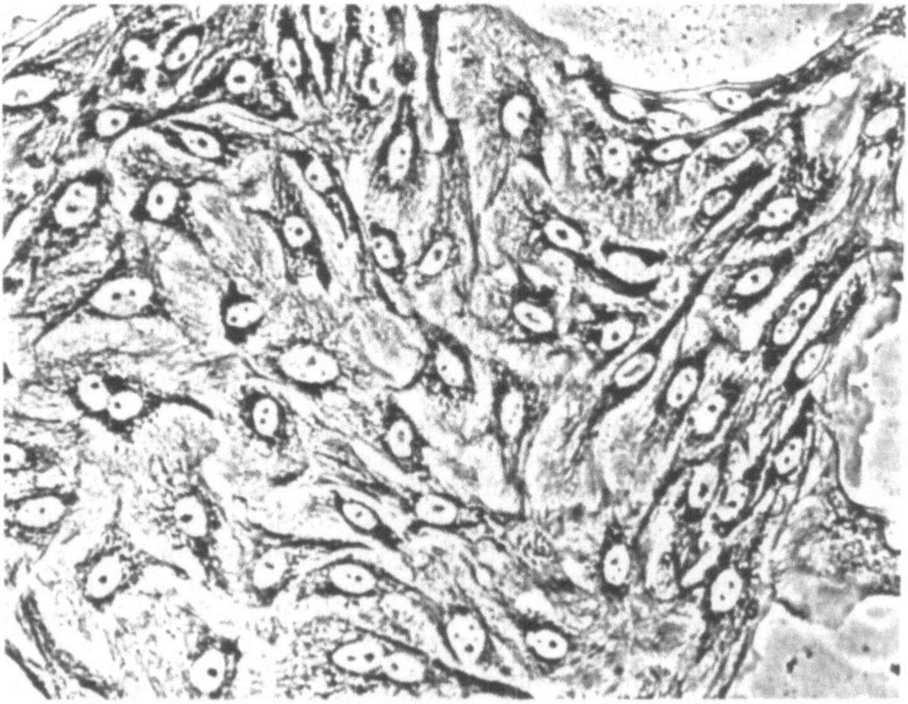

**Fig. 3.4.** Biotin/avitin staining, demonstrating the presence of cytokeratin in cells (×220).

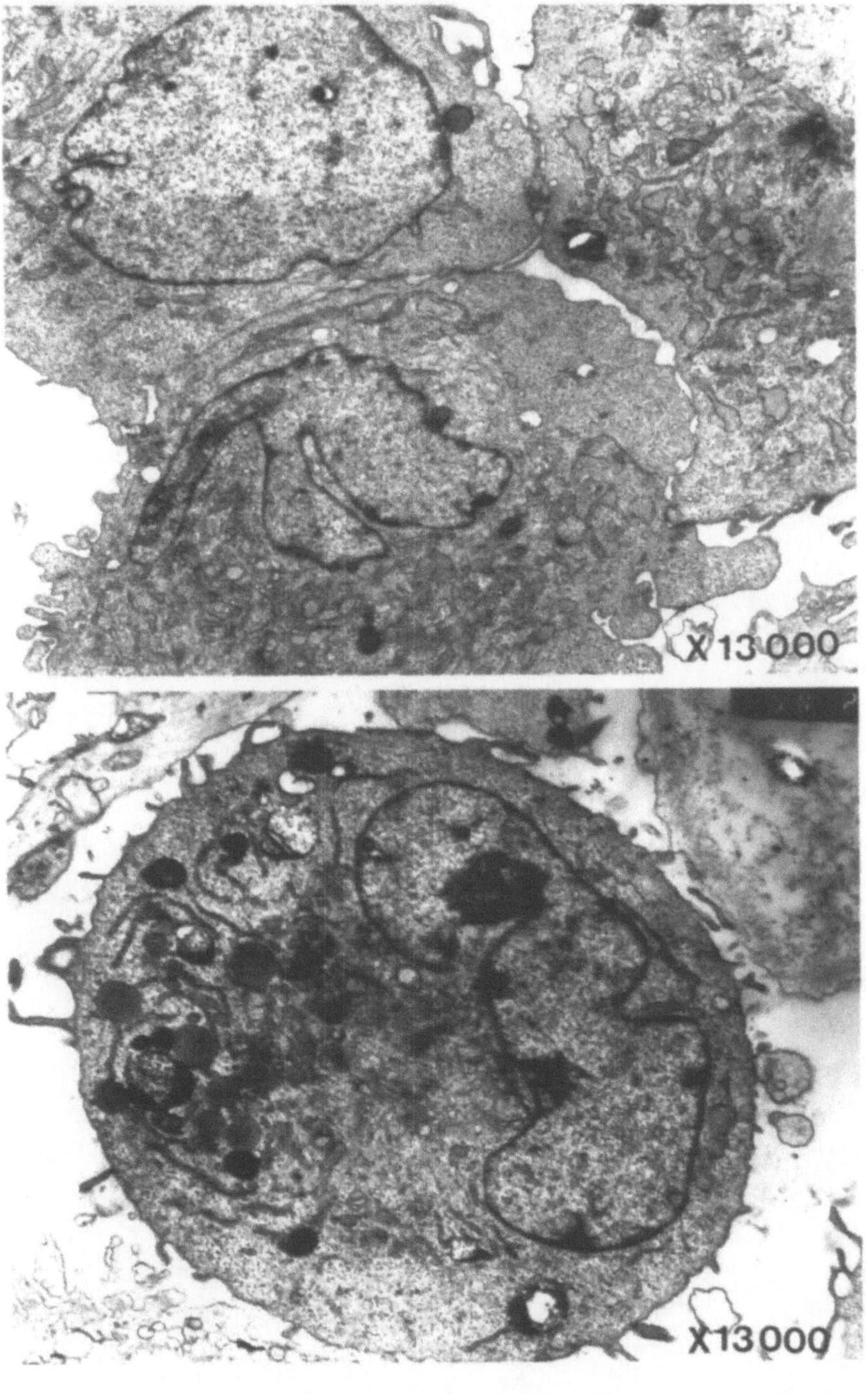


**Fig. 3.5a,b,c.** Transmission electron microscopy of subcultured cells, demonstrating the presence of reticulate nucleoli, numerous mitochondria, abundant endoplasmic reticulum, electron-dense granules and lipid droplets (×13 000). (*continued on next page*)

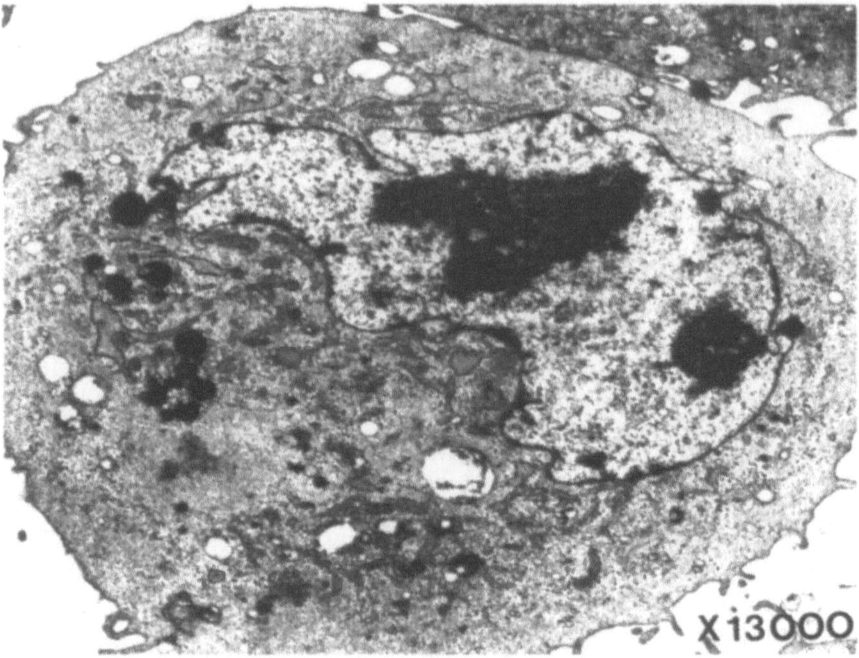


**Fig. 3.5** (*continued*)

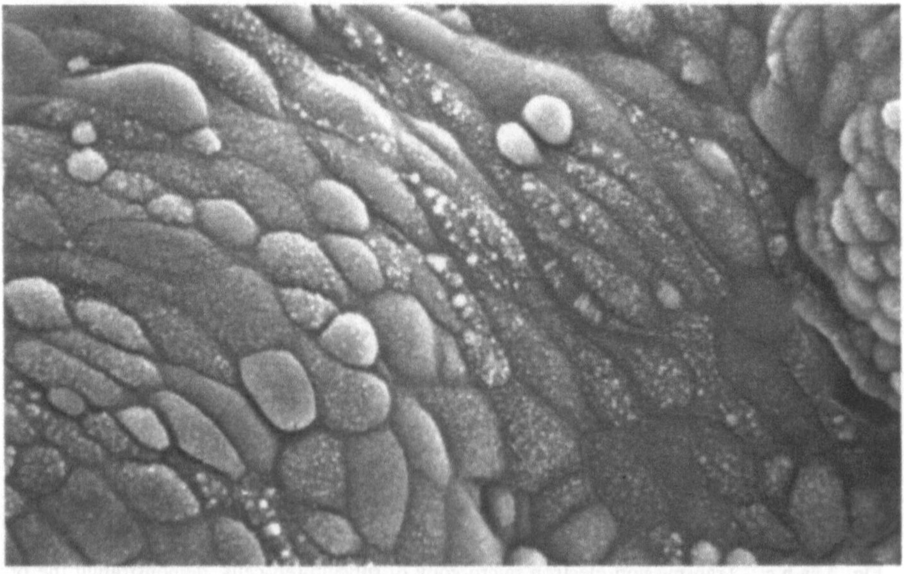

**Fig. 3.6.** Scanning electron microscopy of polarised epithelial cells (×900).

## Polarised Epithelial Cell Culture

In order to develop polarised epithelial cell culture Millicell PC (Millipore Corp., Bedford, MA) was treated with 50-$\mu$l basal lamina extract, Matrigel (Collaborative Research, Bedford, MA) to cover and gel on its upper surface. This Millicell/Matrigel insert was then transferred to a 24-well flat-bottomed plastic tissue culture plate (Falcon Plastics, Los Angeles, CA) creating two compartments. 300 $\mu$l of culture medium was added into the lower compartment created in the system by Millicell. Fallopian tube epithelial cells which were removed by trypsinisation from subcultures were seeded into the upper compartment of the system in 150 $\mu$l of culture medium. In this study, subcultures 1, 4 and 7 were used to develop polarised cells in 11 cases.

## Current Success Rates

With these methods, we have established that 98% of cells in primary culture, and 80% on Day 40, were of epithelial origin (Kervancioglu et al. 1992). The reported life span of cultures ranges from 21 days (Takeuchi et al. 1991) to 60 days (Kervancioglu et al. 1992). Ciliated cells have only been identified in primary culture and disappear after the first passage (Bongso et al. 1989a; Henrikson et al. 1990). It is unclear whether these cells simply lose their cilia in subculture, or die. Ouhibi et al. (1989) observed that the maximum number of ciliated cells occurred in the primary culture of cells obtained during the periovulatory phase of the ovarian cycle. We have demonstrated that ciliated cells continue to proliferate when the tissue in a primary culture is removed after 7–10 days and the primary culture is repeated using this tissue in fresh medium. This suggests that the growth of ciliated cells may be dependent on some factor present in the fallopian tube (Kervancioglu et al. 1992).

There appears to be no difference between the in vitro growth rate of epithelial cells obtained during the follicular and luteal phases of the ovarian cycle (Takeuchi et al. 1991). The addition of oestrogen, fibroblast growth factor, insulin and transferrin had no stimulatory effect on in vitro cell growth. However, when progesterone was added cell growth tended to be inhibited (Takeuchi et al. 1991).

## Coculture of Epithelial Cells with Gametes and Embryos

There are many theoretical reasons why coculture may be of benefit to gametes and the pre-embryo. The epithelial cells may secrete specific factors and there is evidence that oviduct secretory cells do continue to secrete proteins in culture (Joshi 1988). Another factor may simply be the contact between the gametes or pre-embryo and the epithelial cells (Allen and Wright 1984). The epithelial cells may provide no active support at all, but simply act as means of metabolising waste products from the micro-environment surrounding the gametes or pre-embryo.

Pollard et al. (1991) have demonstrated that bovine sperm viability and fertilising capacity in an oviduct cell culture can be preserved for a significantly longer period (30 h) when compared with sperm incubated with medium alone or cocultured with tracheal epithelial cells. When the movement characteristics and hyperactivation of human sperm cocultured with different epithelial cells were studied, there was a higher rate of hyperactivation than in sperm cocultured with monkey kidney (Vero) cells or in control medium.

Coculture of sheep embryos with oviductal cells yields 42% of embryos in the expanded blastocyst stage, while only 4.5% reach this stage when cocultured with fibroblasts (Gandolfi and Moor 1987). In human studies, an increased rate of blastocyst formation has been demonstrated when embryos are cocultured with human ampullary epithelial cells (Bongso et al. 1989b). We have studied fertilisation and blastocyst formation rates when sperm and oocytes were cocultured with a human ampullary epithelial cell culture and compared the results with conventional medium alone. Neither the fertilisation nor cleavage rate was increased in coculture; however, the blastocyst formation rate was significantly increased in coculture (Fig. 3.7).

To determine whether this phenomenon is specific to the oviduct epithelial cell, coculture with other epithelial cells (Vero or bovine kidney) has been compared in mice and humans (Menezo et al. 1990; Ouhibi et al. 1990). Both these studies reported a higher blastocyst formation rate when cocultured embryos were compared with those in conventional media. Thus the beneficial effects of coculture may not be specific to oviduct epithelial cells.

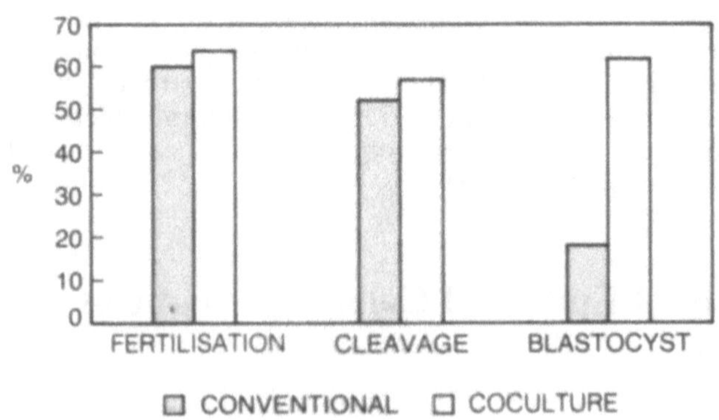


**Fig. 3.7.** Fertilisation, cleavage and blastocyst formation in conventional culture and coculture (n = 147).

## Conclusions

The epithelial layer of the fallopian tube displays morphological changes in response to the endocrine environment of the ovarian cycle. The secretory cells release their contents into the tubal lumen during the luteal phase when fertilisation and early embryo development occur. This has suggested that the epithelium may play an active role.

Human oviduct epithelial cells can be cultured in vitro using readily available media. These cultures can be maintained for up to 60 days.

Coculture of embryos with a fallopian tube epithelial cell culture appears to facilitate embryonic growth to the blastocyst stage. Further controlled studies comparing coculture of sperm, oocytes and embryos with fallopian tube epithelial cells and epithelial cells of non-müllerian, or non-human, origin will be required to determine if the facilitation of embryo growth is specific to the human tubal epithelial cell. Polarised cells may have an advantage over the non-polarised cells, as they resemble morphology in vivo, so that studies of cell function and coculture work may be more appropriate with them.

## References


Allen RL, Wright RW (1984) In vitro development of porcine embryos in coculture with endometrial cell monolayers or culture supernatants. J Anim Sci 59:1657–1661

Batra S, Helm G, Owman C, Sjöberg N-O, Walles B (1980) Female sex steroid concentrations in the ampullary and isthmic regions of the human fallopian tube and their relationship to plasma concentrations during menstrual cycle. Am J Obstet Gynecol 136:986–991

Blandau RJ (1969) Gamete transport – comparative aspects. In: Hafez ESE, Blandau RJ (eds) The mammalian oviduct. University of Chicago Press, Chicago, pp 129–162

Blandau RJ, Verdugo P (1976) An overview of gamete transport – comparative effects. In: Harper MJK, Pauerstein CJ, Adams CE, Coutinho EM, Croxatto HB, Paton DM (eds) Symposium on ovum transport and fertility regulation. Scriptor, Copenhagen, pp 138–146

Bongso A, Ng SC, Sathananthan AH, Ng PL, Rauff M, Ratnam SS (1989a) Establishment of human ampullary cell cultures. Hum Reprod 4:486–494

Bongso A, Ng SC, Sathananthan AH, Ng PL, Rauff M, Ratnam SS (1989b) Improved quality of human embryos when co-cultured with human ampullary cells. Hum Reprod 4:706–713

Borell U, Nilsson O, Westman A (1957) Ciliary activity in the rabbit fallopian tube during oestrus and after copulation. Acta Obstet Gynecol Scand 36:22–28

Brenner RM (1969) Renewal of oviduct cilia during the menstrual cycle in the rhesus monkey. Fertil Steril 20:599–611

Byres SW, Hadley MA, Djakiew D, Dym M (1986) Growth and characterisation of polarised monolayers of epididymal epithelial cells and Sertoli cells in dual environmental chambers. Journal of Andrology 7:59–68

Cai XQ, Marik JJ (1990) Comparison of the effects on penetration capacity of human spermatozoa between using Ham's F-10 medium and a medium based on the composition of human tubal fluid. Andrologia 22:539–542

Carson DD, Tang JP, Julian J, Glasser SR (1988) Vectorial secretion of proteoglycans by polarized rat uterine epithelial cells. J Cell Biol 107:2425–2435

Critoph FN, Dennis KJ (1977) The cellular composition of the human oviduct epithelium. Br J Obstet Gynaecol 84:219–221

Cummins JM, Breen TM, Fuller FM, Harrison KL, Wilson LM, Hennessey JS, Shaw JM, Shaw G (1986) Comparison of two media in a human in vitro fertilization program: lack of significant differences in pregnancy rate. J In Vitro Fertil Embryo Transfer 3:326–328

Devoto L, Soto E, Magofke AM, Sierralta W (1980) Unconjugated steroids in the fallopian tube and peripheral blood during the normal menstrual cycle. Fertil Steril 33:613–617

Ferenczy A, Richart RM, Agate FJ, Purkerson ML, Dempsey EW (1972) Scanning electron microscopy of the human fallopian tube. Science 175:783–784

Fredricks CM (1986) Morphological and functional aspects of the oviductal epithelium. In: Siegler AM (ed) The fallopian tube: basic studies and clinical contributions. Futura Publishing, New York, pp 67–80

Freshney RI (1987) Culture of animal cells. A manual of basic technique. Alan R Liss, Inc., New York, pp 107–127

Gandolfi F, Moor RM (1987) Stimulation of early embryonic development in the sheep by co-culture with oviduct epithelial cells. J Reprod Fertil 81:23–28

Gandolfi F, Brevini TA, Richardson L, Brown CR, Moor RM (1989) Characterization of proteins secreted by sheep oviduct epithelial cells and their function in embryonic development. Development 106:303–312

Gilbert SF, Migeon BR (1975) D-Valine as a selective agent for normal human and rodent epithelial cells in culture. Cell 5:11–17

Gospodarowicz D, Delgado D, Vlodavsky I (1980) Permissive effect of the ECM on cell proliferation in vitro. Proc Natl Acad Sci, USA 77:4094–4098

Hadley MA, Byres SW, Suarez-Quian CA, Kleinman HK, Dym M (1985) Extracellular matrix regulated Sertoli cell differentiation, testicular cord formation and germ cell development in vitro. J Cell Biol 101:1511–1522

Henriksen T, Tanbo T, Abyholm T, Oppedal BR, Clussen OP, Hovig T (1990) Epithelial cells from human fallopian tube in culture. Hum Reprod 5:25–31

Joshi MS (1988) Isolation, cell culture and immunocytochemical characterization of oviduct epithelial cells of the cow. J Reprod Fertil 83:249–261

Jung-Testas I, Garcia T, Baulieu EE (1986) Steroid hormones induce cell proliferation and specific protein synthesis in primary chick oviduct cultures. J Steroid Biochem 24:273–279

Kervancioglu ME, Martin J, Maguiness SD, Djahanbakhch O (1992) A simple technique for the culture and subculture of human fallopian tube epithelial cells. Br J Obs Gynae 99:700

Kutteh WH, Hatch KD, Blackwell RE, Mestecky J (1988) Secretory immune system of the female reproductive tract. I. Immunoglobulin and secretory component-containing cells. Obstetric Gynecol 71:56–60

Lillie JH, MacCallum DK, Jepsen A (1980) Fine structure of subcultivated stratified squamous epithelium grown on collagen rafts. Exp Cell Res 125:153–165

Lippes J, Wagh PV (1989) Human oviductal (hOF) proteins. IV. Evidence for hOF proteins binding to human sperm. Fertil Steril 51:89–94

Lippes J, Krasner J, Alfonso LA, Dacalos ED, Lucero R (1981) Human oviductal fluid proteins. Fertil Steril 36:623–629

Ludwig H, Metzer H (1976) The human female reproductive tract. A scanning electron microscopic atlas. Springer-Verlag, Heidelberg, pp 79–105

McComb P, Langley L, Villalon M, Verdugo P (1986) The oviductal cilia and Kartagener's syndrome. Fertil Steril 46:412–416

Menezo YJR, Guerin JF, Czyba JC (1990) Improvement of human early embryo development in vitro by coculture on monolayers of Vero cells. Biol Reprod 42:301–306

Ouhibi N, Menezo Y, Benet G, Nicollet B (1989) Culture of epithelial cells derived from the oviduct of different species. Hum Reprod 4:229–235

Ouhibi N, Hamidi J, Guillaud J, Menezo Y (1990) Co-culture of 1-cell mouse embryos on different cell supports. Hum Reprod 5:737–743

Parrish JJ, Susko-Parrish JL, Handrow RR, Sims MM, First NL (1989) Capacitation of bovine spermatozoa by oviduct fluid. Biol Reprod 40:1020–1025

Patek E, Nilsson L, Johannisson E (1972a) Scanning electron microscopic study of the human fallopian tube. Report I. The proliferative and secretory stages. Fertil Steril 23:459–465

Patek E, Nilsson L, Johannisson E (1972b) Scanning electron microscopic study of the human fallopian tube. Report II. Fetal life, reproductive life, and menopause. Fertil Steril 23:719–733

Pauerstein CJ (1975) Clinical implications of oviductal physiology and biochemistry. Gynecol Invest 6:253–264

Pollard JW, Plante C, King WA, Hansen PJ, Betteridge KJ, Suarez SS (1991) Fertilizing capacity of bovine sperm may be maintained by binding to epithelial cells. Biol Reprod 44:102–107

Pollow K, Intraphuvasak J, Manz B, Grill H-J, Pollow B (1981) A comparison of cytoplasmic and nuclear estradiol and progesterone receptors in human fallopian tube and endometrial tissue. Fertil Steril 36:615–622

Quinn P, Kerin JF, Warnes GM (1985) Improved pregnancy rate in human in vitro fertilization with the use of a medium based on the composition of human tubal fluid. Fertil Steril 44:493–498

Takeuchi K, Maruyama I, Yamamoto S, Oki T, Nagata Y (1991) Isolation and monolayer culture of human fallopian tube epithelial cells. In Vitro Cell Dev Biol 27:720–724

Verhage HG, Bareither ML, Jaffe RC, Akbar M (1979) Cyclic changes in ciliation, secretion and cell height of the oviductal epithelium in woman. Am J Anat 156:505–510

Wagh PV, Lippes J (1989) Human oviductal proteins. III. Identification and partial purification. Fertil Steril 51:81–88

Chapter 4

# Biochemistry of Tubal Secretions

H.J. Leese, I.A. Brewis, L.J. Edwards, S.M. Gray, L.S. Skiera and R.M.L. Winston

This review will be concerned with the tubal secretion of small molecules important in the nutrition of gametes and preimplantation embryos: principally, pyruvate, lactate, glucose and amino acids. A variety of experimental approaches will be described with the emphasis on work on the human wherever possible.

Pyruvate is consumed by unfertilised and fertilised mouse oocytes and is a constituent of all culture media for the mammalian embryo. Lactate acts synergistically with pyruvate in promoting the development of 2-cell mouse embryos. Glucose is utilised in the later preimplantation stages in the mouse, rabbit, sheep, cow, rat and human (Leese 1991a), and is converted, in some cases completely, to lactate (Gardner and Leese 1990; Gott et al. 1990a; Brison and Leese 1991). Amino acids, particularly glutamine, are consumed in increasing quantities as preimplantation development progresses (Gardner et al. 1989). Sperm may use glucose, pyruvate and lactate and certain amino acids as respiratory substrates. They may also convert glucose to lactate anaerobically.

The nutrients listed above are ultimately derived from the blood (Leese 1988), and are potentially metabolic substrates for adult mammalian tissues. The ciliated and non-ciliated (secretory) cells which line the fallopian tube therefore face the problem of having to take up such molecules at their basal poles and secrete them into the lumen without consuming them *en route*. Little is known about how this is accomplished. The same dilemma is faced by the cells which line tissues such as the small intestine and kidney tubule, which have to absorb nutrients into the blood without metabolising them to any great degree. It is, therefore, of interest to examine the metabolism of the fallopian tube, in particular the requirement for nutrients, in an attempt to discover how this relates to the secretory function.

## The Oxygen Consumption of the Fallopian Tube

A useful parameter of the overall metabolic capacity of a tissue is its oxygen consumption. In order to measure optimal rates of oxygen consumption in vitro, it is necessary to remove tissues from the animal as rapidly as possible, slice them thinly and incubate them in well-stirred and oxygenated medium (Leese et al. 1981). These conditions were satisfied in the study of Brewis et al. (1992) in which small pieces of human fimbrial mucosa (2–10 mg fresh wt) were removed from women undergoing tubal microsurgery to treat infertility. The pieces were transferred within 1 min of removal from the patient into an incubation vessel containing a Clark electrode for measurement of their oxygen consumption. Results, expressed as $Q_{O_2}$ ie. $\mu lO_2$/mg dry wt/h, plotted against the day of the menstrual cycle, are given in Fig. 4.1. There was considerable variation in the data with a mean value of 3.4 $\mu$l/mg dry wt/h, similar to that reported by Mastroianni et al. (1958), and typical of a metabolically quiescent tissue. There was a suggestion of variation with endocrine state, but further data would be required to confirm this. Whole slices of rabbit and mouse oviduct have $Q_{O_2}$ values slightly higher than those of the human endosalpinx: 5.5 $\mu$l/mg dry wt/h (Leese et al. 1981; Edwards and Leese, unpublished). The ATP content of rabbit oviduct slices (7.7 and 5.1 $\mu$mol/g dry wt for ampulla and isthmus respectively (Leese et al. 1981) is also consistent with the relatively low metabolic activity of the tube. The next question to consider is the nature of the fuel(s) used by the endosalpinx.

## The Role of Glucose

The experiments on human tubal mucosa were therefore repeated in the presence of potential metabolic substrates. 1 mM glutamine and 1 mM acetoacetate reduced the $Q_{O_2}$, while 5.55 mM glucose raised it by about 50% (Fig. 4.2). We have obtained qualitatively similar data for rabbit oviduct tissue slices, both from the ampulla and isthmus. The response to glucose was investigated in more detail in the rabbit oviduct, since fresh tissue was more readily available from this source than from the human.

In this work, a preparation of epithelial cells of rabbit oviduct was used, devoid of contaminating stromal or myometrial cells. The method is briefly described below in the section *Glucose and lactate*. At low concentrations, glucose stimulated the oxygen uptake of the cells, but beyond the physiological concentration of 5.55 mM (1 mg/ml), the respiration was inhibited; a so-called Crabtree effect (Fig. 4.3).

Further evidence for a key role for glucose in sustaining the metabolism of human endosalpinx was obtained from measurements of the activities of four enzymes thought to have a regulatory role in the energy metabolism of other tissues: hexokinase (HK), 6-phosphofructokinase (PFK), glycogen phosphorylase and 2-oxoglutarate dehydrogenase (Brewis et al. 1992).

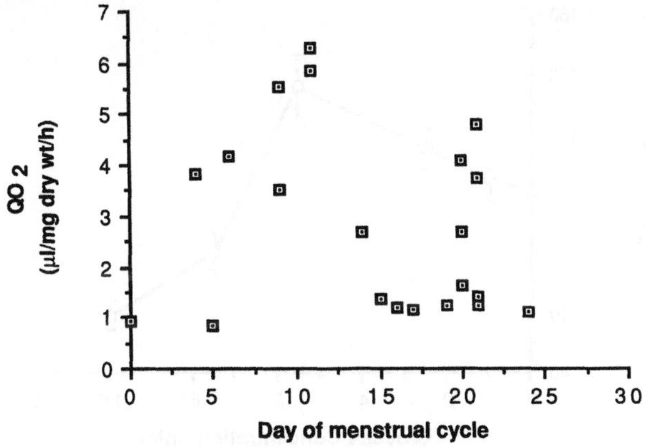


**Fig. 4.1.** Oxygen consumption of thin slices of fimbrial mucosa removed on different days of the menstrual cycle. Values are $\mu lO_2$ consumed/mg dry wt/h.

Hexokinase had the highest activity, followed by 2-oxoglutarate dehydrogenase. PFK and glycogen phosphorylase had low activities. The relative activities were consistent with glucose being a major respiratory substrate for human endosalpinx. This conclusion was reinforced by the finding that very little lactate was formed by isolated fimbrial mucosa during the experiments to measure $Q_{O_2}$.

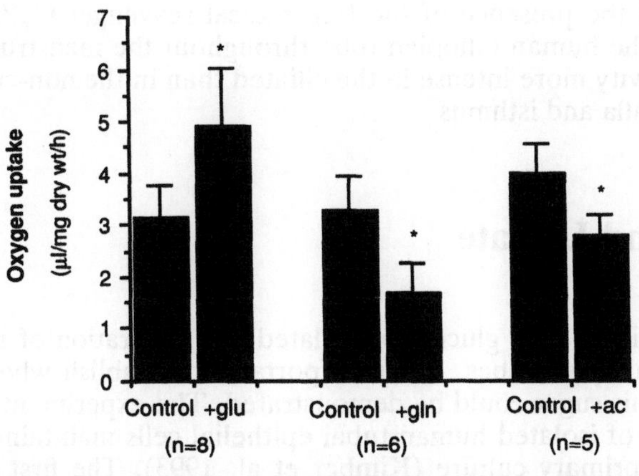


**Fig. 4.2.** Effect of 5.55 mM glucose (n = 8), 1 mM glutamine (n = 6) and 1 mM acetoacetate (n = 5) on oxygen consumption of human endosalpinx. Values are means ± SEM; n: the number of determinations. *Significantly different ($p < 0.05$) from control using paired t-tests based on the differences for each patient. Reproduced with permission from Brewis, Winston, Leese (1992) Journal of Reproduction and Fertility. Journals of Reproduction and Fertility Ltd. Cambridge, UK.

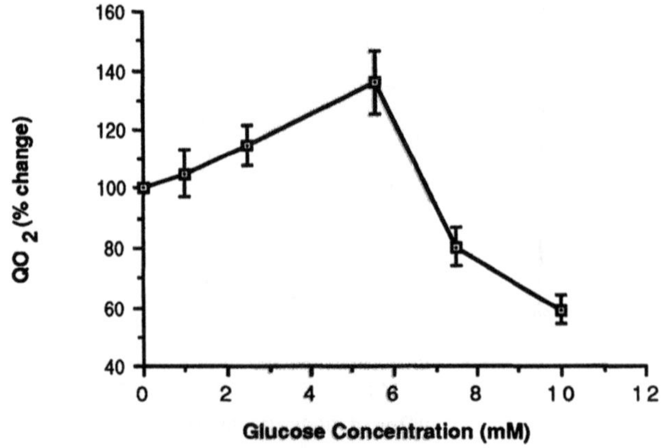


**Fig. 4.3.** Effect of increasing glucose concentration on the oxygen consumption ($Q_{O_2}$) by isolated rabbit oviduct epithelial cells. Values, which are means of at least 6 determinations, are expressed as per cent change from the control in the absence of glucose.

### Oxygen Free Radicals

Since the fallopian tube has an aerobic metabolism, it is worth considering how it protects itself from the potentially harmful effects of oxygen free radicals. Interest in this topic has been raised by reports that the block to the development of 2-cell mouse embryos in vitro may, to some extent, be caused by toxic oxygen species and relieved by free radical scavengers (Loutradis et al. 1987; Noda et al. 1989; Nasr-Esfahani et al. 1990; Legge and Sellens 1991). It is, therefore, of significance that Narimoto et al. (1991) have reported the presence of the free radical scavenger CuZn superoxide dismutase in the human fallopian tube throughout the menstrual cycle, with immunoreactivity more intense in the ciliated than in the non-ciliated cells in both the ampulla and isthmus.

## Glucose and Lactate

Having established that glucose stimulated the respiration of rabbit, mouse and human fallopian tubes, it was important to establish whether the *consumption* of this sugar could be demonstrated. The experimental system was a preparation of isolated human tubal epithelial cells maintained as a polarised layer in primary culture (Kimber et al. 1993). The first phase of this technique involved the isolation of the epithelial cells by enzymic digestion. The cells were plated onto collagen-coated inserts in tissue culture wells, in which situation they form tight junctions with one another establishing a polarised confluent monolayer (Dickens et al. 1993). The preparation enables the consumption of glucose and its conversion to lactate to be measured. The results shown in Fig. 4.4 indicated that glucose was consumed at

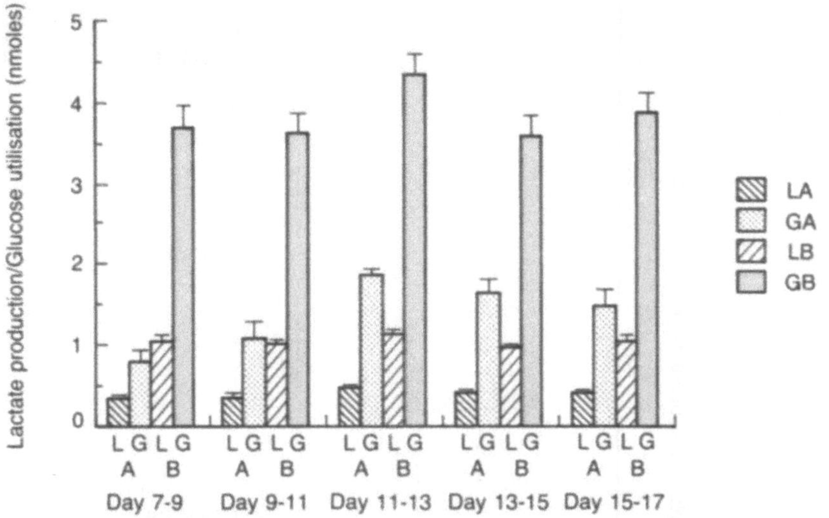


**Fig. 4.4.** Glucose utilisation (G) and lactate production (L) by human Fallopian tubal epithelial cells maintained as a polarised layer in primary culture. Values (nmoles) are for successive 2-day culture periods. (A) and (B) refer to media bathing the apical and basal sides of the cells respectively.

a steady rate for at least 17 days following cell isolation and that it was taken up preferentially from the basal side of the cells (the blood side in vivo) as might be expected. Lactate also appeared preferentially in this compartment, though a significant amount was found on the apical side, where it could act as a substrate for sperm and early preimplantation embryos. In this metabolic experiment, glucose was initially present at high concentration (16.5 mM) on both sides of the cell preparation, precluding the detection of net glucose transport. However, the method may be used to study the transport of glucose across the epithelium following sugar addition to the apical or basal side only.

Nutrient transport experiments were carried out with a more physiological preparation of the rabbit oviduct, involving vascular and luminal perfusion (Leese and Gray 1985). In this technique, the ovarian artery is cannulated and perfused in a single pass with Medium 199 supplemented with bovine serum albumin and antibiotics, and gassed with 95%$O_2$/5%$CO_2$. At the same time, the lumen is cannulated at its fimbrial and uterine ends and perfused with recirculated Krebs–Ringer bicarbonate medium.

When pyruvate, glucose, lactate and the passive marker sucrose are added at equal concentrations to the vascular medium, they appear in the lumen at widely different rates, not explicable in terms of their differing molecular weights and indicating that these nutrients are transported selectively (Fig. 4.5). In their absence in the vascular compartment, only small amounts of these nutrients are detected in the lumen, suggesting they are normally derived from the blood. This conclusion has to be provisional since the experiment necessitated perfusing the vascular compartment with substrate-

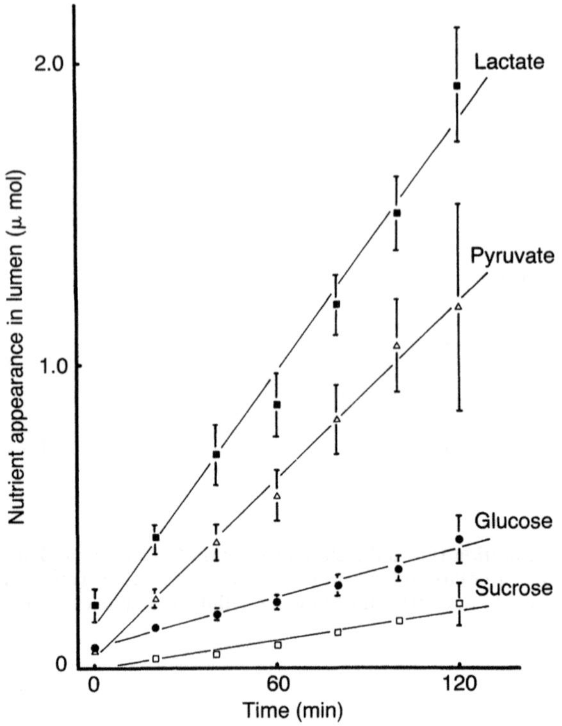


**Fig. 4.5.** Time course of appearance of lactate, pyruvate, glucose and sucrose in the lumen of the vascularly-perfused rabbit oviduct. Each compound was added to the vascular medium at an initial concentration of 5 mM. Values are means ± SEM of at least 8 determinations. Reproduced, with permission, from Leese and Gray (1985) American Journal of Physiology 248:E624–E632. The American Physiological Society, Bethesda, Maryland, USA.

free Krebs–Ringer bicarbonate medium, which is less physiological than albumin-supplemented Medium 199.

Luminal lactate appeared to have a dual origin. About 75% was derived from vascular glucose, with the remaining 25% coming from vascular lactate. The proportion derived from glucose was higher than in the preparation of polarised epithelial cells from the human endosalpinx. It is possible that some lactate may have been derived by metabolism in the myosalpinx and the stroma, both of which were present in the vascularly-perfused preparation, but not the epithelial cell preparation.

## The Effect of Ovulation

When rabbit oviducts were taken 3 days after mating, the secretion of nutrients into the lumen of the vascularly-perfused preparation was considerably reduced. Data obtained for rabbit oviducts perfused through the lumen in vivo indicated a 50% reduction post-ovulation (Leese and Aldridge 1979). The physiological significance of these observations is unclear. On the third day after mating, rabbit embryos are found predominantly in the isthmus, whereas the bulk of oviduct fluid is formed in the ampulla. It is possible that changes in overall secretory rates are largely a reflection of events in the ampulla and, as such, may mask differences in the isthmus.

### Conclusion: Glucose and Lactate in Oviduct Fluid

Glucose is the major energy substrate for human endosalpinx and rabbit oviduct epithelial cells. The glucose originates in the blood and a proportion of that which enters the cells is secreted into the lumen. A further proportion is converted to lactate, some of which may also enter the lumen.

The end result of these transport and metabolic events is the presence of glucose and lactate in human tubal fluid. Their concentrations in neat samples taken during tubal surgery were 1.0 mM and 2.16 mM respectively. These values were close to those obtained by Gott et al. (1990a) for human hydrosalpinx fluid.

## Amino Acids

Leese et al. (1979) found that a mixture of amino acids appeared in saline medium recirculated through the lumen of the rabbit oviduct in vivo. The amino acids appeared at differing rates with respect to their plasma concentrations: glycine had the highest rate, followed by alanine. There was no evidence for the active transport of amino acids from blood to lumen. The end product of nitrogen metabolism, urea, which is readily diffusible, reached the same concentration in the lumen as the blood. Substantially similar results for amino acids were obtained with the vascularly-perfused rabbit oviduct preparation. When a physiological mixture was added to the vascular compartment, the amino acids appeared at differing rates (Fig. 4.6), which, as in the case of glucose and lactate, were reduced 3 days following ovulation. Glycine and alanine were again transported to the greatest extent, a result in agreement with the data of Miller and Schultz (1987).

## Pyruvate

Pyruvate appeared in saline medium recirculated through the lumen of the rabbit oviduct in vivo (Leese and Aldridge 1979). The rate of appearance was approximately halved in oviducts 3 days post-ovulation; a slightly greater reduction than was found in the vascularly-perfused preparation (Leese and Gray 1985). In rabbits and other partial and full ruminants, pyruvate may also be derived from the short-chain fatty acid propionate (Leese 1980). A further source of pyruvate is the cumulus mass which surrounds the ovulated oocyte(s). Leese and Barton (1985) showed that whole

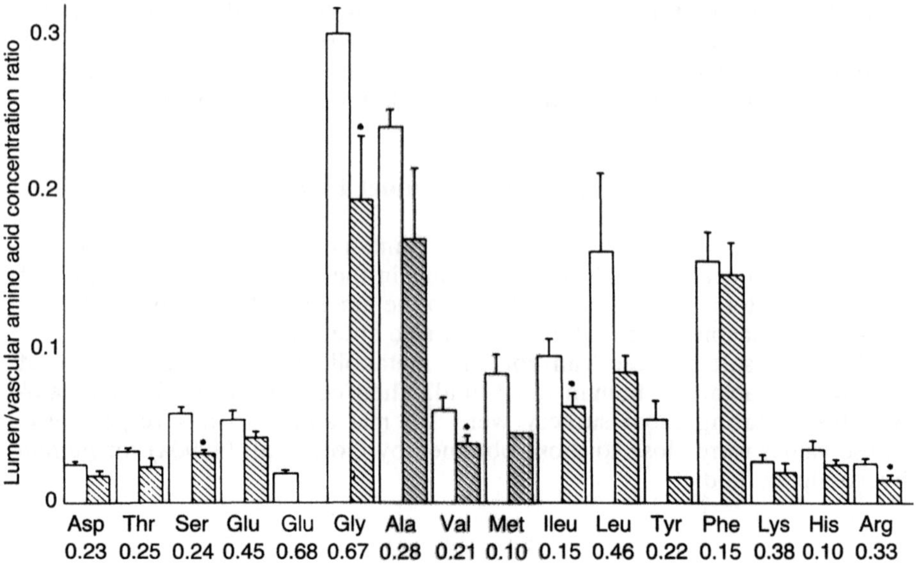


**Fig. 4.6.** Effect of ovulation on appearance of amino acids in lumen of the perfused rabbit oviduct. Open bars represent lumen-to-vascular amino-acid concentration ratios for oviducts from oestrous rabbits. Values are means ± SEM of at least 8 determinations. Hatched bars represent lumen-to-vascular amino-acid concentration ratios for oviducts from rabbits given human chorionic gonadotrophin 3 days previously. Values are means ± SEM of at least 4 determinations. Glutamine post-ovulation was not determined. *Statistically significant ($p < 0.05$) difference between mean values for oestrous and postovulation oviducts. Concentration of each amino acid in vascular medium in mM is given below its abbreviation. Reproduced with permission from Leese and Gray (1985) American Journal of Physiology 248:E624–E632. The American Physiological Society, Bethesda, Maryland, USA.

cumulus masses and isolated cumulus cells from the mouse could form pyruvate from glucose and lactate. That pyruvate from this source might have some physiological significance is evident from the data of Gardner and Leese (1990), who showed that the pyruvate concentration in the vicinity of the mouse cumulus mass, at 0.37 mM, was higher than that in its absence (0.14 mM). Human cumulus masses are also net producers of pyruvate (Ahuja 1988). Leese (1991b) has speculated that pyruvate might act as a free-radical scavenger as well as a nutrient for sperm and unfertilised and fertilised oocytes. The pyruvate concentration in neat samples of human tubal fluid was 0.24 mM, close to the concentration in human hydrosalpinx fluid (Gott et al. 1990b).

## Conclusion

Fig. 4.7 summarises the origins of pyruvate, glucose and lactate in the tubal lumen at fertilisation. When compared with the detailed, quantitative pic-

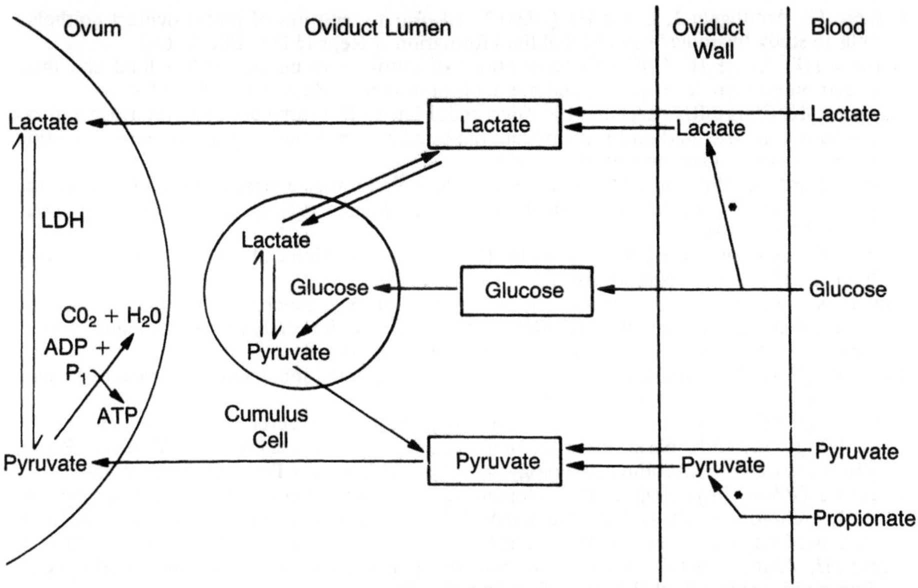


**Fig. 4.7.** Diagrammatic respresentation of the sources of pyruvate available at fertilisation. Reproduced with permission from Leese and Barton (1985) Journal of Experimental Zoology 234:231–236. Alan R Liss, New York.

tures which could be presented for the transport of molecules across other epithelial tissues, such as the small intestine, kidney tubule and pancreas, Fig. 4.7 amounts to a low level of information. A major reason for this state of biochemical neglect has been the apparent success of human in vitro fertilisation and embryo transfer procedures, which have tended to relegate the tube to the status of a passive conduit for gametes and early embryos. Happily, a renaissance has set in, and the availability of methods and approaches successfully applied to other tissues will ensure that tubal biochemistry develops as a topic in its own right.

*Acknowledgements.* The authors' studies reported in this review were supported by The Medical Research Council, The Science and Engineering Research Council, The Wellcome Trust and Birthright.

# References

Ahuja KK (1988) Fertilisation: the importance of scientific research to clinical practice. Br J Family Planning 13:18–24

Brewis IA, Winston RML, Leese HJ (1992) Energy metabolism of the human fallopian tube. J Reprod Fert 95:257–262

Brison DR, Leese HJ (1991) Energy metabolism in late preimplantation rat embryos. J Reprod Fert 93:245–251

Dickens CJ, Southgate J, Leese HJ (1993) Used primary cultures of rabbit oviduct epithelial cells to study the ionic basis of tubal fluid formation. J Reprod Fert 98:603–610
Gardner DK, Leese HJ (1990) Concentrations of nutrients in mouse oviduct fluid and their effects on embryo development and metabolism in vitro. J Reprod Fert 88:361–368
Gardner DK, Clarke RN, Lechene CP, Biggers JD (1989) Development of a noninvasive ultramicrofluorometric method for measuring the uptake of glutamine by single preimplantation mouse embryos. Gamete Res 24:427–438
Gott A, Hardy K, Winston RML, Leese HJ (1990a) Non-invasive measurement of glucose and pyruvate uptake and lactate production by single human preimplantation embryos. Hum Reprod 5:104–108
Gott A, Hardy K, Winston RML, Leese HJ (1990b) The nutrition and environment of the early human embryo. Proc Nat Soc 49:2A
Kimber SJ, Waterhouse R, Lindenberg MD (1993) In vitro models for implantation of the mammalian embryo. In: Bavister BD (ed) Preimplantation embryo development. Serono Symposia USA. Springer-Verlag, New York, pp 244–263.
Leese HJ (1980) The stimulation of pyruvate appearance in the rabbit oviduct lumen by sodium propionate. J Reprod Fert 59:421–424
Leese HJ (1988) The formation and function of oviduct fluid. J Reprod Fert 82:843–856
Leese HJ (1991a) Metabolism of the preimplantation mammalian embryo. In: Milligan SR (ed) Oxford reviews of reproductive biology, 13. Oxford University Press, Oxford, pp 35–72
Leese HJ (1991b) Physiology of the fallopian tube: the provision of nutrients for oocytes and early embryos. In: Evers JHL, Heineman MJ (eds) From ovulation to implantation, International Congress Series No 917, Excerpta Medica. Elsevier Science Publishers, pp 121–126
Leese HJ, Aldridge S (1979) The movement of pyruvate, lactate and lactate dehydrogenase into rabbit oviduct fluid. J Reprod Fert 56:619–622
Leese HJ, Barton AM (1985) Production of pyruvate by isolated cumulus cells. J Exp Zool 234:231–236
Leese HJ, Gray SM (1985) Vascular perfusion: a novel means of studying oviduct function. Am J Physiol 248:E624–E632
Leese HJ, Aldridge S, Jeffries KS (1979) The movement of amino acids into rabbit oviduct fluid. J Reprod Fert 56:623–626
Leese HJ, Humpherson PG, Jeffries KS (1981) Two preparations for the study of the isolated rabbit oviduct. J Reprod Fert 63:249–256
Legge M, Sellens MH (1991) Free radical scavengers ameliorate the 2-cell block in mouse embryo culture. Hum Reprod 6:867–871
Loutradis D, John D, Kiessling AA (1987) Hypoxanthine causes a 2-cell block in random-bred mouse embryos. Biol Reprod 37:311–316
Mastroianni L Jr, Winternitz WW, Lowi NP (1958) The in vitro metabolism of the human endosalpinx. Fertil Steril 9:500–509
Miller JGO, Schultz GA (1987) Amino acid content of preimplantation rabbit embryos and fluids of the reproductive tract. Biol Reprod 36:125–129
Narimoto K, Noda Y, Shiotani M et al. (1991) Role of superoxide dismutase in the fallopian tube function: immunohistochemical assessment of superoxide dismutase in the fallopian tube. Acta Histochem Cytochem 24:85–91
Nasr-Esfahani MH, Aitken JR, Johnson MH (1990) Hydrogen peroxide levels in mouse oocytes and early cleavage stage embryos developed in vitro and in vivo. Development 109:501–507
Noda Y, Matsumoto H, Umaoka Y, Tatsumi K, Mori T (1989) Effects of superoxide dismutase on 2-cell block in mouse embryos cultured in vitro. Cell Diff Devel 27:S16

Chapter 5

# Oviduct Proteins

S.D. Maguiness, K. Shrimanker, O. Djahanbakhch and J.G. Grudzinskas

## Introduction

The oviduct has many roles in the process of natural conception, beginning with retrieval of the oocyte released by the ruptured ovarian follicle, and facilitation of the final maturation of sperm which have passed through the uterus (Adams and Chang 1962; Bedford 1968; Hunter and Hall 1974). Both male and female gametes are transported in the oviduct, and meet within well-defined time limits which are species-dependent (Andersen 1927; Harper 1961a,b; Blandau 1969; Boling 1969; Hunter 1974; Blandau and Verdugo 1976; Croxatto and Ortiz 1975; Pauerstein 1975; Eddy et al. 1976). Fertilisation takes place at the isthmic-ampullary junction and the pre-embryo is then transported to the uterine cavity at the optimum time for nidation. While in the oviduct, early development of the mouse pre-embryo appears to be enhanced (Bowman and McLaren 1970; Harlow and Quinn 1982). This may also be the case in humans and has led to studies to determine whether it is beneficial for pre-embryos to be cocultured with oviduct epithelial cell cultures (Bongso et al. 1990). During reproductive events in the oviduct the male gametes and pre-embryo, which are antigenically different from the female host, do not appear to be affected by the maternal immune system. The mechanism of this is unknown.

Currently our ability to test the function of the fallopian tube is synonymous with the demonstration of tubal patency and a normal appearance at endoscopy (Blackwell 1989; Maguiness et al. 1992a). The factors controlling gamete and pre-embryo movement, maturation, and interaction with the maternal immune system, are poorly understood. The ability to draw conclusions from animal studies which may be relevant to human reproduction has been hampered by the fact that mammalian species have different reproductive plans determined by their environment; therefore the findings from the oviduct in one species cannot form a model for another (Verdugo 1986). It is important to interpret any investigation with respect to the animal species studied.

For many years studies have been conducted to determine both the qualitative and quantitative nature of proteins present in oviduct fluid and tissue in order to determine their role in normal reproduction. More recently, studies have been performed to establish which proteins are specifically synthesised by the cells of the oviduct. This chapter summarises current knowledge of factors in the oviduct environment which may have a role in the endocrine and paracrine control of reproductive events within the oviduct lumen and discusses the advantages and disadvantages of each approach. We will follow the example of Leese (1988) and use the term oviduct when referring to mammalian studies, reserving the term fallopian tube for specifically human studies.

# Oviduct Fluid

It is not easy to sample oviduct fluid for study in normal human subjects in vivo. To investigate the oviduct environment, various workers have therefore tried to develop effective methods of collecting oviduct fluid. The simplest is to flush the oviduct lumen. While this method had the advantage of minimising trauma, the volume collected is small and the fluid may be contaminated by blood (Oliphant 1986). Woskressensky (1891) demonstrated that fluid would accumulate in the rabbit oviduct when its ends were ligated. By tying a cannula into the infundibulum and vertically orientating its end, Bishop (1956) studied changes in the rate and pressure of secretion during various oestrus states and in pregnancy. The major problem is that the extent to which pressure affects transudation from serum and secretion by tubal epithelium has not been determined.

The effects of increased pressure can be minimised by exteriorisation of the cannula to allow intermittent aspiration (Feigelson and Kay 1972; Riddick 1975). This method allows increased amounts of fluid to be collected. Criticisms of this method are that the negative pressure exerted during aspiration may induce movement of plasma across the epithelial layer, while the duration of the collection increases the chances of infection and contamination of the fluid.

Continuous flow collections have been developed in which the oviductal fluid is refrigerated as it is collected to provide better storage (Clewe and Mastroianni 1960; Mastroianni and Jones 1965; Mastroianni et al. 1970). Variations on this methodology have been used to study human tubal secretions (Lippes et al. 1972; Shams et al. 1977). However, secretions have to traverse a long tube, representing many hours of secretion, and infection is still a potential problem. Hamner and Williams (1965) developed an intraperitoneal flask collection method for use in animals, which included a "Pasteur loop" in an attempt to limit bacterial contamination. The flask is designed to allow filtered air to enter during aspiration, thereby eliminating negative pressure effects.

All of these collection methods have fundamental shortcomings. Surgery, the presence of the catheter, negative pressure applied to withdraw the fluid, may all affect the volume and the production and constitution of secretions. It is also difficult to investigate each anatomical section of the oviduct. These factors must be taken into account when interpreting the following experimental data.

## Protein Concentration

The range of protein concentrations in oviduct fluid has been reported as 2.2–8.0 mg/ml for the rabbit (Holmdahl and Mastroianni 1965; Iritani et al. 1971; Oliphant et al. 1978), 9.3–30.0 mg/ml for sheep (Restall and Wales 1966) and 1.0–18.0 mg/ml for humans (Lippes et al. 1972, 1981; David et al. 1973). The variable results in each species probably reflect different study methodologies. Overall, the total concentration of protein in oviduct fluid is lower than that of the corresponding serum, providing evidence for selective passage of macromolecules (Glass and McClure 1965; Glass 1969). Oliphant et al. (1978) suggested that the ability of macromolecules to enter rabbit oviduct fluid was inversely proportional to their molecular weight. However, lactate can achieve 50% (Leese et al. 1979), and the complement component, C3, 17% of serum concentrations (Oliphant et al. 1978) suggesting that molecular size is not the only factor affecting protein movement into the oviduct fluid. The low protein concentrations led Roberts et al. (1975) to suggest that transudation of fluid might account for only a small portion of oviduct fluid, the bulk of the aqueous phase being from an active secretory process.

David et al. (1969) demonstrated that the concentration of protein in the ampulla of the rabbit oviduct was less than that in the isthmus. However, since much more fluid was secreted into the ampulla, the total amount of protein transferred was higher.

When the proteins in oviduct fluid are separated according to their molecular mass using gel electrophoresis the patterns are similar to the corresponding serum, with the most abundant proteins being albumin and IgG (Oliphant et al. 1978). The major studies of oviduct fluid protein content are listed in Table 5.1.

## Oviduct Fluid-Specific Proteins

Immunoelectrophoresis of oviduct fluid has suggested the presence of unique proteins which may have been synthesised and secreted by the oviduct, e.g., specific $\beta$-glycoproteins, in humans (Moghissi 1970), monkeys (Mastroianni et al. 1970) and sheep (Roberts et al. 1976). Immunoaffinity adsorption has been used to separate these proteins from those derived from serum in human tubal fluid (Lippes and Wagh 1989; Wagh and Lippes 1989). These studies report a series of proteins, one of which (molecular mass

**Table 5.1.** Studies to determine the protein content of oviduct fluid, listed in chronological order (SDS = sodium dodecyl sulphate; PAGE = polyacrylamide gel electrophoresis; kDa = Daltons × 1000)

| Author | Animal | Methodology | Main findings |
|---|---|---|---|
| Marcus and Saravis (1965) | Monkey | 1-dimensional PAGE | No difference between serum and oviduct fluid |
| Mastroianni et al. (1970) | Monkey | 1-dimensional PAGE | Additional protein present during the luteal phase |
| Moghissi (1970) | Human | Immunoelectrophoresis | 15 serum proteins present, no IgM<br>1 tubal specific $\beta$-globulin |
| Kay and Feigelson (1972) | Rabbit | 1-dimensional PAGE | 2 additional protein bands appeared during pregnancy |
| Hanscom and Oliphant (1976) | Rabbit | Radiolabelled amino acid incorporation<br>1-dimensional PAGE | 2 progesterone-dependent proteins, 45, 72 kDa |
| Stone et al. (1977) | Rabbit | Immunodiffusion | 2–3 reproductive-tract-specific proteins, ? uteroglobulin |
| Lippes et al. (1981) | Human | Immunoelectrophoresis | Variation in protein content in albumin and $\beta$-globulin region for 4–5 days after ovulation |
| Sutton et al. (1984) | Sheep | 1-dimensional PAGE | 80–90 kDa protein present on oestrus days 1–5. Increase in 100 kDa protein after onset of oestrus |
| Wagh and Lippes (1989) | Human | Immunoaffinity gel<br>DEAE-chromatography<br>SDS-PAGE | 4 proteins, 44–150 kDa which bind to the body and/or head of sperm |

54000 Daltons) has been shown to bind to the head of spermatozoa. The ratio of oviduct fluid proteins from serum transudate, and those presumed to be specifically synthesised and secreted by the oviduct is reported to vary during the ovarian cycle (Mastroianni et al. 1970; Brackett and Mastroianni 1974).

## Glycoproteins

Studies of sulphated mucopolysaccharides and mucoproteins in oviduct fluid suggest that they may originate from granules in the secretory epithelium of the oviducts (Shapiro et al. 1971; Hanscom and Oliphant 1976; Barr and Oliphant 1981), and that they form the mucin coat which surrounds the zona pellucida of the rabbit ovum (Greenwald 1958).

Sutton et al. (1984) reported variation in the glycoprotein content of sheep oviduct fluid during the oestrus cycle, analysed on one-dimensional sodium dodecyl sulphate polyacrylamide gel electrophoresis (SDS-PAGE). A glycoprotein of molecular mass 80000–90000 Daltons was found in the oviduct fluid for 3–6 days of each oestrus cycle. It appeared either on the first day of oestrus or on the following day, coinciding with the high rate of flow of oviduct fluid. Sutton et al. (1986) have subsequently ascribed the protein a molecular mass of 70000–90000 Daltons, and demonstrated that it had the ability to bind to spermatozoa. Electrophoresis of human fallopian tube fluid collected at the time of ovulation and up to 5 days after has revealed the presence of proteins which migrated with the albumin and $\beta$-globulin regions (Lippes et al. 1981).

Greenwald (1962) suggested that the rabbit embryo had a decreased ability to develop and implant if the amount of mucin was reduced. However the fact that embryos with reduced mucin can develop and implant, as well as the success of in vitro fertilisation, suggest that oviduct secretions are not essential but rather facilitate the reproductive process (Oliphant 1986). An example of this may be the inactivation of an embryonic inhibiting peptide thought to enter oviduct fluid from serum (Stone et al. 1977). A complement inhibitor which has also been identified in rabbit oviduct fluid is a sulphated glycoprotein that can protect both sperm and embryos from the maternal humoral immune system (Oliphant et al. 1984; Oliphant 1986).

## Oviduct Tissue Protein Content

Secretory granules in the oviduct epithelium stain under conditions expected for acidic mucopolysaccharides or mucoproteins (Lillie 1949; Hadek 1955; Zachariae 1958). This group of proteins has been extensively investigated because the granules exhibit staining characteristics similar to glycoproteins in oviduct fluid. The major studies to determine which proteins are present in oviduct tissue are listed in Table 5.2. These studies do not provide any information about the site of synthesis of proteins which could have reached the oviduct from serum.

There is variation in both the qualitative and quantitative nature of sulphated glycoproteins between the isthmus and ampulla of rabbit oviducts (Oliphant et al. 1984; Hyde and Black 1986). Using immunohistochemical localisation and radioimmunoassay, Pregnancy Associated Placental Protein-A, PAPP-A (Sjöberg et al. 1986), and Placental Protein 5, PP5 (Butzow 1989) have been demonstrated in the human fallopian tube. This methodology, refined by the use of gel filtration, has also identified the presence of Placental Protein 10, PP10 (Tiitinen et al. 1986) and a major secretory protein of the endometrium, Placental Protein 14, PP14 (Julkunen et al. 1986) which is reported to have immunosuppressive properties (Bolton et al. 1987; Okamoto et al. cited in Seppälä et al. 1991). The presence of PP14 has also been reported using monoclonal antibodies and immunohistochemical localisation (Waites et al. 1990). All of these proteins are present in serum and may reach the tubal secretions from that compartment.

In animal studies, granules with the staining characteristics of acidic mucopolysaccharides or mucoproteins appear under the influence of exogenous oestrogen, and are released when progesterone is administered (Greenwald 1958; Brower and Anderson 1969; Lambert et al. 1973). During the ovarian cycle changes in the tissue content of both PAPP-A and PP14 are observed. The PAPP-A content was higher in the follicular phase (Sjöberg et al. 1986). The tissue content of PP14 was found to be higher in the luteal phase of the menstrual cycle, but this difference only reached statistical significance in the fimbrial region of the tube (Julkunen et al. 1986).

**Table 5.2.** Studies to determine the protein content of oviduct tissue listed in chronological order (PAGE = polyacrylamide gel electrophoresis; kDa = Daltons × 1000; SDS = sodium dodecyl sulphate)

| Author | Animal | Methodology | Main findings |
|---|---|---|---|
| Barr and Oliphant (1981) | Rabbit | Radiolabelled amino acid incorporation, tissue homogenisation, disc gel electrophoresis, 1-dimensional PAGE | 2 sulphated protein components |
| Oliphant and Ross (1982) | Rabbit | Radiolabelled amino acid incorporation, gel filtration, ion exchange chromatography, SDS-PAGE | 3 sulphated glycoproteins > 200 kDa |
| Oliphant et al. (1984) | Rabbit | Radiolabelled amino acid incorporation, immunohistochemical localisation | Oestrogen primed cells incorporate radiolabel into secretory granules in epithelial cells |
| Sjöberg et al. (1986) | Human | Immunohistochemistry | PAPP-A: Fimbrial content higher during luteal phase |
| Tiitinen et al. (1986) | Human | Immunohistochemistry<br>Gel filtration<br>Radioimmunoassay | PP10: No anatomical variation<br>No ovarian cycle variation |
| Julkunen et al. (1986) | Human | Immunohistochemistry<br>Gel filtration<br>Radioimmunoassay | PP14: Fimbrial content increased in luteal phase |
| Butzow (1989) | Human | Immunohistochemistry<br>Radioimmunoassay | PP5: Present in epithelial cells<br>No anatomical variation |
| Waites et al. (1990) | Human | Monoclonal antibodies<br>Immunochemical localisation | α2-PEG (PP14): Present in epithelial cells in late luteal phase |

In early pregnancy, the mouse oviduct released specific proteins only in association with the presence of an embryo (Nieder and Macon 1987). These proteins were similar to embryo-dependent proteins found in the uterus and had a characteristic pattern in different portions of the reproductive tract, possibly reflecting different roles for each area.

Kapur and Johnson (1986) demonstrated that a 215 000-Dalton glycoprotein was released by the mouse oviduct and selectively sequestered into the perivitelline space of oocytes and embryos. They postulated that this protein was involved in the creation of a specialised microenvironment for fertilisation and early embryo development. A similar phenomenon in the hamster has been reported by Léveillé et al. (1987) who demonstrated uptake of an oviduct-derived component by the zona pellucida.

# Secretory Proteins

The capacity of a tissue to synthesis a protein can be examined by incorporation of a radiolabelled amino acid, followed by separation of the newly synthesised proteins by polyacrylamide gel electrophoresis (PAGE) (Laemmli 1970). In vitro de novo synthesis of protein can then be detected by the pattern of incorporation of the radioactivity. The proteins are normally run under reducing conditions, i.e., large molecules are broken down into their constituent monomers and analysed by SDS-PAGE electrophoresis. Of published studies on the oviduct (Table 5.3), only three have been concerned with the human.

A criticism of most studies of incorporation of radiolabel into the oviduct is that details of control experiments have not been given (Maguiness et al. 1992b). A tissue culture well containing the enzyme inhibitor cycloheximide should produce no radiolabelled protein. This discriminates between the active process of secretion and the passive process of release. A well containing no tissue controls for protein production by bacterial contamination (Tabaqchali et al. 1987).

The culture medium should be changed after an initial equilibration period. The culture media of 7.5% of samples contained detectable PP14 after 3 h of incubation (Maguiness et al. 1991), some of which may have arisen from residual serum contained in the tissue. Protein synthesis by cultures of epithelial cells, mucosal cells and cells from the full thickness of the tubal wall cannot be directly compared because of the possibility of paracrine influence remaining in vitro.

Oliphant and Ross (1982) studied the incorporation of radiolabelled amino acids into proteins synthesised by epithelial cell suspensions of rabbit oviduct and oviduct fluid. Fractionation and gel filtration indicated that both tubal fluid and epithelium contained three mucoproteins of high molecular weight (>200 000 Daltons). SDS–PAGE revealed a 71 000-Dalton sulphated subunit and a 32 000-Dalton non-sulphated subunit. Ouchterlony analysis of these proteins demonstrated complete homology between the oviductal components separated by DEAE chromatography.

In a study comparing de novo synthesis of proteins by different sections of the fallopian tube and endometrium, Maguiness et al. (1993) noted two proteins with a molecular mass of 17 000 Daltons and 25 000 Daltons, synthesised by each section of the fallopian tube, but not by endometrium from the same source or controls. In studies of fallopian tube mucosa from postmenopausal women the 17 000-Dalton protein was absent, suggesting that its synthesis might be dependent on ovarian function. On a Western blot the 25 000-Dalton protein was immunochemically identical to $\kappa$ immunoglobulin light chain. There was none of this protein in the endometrium, agreeing with studies which suggest that immunoglobulin is not present in endometrial tissue in the non-inflammatory state (Hurlimann et al. 1978).

Hyde and Black (1986) used in vitro radiolabelled amino acid incorporation in a short-term explant system of rabbit oviduct tissue to provide evidence for anatomical variation in secretion of proteins. The ampulla secreted the greatest total amount of protein while the major protein constituent, which had a molecular mass of 66 000 Daltons, was secreted by both sections. Using similar methodology, differential synthesis and secretion of proteins in different sections of the baboon oviduct was observed by Fazleabas and Verhage (1986, 1988). Oestrogen-dependent synthesis of both acidic (100 000–120 000 Daltons) and basic (120 000–130 000 Daltons) proteins was observed. While both the acidic and basic proteins were secreted by the ampulla, the acidic protein was dominant in the fimbria and the basic protein dominant in the isthmus. In addition Fazleabas and Verhage found that the fimbria synthesised a protein with a mass of 110 000 Daltons.

**Table 5.3.** Studies to determine protein synthesis and secretion/release by the cellular constituents of the oviduct, listed in chronological order (SDS = sodium dodecyl sulphate; PAGE = polyacrylamide gel electrophoresis; kDa = Daltons × 1000)

| Author | Animal | Methodology | Main findings |
|---|---|---|---|
| Hyde and Black (1986) | Rabbit | Radiolabelled amino acid incorporation<br>Short-term explant SDS-PAGE | Protein synthesis by ampulla > isthmus Major protein produced = 66 kDa, 92 kDa protein and multiple proteins < 66 kDa also synthesised |
| Fazleabas and Verhage (1986) | Baboon | Radiolabelled amino acid incorporation<br>Short-term explant<br>1&2-dimensional PAGE | Oviduct-specific proteins, 16, 88, 130 kDa, 130 kDa protein only present in follicular phase |
| Nieder and Macon (1987) | Mouse | Radiolabelled amino acid incorporation<br>Short-term explant<br>1&2-dimensional PAGE | Day 4–5 of pregnancy – uterus: protein synthesis altered by presence of embryo in oviduct, – oviduct: same change but not dependent on presence of embryo. |
| Malayer et al. (1988) | Cow | Radiolabelled amino acid incorporation<br>Short-term explant<br>1&2-dimensional PAGE | 4 major protein groups, 97, 85–97, 55, 30 kDa, synthesised by ampulla and isthmus during oestrus and early dioestrus |
| Fazleabas and Verhage (1988) | Baboon | Radiolabelled amino acid incorporation<br>Short-term explant<br>2-dimensional PAGE | 2 oestrogen-dependent proteins, 100-130 kDa, acidic protein content > fimbria, basic protein content > isthmus, 110 kDa protein produced by fimbria |
| Verhage et al. (1988) | Human | Radiolabelled amino acid incorporation<br>Short-term explant<br>1&2-dimensional PAGE<br>Immunochemical reaction on Western blot | Mid-region of tube studied during ovarian cycle & postpartum. 2 proteins 120–130 kDa synthesised mid-cycle. PP4 & PP7 synthesised throughout cycle, PP14 in late luteal phase |
| Buhi et al (1989a) | Pig | Radiolabelled amino acid incorporation<br>Short-term explant<br>1-dimensional PAGE | Radiolabelled amino acid incorporation rate: ampulla > isthmus, & faster in association with high oestrogen levels.<br>Proestrus/oestrus/metoestrus: 3 oviduct-specific proteins synthesised, 335, 115, 85 kDa<br>Dioestrus: 2 oviduct-specific proteins synthesised, 20, 60 kDa |
| Buhi et al. (1989b) | Human | Radiolabelled amino acid incorporation<br>Short-term explant<br>2-dimensional PAGE | Cross-section of ampulla studied postpartum. Synthesis of IgA, IgG & 2 polypeptide subunit complexes identified with a serum protein map |
| Maguiness et al. (1991, 1993) | Human | Radiolabelled amino acid incorporation<br>Short-term explant<br>1-dimensional PAGE<br>Immunochemical reaction on Western blot | Mucosa of isthmus, ampulla & fimbria studied.<br>PP14 synthesised throughout ovarian cycle, no variation, $\kappa$ light chain Ig synthesis identified immunochemically, 17 kDa protein synthesised by each section of the fallopian tube throughout the ovarian cycle, not postmenopause |

Differential production and release of proteins has been reported during the oestrus cycle of cows (Malayer et al. 1988), pigs (Buhi et al. 1989a) and baboons (Fazleabas and Verhage 1986, 1988). De novo synthesis of proteins by the ampulla of the human fallopian tube using radiolabel incorporation studies, varies during the ovarian cycle (Verhage et al. 1988). Gel electrophoresis revealed a major diffuse band of 120 000–130 000 Daltons in the peri-ovulatory period (day 8–16 of the menstrual cycle) which was barely detectable at other stages of the cycle.

Placental Protein 4 and Placental Protein 7 are released throughout the ovarian cycle and Placental Protein 14 (PP14) only in the late luteal phase (Verhage et al. 1988). Maguiness et al. (1991) observed that PP14 was synthesised and secreted in vitro by tubal mucosa explants at all stages of the ovarian cycle. In this study there was no difference in the amount of PP14 as measured by radioimmunoassay between the anatomical sections of the fallopian tube or the right and left fallopian tubes at different stages of the ovarian cycle. This study also demonstrated an immunochemical reaction to PP14 on Western blots obtained throughout the ovarian cycle (Maguiness et al. 1991). Since PP14 is only present in significant amounts in tubal mucosa in the late luteal phase (Waites et al. 1990) it could be postulated that mucosal cells can synthesise PP14 throughout the ovarian cycle, but that this protein is stored rather than released during the follicular phase.

The mouse uterus changes its pattern of protein secretion during the fourth and fifth day of pregnancy when an embryo is present (Nieder and Macon 1987). While the oviduct secretions inhibited these uterine embryo-dependent proteins, their appearance was not influenced by the presence of embryos during the first 3 days of pregnancy.

Buhi et al. (1989b) used a short-term explant culture system to demonstrate de novo synthesis and release of proteins by tissue samples from the isthmus and ampulla of the post-partum fallopian tube. Using a serum protein map (Anderson and Anderson 1977) this group identified IgA And IgG as the major proteins produced by the ampulla, which also synthesised two complexes of acidic ($PI < 5$) polypeptide subunits. The isthmus released two families of proteins with a molecular mass of 51 000 Daltons and 60 000 Daltons. These appeared in only trace amounts.

# Conclusions

The oviduct synthesises and secretes both specific proteins and proteins of general Müllerian origin, some of which vary according to anatomical site, stage of the oestrus or ovarian cycle, and during pregnancy. There are as yet few results from systematic, controlled studies of specific protein synthesis and secretion in normal human fallopian tube and there are no simple assays to measure proteins specific to it. Such assays are essential for evaluation of these substances as markers of fallopian tube function. For clinicians these phenomena will be important both for the possible development of new methods of contraception and in the assessment of subfertile women who do not have an anatomical tubal factor. Furthermore, this information may facilitate better selection of patients in assisted conception programmes which utilise the tubal environment (gamete intrafallopian transfer, tubal embryo transfer) rather than techniques which by-pass the fallopian tube.

# References


Adams CE, Chang MC (1962) Capacitation of rabbit spermatozoa in the fallopian tube and in the uterus. J Exp Zool 15:159–166

Andersen DH (1927) The rate of passage of the mammalian ovum through various portions of the fallopian tube. Am J Physiol 82:557–569

Anderson L, Anderson NG (1977) High resolution two dimensional electrophoresis of human plasma proteins. Proc Natl Acad Sci USA 74:5421–5425

Barr SH, Oliphant G (1981) Sulphate incorporation into macro-molecules produced by cultured oviductal epithelium. Biol Reprod 24:852–858

Bedford JM (1968) Importance of the fallopian tube for capacitation in the rabbit. Proc 6th Int Congr Anim Reprod, Paris 1:35–37

Bishop DW (1956) Active secretion in the rabbit oviduct. Am J Physiol 187:347–352

Blackwell RE (1989) The infertility workup and diagnosis. J Reprod Med 34:81–85

Blandau RJ (1969) Gamete transport – comparative aspects. In: Hafez ESE, Blandau RJ (eds) The mammalian oviduct. University of Chicago Press, Chicago, pp 129–162

Blandau RJ, Verdugo P (1976) An overview of gamete transport – comparative effects. In: Harper MJK, Pauerstein CJ (eds) Symposium on ovum transport and fertility regulation. Scriptor, Copenhagen, pp 138–146

Boling JL (1969) Endocrinology of oviductal musculature. In: Hafez ESE, Blandau RJ (eds) The mammalian oviduct. Chicago, University of Chicago Press, Chicago, pp 163–181

Bolton AE et al. (1987) Identification of placental protein 14 as an immunosuppressive factor in human reproduction. Lancet 1:593–595

Bongso A, Ng SC, Ratnam SS (1990) Co-cultures: their relevance to assisted reproduction. Hum Reprod 5:893–900

Bowman GM, McLaren A (1970) Cleavage rate of mouse embryos in vivo and in vitro. J Embryol Exp Morph 24:203–207

Brackett BG, Mastroianni L (1974) Composition of oviductal fluid. In: Johnson AD, Foley CW (eds) The oviduct and its functions. Academic Press, New York, pp 135–159

Brower LK, Anderson E (1969) Cytological events associated with the secretory process in the rabbit oviduct. Biol Reprod 1:130–148

Buhi WC, Vallet JL, Bazer FW (1989a) De novo synthesis and release of polypeptides from cyclic and early pregnant porcine oviductal tissue in explant culture. J Exp Zool 252:79–88

Buhi WC, Van Wert JW, Alvarez IM, Dones-Smith MM, Bernhisel MA (1989b) Synthesis and secretion of proteins by postpartum human oviductal tissue in culture. Fertil Steril 51:75–80

Butzow R (1989) The human fallopian tube contains placental protein 5. Hum Reprod 4:17–20

Clewe TH, Mastroianni L (1960) A method for continuous volumetric collection of oviduct secretions. J Reprod Fertil 1:146–150

Croxatto HB, Ortiz ME (1975) Egg transport in the fallopian tube. Gynaecol Invest 6:215–225

David A, Brackett BG, Garcia CR, Mastroianni L (1969) Composition of rabbit oviduct fluid in ligated segments of the fallopian tube. J Reprod Fertil 19:285–289

David A, Serr DM, Czernobilsky B (1973) Chemical composition of human oviduct fluid. Fertil Steril 24:435–439

Eddy CA, Garcia RG, Kraemer DC, Pauerstein CJ (1976) Ovum transport in non-human primates. In: Harper MJK, Pauerstein CJ (eds) Symposium on ovum transport and fertility regulation. Scriptor, Copenhagen, pp 447–453

Fazleabas AT, Verhage HG (1986) The detection of oviduct-specific proteins in the baboon (*Papio anubis*). Biol Reprod 35:455–462

Fazleabas AT, Verhage HG (1988) The in vitro synthesis of estrogen-dependent proteins by the baboon (*Papio anubis*) oviduct. Endocrinology 123:552–558

Feigelson M, Kay E (1972) Protein patterns of rabbit oviductal fluid. Biol Reprod 6:244–252

Glass LE (1969) Immunocytological studies of the mouse oviduct. In: Hafez ESE, Blandau RJ (eds) The mammalian oviduct. University of Chicago Press, Chicago, pp 459–476
Glass LE, McClure TR (1965) Postnatal development of the mouse oviduct: transfer of serum antigens to the tubal epithelium. In: Wolstenholme GEW (ed) Preimplantation stages of pregnancy. Little, Brown & Co., Boston, pp 294–321
Greenwald GS (1958) Endocrine regulation of the secretion of mucin in the tubal epithelium of the rabbit. Anat Rec 130:477–495
Greenwald GS (1962) The role of the mucin layer in the development of the rabbit blastocyst. Anat Rec 142:407–415
Hadek R (1955) The secretory process in the sheep's oviduct. Anat Rec 121:187–201
Hamner CE, Williams W (1965) Composition of rabbit oviductal secretions. Fertil Steril 16:170–176
Hanscom DR, Oliphant G (1976) Hormonal regulation of incorporation of 35S into macromolecules of oviduct fluid. Biol Reprod 14:599–604
Harlow GM, Quinn P (1982) Development of preimplantation mouse embryos in vivo and in vitro. Aust J Biol Sci 35:187–193
Harper MJK (1961a) The mechanisms involved in the movement of newly ovulated eggs through the ampulla of the rabbit fallopian tube. J Reprod Fertil 2:522–524
Harper MJK (1961b) Egg movement through the ampullar region of the fallopian tube of the rabbit. Proc 4th Int Congr Anim Reprod, The Hague, pp 375–380
Holmdahl TH, Mastroianni L (1965) Continuous collection of rabbit oviduct secretions at low temperature. Fertil Steril 16:587–595
Hunter RHF (1974) Chronological and cytological details of fertilisation and early embryonic development in the domestic pig, *Sus scrofa*. Anat Rec 178:169–186
Hunter RHF, Hall JP (1974) Capacitation of boar spermatozoa: synergism between uterine and tubal environments. J Exp Zool 188:203–214
Hurlimann J, Dayal R, Gloor E (1978) Immunoglobulins and secretory component in endometrium and cervix. Virchows Arch A Path Anat Histol 377:211–223
Hyde BA, Black DL (1986) Synthesis and secretion of sulphated glycoproteins by rabbit oviduct explants in vitro. J Reprod Fertil 78:83–91
Iritani A, Nishikawa Y, Gomes WR, Van Demark NL (1971) Secretion rates and chemical composition of oviduct and uterine fluids in rabbits. J Anim Sci 33:829–835
Julkunen M, Wahlstrom T, Seppälä M (1986) Human fallopian tube contains placental protein 14. Am J Obstet Gynecol 154:1076–1079
Kapur RP, Johnson LV (1986) Selective sequestration of an oviduct fluid glycoprotein in the perivitelline space of mouse oocytes and embryos. J Exp Zool 238:249–260
Kay E, Feigelson M (1972) An estrogen modulated protein in rabbit oviduct fluid. Acta Biochim Biophys 271:436–441
Laemmli UK (1970) Cleavage of structural proteins during the assembly of the head of bacteriophage T4. Nature 227:680–685
Lambert JC, Hamner CE, Gemmill CL (1973) Ultrastructural study of secretion in the rabbit oviduct under different hormonal influences. Fed Proc 32: Abstract 13
Leese HJ (1988) The formation and function of oviduct fluid. J Reprod Fert 82:843–856
Leese HJ, Aldridge S, Jeffries KS (1979) The movement of amino acids into rabbit oviductal fluid. J Reprod Fertil 56:623–626
Léveillé MC, Roberts KD, Chevalier S, Chapdelaine A, Beau G (1987) Uptake of oviductal antigen by the hamster zona pellucida. Biol Reprod 36:227–238
Lillie RD (1949) Studies on the histochemistry of normal and pathological mucins in man and in laboratory animals. Bull Int Assoc Med Mus 29:1–53
Lippes J, Wagh PV (1989) Human oviductal fluid (hOF) proteins. IV. Evidence for hOF proteins binding to human sperm. Fertil Steril 51:89–94
Lippes J, Enders RG, Pragay DA, Bartholomew WR (1972) The collection and analysis of human fallopian tube fluid. Contraception 5:85–103
Lippes J, Krasner J, Alfonso LA, Dacalos ED, Lucero R (1981) Human oviductal fluid proteins. Fertil Steril 36:623–629
Maguiness SD, Shrimanker K, Djahanbakhch O, Grudzinskas JG (1991) PP14 and total protein production by short term explants of fallopian tube epithelium. Human Reproduction 6: Suppl 1 (ESHRE), abstract 78
Maguiness SD, Djahanbakhch O, Grudzinskas JG (1992a) Assessment of the fallopian tube. Obstet Gynecol Survey 47:587–603

Maguiness SD, Shrimanker K, Djahanbakhch O, Grudzinskas JG (1992b) Oviduct proteins. Contemp Rev Obstet Gynaecol 4:42–50
Maguiness SD, Shrimanker K, Djahanbakhch O, Grudzinskas JG (1993) The identification of two new fallopian tube proteins (TEP-1 and TEP-2). Hum Reprod 8:1199–1202
Malayer JR, Hansen PJ, Buhi WC (1988) Secretion of proteins by cultured bovine oviducts collected from estrus through early diestrus. J Exp Zool 248:345–353
Marcus SL, Saravis CA (1965) Oviduct fluid in the Rhesus monkey: a study of its protein components and its origin. Fertil Steril 16:785–794
Mastroianni L, Jones R (1965) Oxygen tension within the rabbit fallopian tube. J Reprod Fertil 9:99–102
Mastroianni L, Urzua M, Stambaugh R (1970) Protein patterns of monkey oviductal fluid before and after ovulation. Fertil Steril 21:817–820
Moghissi KS (1970) Human fallopian tube fluid. I. Protein composition. Fertil Steril 21:821–829
Nieder GL, Macon GR (1987) Uterine and oviductal protein secretion during early pregnancy in the mouse. J Reprod Fertil 81:287–294
Oliphant G (1986) Biochemistry and immunology of oviductal fluid. In: Siegler AM (ed) The fallopian tube: basic studies and clinical contributions. Futura Publishing Company, Mount Kisco, pp 129–145
Oliphant G, Ross PR (1982) Demonstration of production and isolation of three sulfated glycoproteins from the rabbit oviduct. Biol Reprod 26:537–544
Oliphant G, Bowling A, Eng LA, Keen S (1978) The permeability of the rabbit oviduct to proteins present in the serum. Biol Reprod 18:516–520
Oliphant G, Cabot C, Ross P, Marta J (1984) Control of the humoral immune system within the rabbit oviduct. Biol Reprod 31:205–212
Pauerstein CJ (1975) Clinical implications of oviductal physiology and biochemistry. Gynecol Invest 6:253–264
Restall BJ, Wales RG (1966) The fallopian tube of sheep. III. The chemical composition of the fluid from the fallopian tube. Austral J Biol Sci 19:687–698
Riddick DH (1975) The composition of rabbit oviductal fluid collected continuously through gestation. J Reprod Fertil 43:563–566
Roberts GP, Parker JM, Symonds HW (1975) Proteins in the luminal fluid from the bovine oviduct. J Reprod Fertil 45:301–313
Roberts GP, Parker JM, Symonds HW (1976) Macromolecular components of genital tract fluids from sheep. J Reprod Fertil 48:431–434
Seppälä M, Angervo M, Koistinen R, Riittinen L, Julkunen M (1991) Human endometrial protein secretion. In: Seppälä M (ed) Factors of importance for implantation, Balliere's Clinical Obstetrics and Gynaecology, London, pp 61–72
Shams A et al. (1977) Human tubal fluid collection via vagina and its quantitative variations during the menstrual cycle. J Reprod Med 18:61–65
Shapiro SS, Jentsch JP, Yard AS (1971) Protein composition of rabbit oviductal fluid. J Reprod Fertil 24:403–408
Sjöberg J, Wahlstrom T, Grudzinskas JG, Sinosich MJ (1986) Demonstration of pregnancy-associated plasma protein-A (PAPP-A)-like material in the fallopian tube. Fertil Steril 45:517–521
Stone SL, Richardson LL, Hamner CE, Oliphant G (1977) Partial characterisation of hormone-mediated inhibition of embryo development in rabbit oviduct fluid. Biol Reprod 16:647–653
Sutton R, Nancarrow CD, Wallace ALC, Rigby NW (1984) Identification of an oestrus-associated glycoprotein in oviductal fluid of the sheep. J Reprod Fertil 72:415–422
Sutton R, Nancarrow CD, Wallace ALC (1986) Oestrogen and seasonal effects on the production of an oestrus-associated glycoprotein in oviductal fluid of sheep. J Reprod Fertil 77:645–653
Tabaqchali S, Silman R, Holland D (1987) Automation in clinical microbiology: a new approach to identifying microorganisms by automated pattern matching of proteins labelled with $^{35}S$ methionine. J Clin Path 40:1070–1087
Tiitinen A, Wahlstrom T, Julkunen M, Seppälä M (1986) The content and immunohistochemical localisation of placental protein 10 (PP10) in the fallopian tube. Br J Obstet Gynaecol 93:924–927
Verdugo P (1986) Functional anatomy of the fallopian tube. In: Insler V, Lunenfeld B (eds) Infertility: male and female. Churchill Livingstone, London, pp 26–55
Verhage HG, Fazleabas AT, Donnelly K (1988) The in vitro synthesis and release of proteins by the human oviduct. Endocrinol 122:1639–1645

Wagh PV, Lippes J (1989) Human oviductal fluid proteins. III. Identification and partial purification. Fertil Steril 51:81–88
Waites GT, Bell SC, Walker RA, Wood PL (1990) Immunohistological distribution of the secretory endometrial protein pregnancy-associated endometrial $\alpha_2$-globulin, a glycosylated $\beta$-lactoglobulin homologue, in the human fetus and adult employing monoclonal antibodies. Hum Reprod 5:105–111
Woskressensky MA (1891) Experimentelle Untersuchungen über die Pyo- und Hydrosalpinxbildung bei den Tieren. Zbl Gynäk, 15:849–860
Zachariae F (1958) Autoradiographic ($^{35}S$) and histochemical studies of sulphomucopolysaccharides in the rabbit uterus, oviduct and vagina. Acta Endocrinol 29:118–134

Chapter 6

# Gamete Transport and Fertilisation

C.L.R. Barratt, M. Williams and M.A. Warren

## Introduction

This chapter will examine the evidence for the interaction of the female reproductive tract and its secretions with spermatozoa, primarily in humans. We will also briefly describe ovum transport, the fertilisation process and possible methods of contraception which may interfere with the process of sperm transport.

A recent review of studies on the dynamics of sperm transport has addressed their limitations (Barratt and Cooke 1991). Furthermore, the reader is referred to texts on sperm selection (Cohen 1991; Birkhead and Moller 1992), significance of white blood cells (Barratt et al. 1990, 1992) and sperm chemotaxis (Coll and Miller 1991).

The isthmus of the oviduct appears to act as a functional reservoir of sperm. Movement of sperm from this region to the ampulla is a highly synchronised event (hamsters: Smith and Yanagimachi 1987, 1991; farm animals: Hunter and Wilmut 1984; Hunter 1987). The oviduct conserves (suppresses) sperm function prior to ovulation and then activates a small proportion of spermatozoa (approximately 1:10 000 in hamsters) to progress to the site of fertilisation. The oviduct also regulates the speed of sperm capacitation. Capacitation proceeds faster when mating occurs after ovulation (Smith and Yanagimachi 1987, 1989, 1990, 1991). Work in humans is very limited and must determine (i) whether storage exists; (ii) the site(s) of such storage; (iii) factors affecting sperm progression; (iv) the functional state of spermatozoa throughout the tract; and (v) the effect of ovulation.

# Sperm Transport and Storage

Sperm transport through the human female reproductive tract involves passage from the hostile environment of the vagina to the cervical mucus, then on to the uterus and fallopian tubes. Transport allows "selected" spermatozoa (probably one in a million) access to the site of fertilisation. Are these sperm "earmarked" for selection at production or does the female tract itself bring about selection (see Barratt and Cooke 1991 for references)?

## The Cervix

Morphologically abnormal sperm experience greater resistance than normal sperm in mucus, thus hampering their entry and progression (Katz et al. 1990). Several days prior to ovulation, sperm transport into cervical mucus is optimal; surprisingly, however, this penetration is reduced at ovulation (Thompson et al. 1993). Thus, there appears to be a critical window of sperm transport prior to ovulation.

When spermatozoa enter the cervix, they elicit an influx of phagocytic cells – the leucocytic cell reaction (LCR) (Barratt et al. 1990). The main cell type involved is the neutrophil (Thompson et al. 1991, 1992). These cells might selectively phagocytose unsuitable spermatozoa and prime the reproductive tract for fertilisation. However, very few phagocytic cells contain spermatozoa fragments. Thus, the well-defined mechanism of sperm phagocytosis in the male tract (Barratt and Cohen 1986, 1987, 1988; Barratt and Cooke 1988; Barratt et al. 1990) remains to be fully documented in the female.

Within the mucus, spermatozoa undergo changes which prepare them for fertilisation. High shear forces remove decapacitation factors (reversible factors which inhibit sperm-fertilising capacity) in humans and animals (Fraser et al. 1990; Oliphant et al. 1985), thus enabling capacitation. In humans, movement of sperm from a slightly alkaline (semen) to acidic (vagina) and then alkaline (mucus) environment brings about cataphoresis, aiding orientation and motility (Miller and Kurzrok 1932). Recovery of sperm from cervical mucus, both in vivo and in vitro, provides evidence for initiation of capacitation as well as conservation of sperm acrosomal status for up to 3 days post insemination (Lambert et al. 1985; Zinaman et al. 1989). Our studies show that spermatozoa recovered from cervical mucus are more heterogeneous than those prepared in media, and that cervical mucus promotes hyperactivated motion (Zhu et al. 1992). Spermatozoa in mucus attain a level of capacitation beyond which a further "stimulus" is required for establishing full fertilising ability. The nature of this "stimulus" is unknown.

## The Uterus

There is very limited knowledge on the role of the uterus in the transport of human spermatozoa (Maathuis and Aitken 1978; Barratt and Cooke 1991). We have developed a technique to recover spermatozoa from the uterus using a Foley catheter. Ten patients were inseminated with donor spermatozoa approximately 24 h after the start of the LH surge and the uterus flushed 4 h later (Williams et al. 1993). Only very low numbers of spermatozoa were recovered (median 43.5; range 0–415). This might be due to sperm endometrial attachment/interaction with incomplete sperm recovery, or a leucocytic reaction as in the cervix (Barratt and Cooke 1991).

Preliminary in vitro data in humans suggests that the uterine environment affects the function of sperm e.g. the acrosome reaction (Zinaman et al. 1988) and capacitation (Kim et al. 1991). However, more comprehensive studies are required to elucidate the role of the uterus on human sperm transport.

## The Oviduct

### *The Environment*

The oviduct consists of epithelium and its appendages (cilia) and the surrounding connective tissues and muscular layers. These all show a gradual change over the length of the tube.

The oviductal epithelium consists of ciliated cells and non-ciliated secretory cells (Figs. 6.1, 6.2). There is variation along the tube (Jansen 1980; Kenemans and Hafez 1984; Tuffrey et al. 1990) with about twice as many ciliated cells in the fimbriae of the infundibulum as in the ampulla or

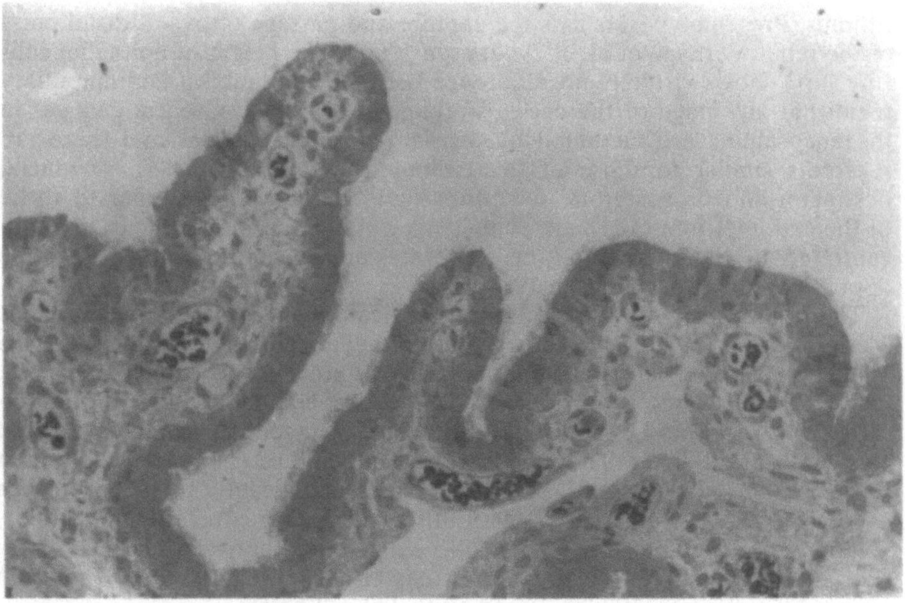

**Fig. 6.1.** Light micrograph of the ampullary region of a human uterine tube stained with toluidine blue. Cilia may be seen on the apical epithelial surface. Blood vessels are common.

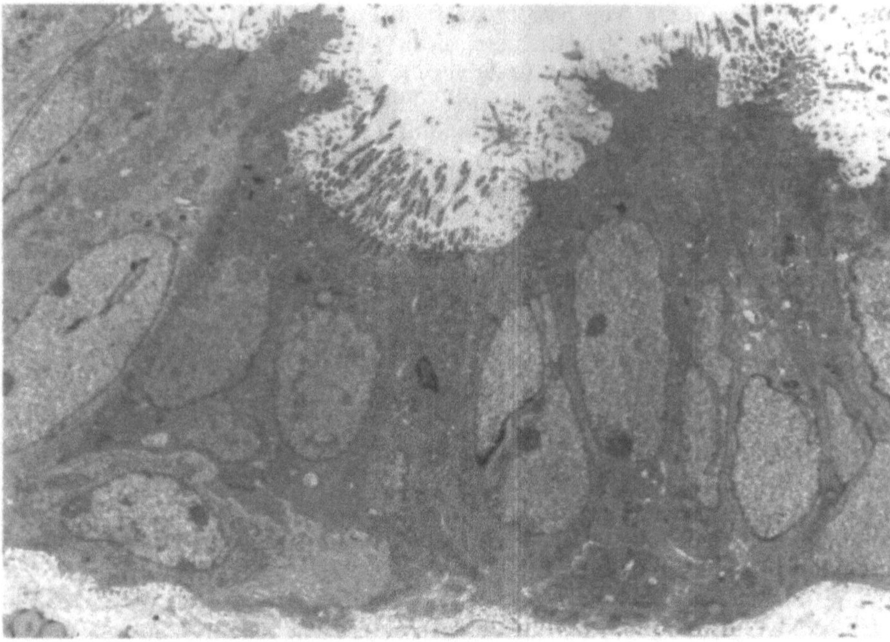

**Fig. 6.2.** Human tubal ampullary cells under the electron microscope have characteristic apical protrusions. Cilia and nuclei are prominent.

isthmus. Presumably, this aids the capture and passage of ova at distal parts of the tube (Verhage et al. 1979; Jansen 1984). The height of epithelial cells (Fig. 6.1) shows virtually no difference between the fimbrial and ampullary regions at any stage of the cycle (Verhage et al. 1979). Cyclical changes in the endosalpinx are mediated by ovarian steroid hormones and there are receptors similar to those of the endometrium (Jansen 1984). Oviductal oestradiol and progesterone receptors have characteristics similar to those of the endometrium (Verhage et al. 1980; Pollow et al. 1981). They are concentrated in the epithelium, with decreasing concentrations as the tube approaches the ovary (Jansen 1984).

There are distinct cyclical morphological changes in oviductal cells. Verhage et al. (1979) have shown that epithelial cell height decreased from 30 $\mu$m during the late follicular phase to 24 $\mu$m by the end of the cycle. These changes were proportional to the levels of circulating oestradiol. Similarly, Kim-Bjorklund et al. (1991) estimated tubal cell height and correlated this with steroid levels. They reported an epithelial cell height of 23.6 $\mu$m at day (LH + O)–day (LH + 3) which decreased significantly to $16.1 \pm 3.4$ $\mu$m by day (LH + 4)–day (LH + 7) with little change thereafter. Significant correlations were seen at day (LH + O)–day (LH + 3) between plasma oestradiol and epithelial cell height, and at day (LH + 4)–day (LH + 7) between corpus luteum oestradiol levels and epithelial cell height.

Verhage et al. (1979) reported that 35% of ampullary cells (Fig. 6.2) and

50% of fimbrial cells were ciliated in the early follicular phase, when oestradiol levels were low (71 ± 20 pg/ml). At this time, the isthmic mucosa was thin, cilia were sparse and there was little secretory material apparent (Jansen 1980). The proportion of ciliated cells increased to reach a peak in the late follicular phase. At this time, secretory material was prominent between the microvilli of secretory cells and sometimes obscured the cilia (Jansen 1980). Jansen (1980) suggested that mucus secreted from the isthmus protects the sperm from the action of the ciliary beating which would otherwise sweep them back to the uterus.

After ovulation, the secretory cells shorten so that the ciliated cells appear to project above them, probably improving their ability to move overlying material (Jansen 1984). By the end of the luteal phase, the cells are uniformly low and the proportion of ciliated cells is at a minimum. All secretory cells undergo a complete cycle of differentiation but only 10%–12% of ciliated cells form new cilia; the remainder simply undergo minor fluctuations in height (Verhage et al. 1979).

Other parts of the oviduct can influence the movement of luminal contents. The tube is surrounded by smooth muscle which receives postganglionic cholinergic innervation at the isthmus. The ganglia are supplied by preganglionic parasympathetic fibres which originate at spinal segments S2 to S4. The ampulla receives terminal branches of the vagus nerve. It is likely that stimulation of these parasympathetic fibres would cause vasodilation of the tubal vascular system (Jansen 1984), but there appears to be no evidence of this. Sympathetic (adrenergic) innervation comes from segments T12 to L2/3 via the inferior mesenteric plexus.

Hormonal influences can also affect contraction of the smooth muscle coat of the tube. In the rabbit, vasoactive intestinal polypeptide, an inhibitor of oviductal motility (Frederichs and Ashton 1982) which acts through adenylate cyclase to potentiate the effect of acetyl choline (Robberecht et al. 1981; Lundberg et al. 1982), is reduced at the time when muscular activity and ciliary beating are increasing (Menghi et al. 1990). This is likely to be combined with an increase in adrenergic impulses (Black 1974) which would further increase tubal motility.

## Sperm Transport and Interaction

There is a paucity of studies on the numbers, distribution, functional status and interaction of sperm with the tubal environment. In an attempt to address this subject, we have developed three experimental approaches:

1. Improvements in techniques to recover spermatozoa from the oviduct and synchronisation of this recovery with ovulation.
2. In vitro examination of reproductive tract fluids e.g. oviductal and follicular fluid on sperm function.
3. Development of in vitro cultures of the ampullary and isthmic portions of the oviduct and coculture with spermatozoa.

Below we summarise the details of these three approaches.

### 1. *In Vivo Transport*

Studies on sperm recovery from the peritoneal cavity have produced conflicting data (Ramsewak et al. 1990); they only determine if spermatozoa can be transported through the oviduct. Many studies examining sperm numbers in the oviduct have experimental limitations; for example, the techniques used to recover sperm are inadequate (e.g. Settlage used a cytocentrifuge which had a recovery rate of only 1%), and the time of ovulation is often not documented (Rubenstein et al. 1951; Ahlgren 1975; Settlage et al. 1973). By using more sophisticated methods of timing and meticulous laboratory techniques, we have ascertained that there are indeed low numbers of spermatozoa in the ampullary oviduct prior to ovulation (ampulla median 55.5, range 0–445; isthmus median 27.0, range 0–128; IMR median 27.0, range 0–124) (Williams et al. 1992, 1993). However, our results are only preliminary as only 10 patients have been examined. Our initial studies using an embryo transfer catheter to recover sperm from the oviduct have been unsuccessful. We are now testing the use of the falloposcope to investigate sperm transport.

### 2. *In Vitro Interaction with Reproductive Tract Fluids*

Both oviductal and follicular fluid have specific effects on sperm function.

*Oviductal Fluid.* Most studies on the interaction between oviductal fluid and spermatozoa have been performed in cows. Bovine oviductal fluid (BOF) maintains sperm motility and capacitates spermatozoa but is not a specific inducer of the acrosome reaction (McNutt and Killian 1991; Parrish et al. 1989). Parrish suggested that the capacitating factor was a heparin-like glycosaminoglycan (GAG) although this remains to be established (Miller and Ax 1990). Fusi and Bronson (1992) have identified fibronectin in human spermatozoa following capacitation. Fibronectin has defined binding sites for heparin which may be exposed during capacitation thus enhancing the ability of the spermatozoa to respond to GAG further to stimulate capacitation. This hypothesis warrants further investigation.

Killian's group have shown that a specific bovine glycoprotein (EAP) maintained sperm motility when added to culture media. Incubation of bovine sperm with ampullary oviductal explants affects the secretion of oviductal proteins, suggesting intimate cell-to-cell communication between the oviduct and spermatozoa (Anderson and Killian 1992). Ellington and colleagues, using transmission electron microscopy, demonstrated a very close apposition between the sperm plasma membrane and uterine tubal cells in culture (Ellington et al. 1991).

The role of oviduct-specific glycoproteins on sperm function remains a mystery. Numerous specific glycoproteins have been identified e.g. bovine (Boice et al. 1990), porcine (Nagai and Moor 1990; Buhi et al. 1989a,b), baboon (Fazleabas and Verhage 1986). Sutton and colleagues demonstrated the binding of glycoproteins to spermatozoa but stated that "the extent, nature or physiological significance of this binding is unknown" (Sutton et al. 1984).

There is a paucity of human studies. Mukherjee and Lippes (1972) used a crude test for the presence of an acrosome and showed that the treatment of rat, mouse and human spermatozoa with tubal fluid led to loss of staining of the acrosome after 4 h. We have studied the effects of oviductal fluid (HOF) and follicular fluid (FF) on sperm kinetics including hyperactivation (HA) and the acrosome reaction (Zhu et al. 1994a,b; De Jorge et al. 1993). HOF maintains sperm motility but in contrast to FF does not induce HA. The low percentage (12%) of HA spermatozoa remained constant over a 9-h incubation period when incubated in HOF. We concluded that HOF maintains a low level of HA whereas FF has a transient stimulatory effect. Oviduct-specific glycoproteins have been identified (Buhi et al. 1989a,b; Verhage et al. 1988; Reuter et al. 1992; Lippes and Wagh 1989) but it is uncertain how they interact with spermatozoa. Lippes and Wagh (1989) suggested, with very little evidence, that they bound to the head to stabilise the acrosome.

In addition to specific glycoproteins, other factors in oviductal fluid are likely to be important for sperm function e.g. metabolites (Burkman et al. 1984). The role of lipoproteins has received attention. Ehrenwald et al. (1990) examined the components of oviductal fluid which support cholesterol efflux. Bovine sperm were incubated with oviductal fluid, the HDL (high density lipoprotein) and albumin fractions. The HDL factors were the main acceptors of cholesterol.

*Follicular Fluid.* There is still some controversy over the effect of follicular fluid (FF) on sperm function (Calvo et al. 1989; Thomas and Meizel 1988; De Jonge et al. 1993; Mortimer and Camenzind 1989). The consensus suggests that follicular fluid can induce the acrosome reaction. Calvo and colleagues (1989) comprehensively investigated this topic. They showed that exposure of capacitated sperm, even to low doses of FF, induces the acrosome reaction. Similar results are now consistently being reported.

Follicular fluid can induce hyperactivation in capacitated spermatozoa (Mbizvo et al. 1990; Zhu et al. 1991). In our study, after 6-h incubation with FF, the levels of HA were above controls, returning to normal after 9 h. Incubation of sperm in FF reduced the proportion of motile spermatozoa after 6 h and 9 h. The factors which stimulate sperm motion are uncertain. Follicular fluid may induce capacitation through an efflux of cholesterol from the plasma membrane of the sperm, an early step in sperm capacitation (Ehrenwald et al. 1988). Ravnik and colleagues (1993) have demonstrated lipid transfer activity (LTA) in human FF which would stimulate capacitation rather than inducing the acrosome reaction.

FF induces a rapid transient increase in calcium in spermatozoa. This may be due to progesterone which, even at low levels (0.05 $\mu$g/ml), can stimulate a rapid transient increase in internal calcium (Blackmore et al. 1990; Thomas and Meizel 1989). Progesterone will also directly stimulate the acrosome reaction and hyperactivation (Mbizvo et al. 1990; De Jonge et al. 1993).

Spermatozoa have to pass through cumulus cells before they reach the zona. In humans, cumulus cells (or their constituents) have been shown to induce the acrosome reaction in vitro (Tesarik et al. 1988; Siiteri et al. 1988; De Jonge et al. 1988; Sullivan et al. 1990). Tesarik and colleagues demonstrated that several high-molecular-weight glycoproteins secreted by the cumulus could bind to human spermatozoa and stimulate conversion of proacrosin to acrosin (Tesarik et al. 1988). Paradoxically, however, enhancement of the acrosome reaction was obtained with low-molecular-weight material (25 kDa) that displayed no proacrosin-converting activity. These results suggest that interaction of different proteins may be necessary for fertilisation.

*Signal Transduction and the Role of Reproductive Tract Fluids.* Signal transduction pathways of the acrosome reaction are poorly understood (Kopf 1990; Zaneveld et al. 1991; Florman and Babcock 1989). In the human, De Jonge and colleagues have provided evidence for the involvement of the diacylglycerol/protein kinase C and the adenylate cyclase pathways in the acrosome reaction in vitro (De Jonge et al. 1991a,b).

Polyphosphoinositide metabolism is active in human spermatozoa (Thomas 1990; Thomas and Meizel 1989; Roldan and Harrison 1989; Harrison and Roldan 1990). In the human, follicular fluid induces the influx of extracellular calcium (Thomas and Meizel 1988), the hydrolysis of phosphoinositides and the acrosome reaction (Thomas 1991). Phosphoinositide hydrolysis is dependent on extracellular calcium and is probably involved in the metabolism of internal calcium (Thomas 1991). This hydrolysis may generate diacylglycerol and activate protein kinase C. Many experiments on signal transduction mechanisms of the AR have used ionophore-induction systems and other compounds which bypass receptor sites on sperm. It is, therefore, difficult to assess the physiological relevance of these studies (see Harrison and Roldan 1990 for detailed discussion). Follicular fluid collected from natural cycle IVF (Barratt et al. 1989) stimulated the acrosome reaction via the PKC and the PKA pathways (De Jonge et al. 1993).

In the human, there are several mechanisms which can induce the acrosome reaction; natural inducers of the reaction can activate more than one of these pathways (De Jonge et al. 1993). However, it is clear that we must use human zona (or recombinant products) in future signal transduction experiments if we are really to understand this complex process.

## 3. *Coculture of Sperm with Oviductal and Uterine Cells*

In the hamster, there appears to be a coordinated, synchronised and dynamic movement of spermatozoa in the oviduct (Smith and Yanagimachi 1987). Sperm remain attached to the isthmic mucosa until they are capacitated, after which a small proportion detach and migrate to the ampulla to fertilise the eggs (Smith and Yanagimachi 1991; Barratt and Cooke 1991).

In vitro studies suggest that the oviductal epithelium of pigs and cows maintains sperm motility and prolongs fertilising ability (Pollard et al. 1991; Suarez et al. 1991; Nagai and Moor 1990).

Coculture models offer an experimental system to investigate the interaction between spermatozoa and the female reproductive tract. Techniques to culture human oviductal tissue are well established. Scanning electron micrographs show that the secretory and ciliated cells are similar to those observed in vivo (Bongso et al. 1991). A positive influence of culturing embryos together with cell monolayers for in-vitro fertilisation has been shown (see Chap. 3).

There is a significantly higher fertilisation rate of human oocytes when spermatozoa are incubated with passaged oviductal cells (Bongso et al. 1991). Unpublished observations indicate an increase in hyperactivated motility in spermatozoa incubated with oviductal cells. This increase in hyperactivation may be responsible for the increased fertilisation rate. There is a threefold increase in the incidence of hyperactivated motility in human spermatozoa incubated with endometrial cells (Guerin et al. 1991). There was no increase in hyperactivation in spermatozoa incubated on Vero cells or conditioned media but there was when the cells were incubated on bovine oviductal cells. Thus, the effect is tissue-specific but not species-specific. Wetzels et al. (1991) showed that incubation of human spermatozoa on Vero-cell monolayers or in conditioned media resulted in a higher percentage of motile cells and velocity compared with controls. Vero cells may stimulate sperm motility by secreting or converting factors in the media. Vero cells secrete proteins but these have not been shown to bind to spermatozoa. In our cultures of the uterine and oviductal epithelium on polarised substrata, we have shown that sperm motility was maintained for significantly longer in cultures but that the levels of hyperactivation were not significantly increased.

## Ovum/Embryo Transport

Ovum maturation within the Graffian follicle takes place within 25–30 h after the onset of the LH surge (Lenton et al. 1988). At ovulation, follicular fluid oestrogen and progesterone concentrations are 800 ng/ml and 12 200 ng/ml respectively (serum midcycle levels; oestrogen 0.3 ng/ml, progesterone 1.0 ng/ml). Thus, at ovulation, the fallopian tube and peritoneal cavity are exposed to high levels of these hormones (approximately 50 $\mu$g progesterone, 5 $\mu$g oestrogen) (Lenton et al. 1988). The ovum is transported into the fallopian tube by the flow of follicular fluid (Harper 1982), aided by the close association between the follicle and fimbria (Jansen 1984). Transperitoneal ovum migration is rare, but cases have been reported (Jansen 1984). Within the fallopian tube, the ovum is in close association with the luminal surface. Movement from the fimbriae to the ampullary-isthmic junction is brought about by tonic and phasic contractions of tubal smooth muscle, which create a to-and-fro motion (net movement towards the uterus) (Verdugo et al. 1976) and cilial beating towards the uterus (Jansen 1984), aided by the cumulus cells surrounding the ovum (Harper 1982). At midcycle, cilial height is at a maximum (Jansen 1984). During the luteal phase, there is an 18% increase in cilia beat as compared to the follicular phase (Critoph and Dennis 1978) thus aiding ovum transport. Lack of muscular contraction or cilial beating (e.g. Kartagener's syndrome) does not prevent fertilisation and pregnancy (Jansen 1984), suggesting that either of these mechanisms is adequate to facilitate ovum transport. In the human, transport from the ovary to the fallopian tube is completed within 7 h or less (Croxatto et al.

1978). Retention within the ampulla lasts approximately 72 h (Croxatto et al. 1978). The ovum remains viable within the ampulla for approximately 24 h. Transport of either a fertilised or unfertilised ovum proceeds similarly from this point (Harper 1982). Embryo/ovum retention ("tubal-blocking") at the ampullary-isthmic junction is brought about by a decreased isthmic luminal diameter due to oedema, increased internal pressure, luminal mucus and decreased isthmic ciliary and contractile activity. These effects occur during oestrogen dominance. As progesterone dominance prevails, i.e., post-ovulation, these effects are antagonised and the block to ovum/embryo transport is removed (Jansen 1980). Decrease in pressure in the isthmic lumen along with the increase in lumen diameter brings about a bulk fluid flow in the direction of the uterus, which, in combination with other transport mechanisms, aids the transport of the ovum/embryo to the uterus. This transport takes only a matter of a few hours; the embryo/ovum is present in the uterus 80 h post-ovulation (Croxatto et al. 1978). The retention of the ovum/embryo at the junction may prevent embryo contact with fertile sperm in the isthmus (Hunter 1987) and allow progesterone dominance to ensure the receptivity of the uterus (Jansen 1984).

Failure of transport can lead to retention of the ovum within the ampulla, allowing blastocyst implantation and tubal ectopic pregnancy to develop. Accelerated ovum transport without retention at the ampullary-isthmic junction leads to premature presence of the embryo within the uterus and a decreased chance of successful implantation (Balmaceda et al. 1992). Failure of transport can be brought about by tubal damage (disease, surgery) or endocrine abnormalities (Jansen 1984).

## Fertilisation

Studies in many mammals now indicate that sperm binding to the zona is a receptor-mediated process (see Wassarman 1992 for an outline). The primary receptor on the zona, at least in pigs and mice (and probably many other mammals) is a glycoprotein – zona glycoprotein 3 (ZP3). There is much confusion about the complementary receptor on the sperm, with several research groups claiming their candidate is the primary molecule. Such candidates include galactosyltransferase (Miller et al. 1992), acrosin (Jones 1990), p95 (Saling 1991; Moore 1990), p56 (Wassarman 1992) and D mannosidase (Cornwall et al. 1991). It is likely, however, that sperm binding to the zona is a multifactorial process. In mice, for example, primary binding is to ZP3 and secondary binding is to ZP2 (Wassarman 1992).

Our knowledge of this process in humans is very sparse. The prime reason for this is the paucity of experimental material e.g. zona. In order to find out more about this process it is necessary to use recombinant molecular biology techniques to recreate artificial zona. Recently, using the cDNA for ZP3 (Professor Dean, NIDDK, USA) we have expressed biologically active recombinant human ZP3. This glycoprotein induces the acrosome reaction to a very high level (see Barratt et al. 1993). We are now in the process of purifying ZP3. This glycoprotein will serve as a useful experimental tool e.g.

determination of the receptor on the sperm, as a biological agonist of the acrosome reaction (maybe this will end the use of ionophores!), and possibly as a potential target for a contraceptive vaccine.

In conclusion, using recombinant molecular biology, combined with our knowledge of gamete physiology, we anticipate obtaining a clear understanding of the human fertilisation process in the near future.

# References


Ahlgren M (1975) Sperm transport to and survival in the human fallopian tube. Gynecologic Investigation 6:206–214

Anderson SH, Killian G (1992) Sperm enhance the secretion of a 35–40 kDa oviductal protein during co-culture. Journal of Androl Suppl 89:40

Balmaceda JP et al. (1992) Embryo implantation rates in oocyte donation: a prospective comparison of tubal versus uterine transfers. Fertil Steril 57:362–365

Barratt CLR, Cohen J (1986) Fate of superfluous sperm products after vasectomy and in the normal male tract of the mouse. J Reprod Fertil 78:1–10

Barratt CLR, Cohen J (1987) Quantitative of sperm disposal and phagocytic cells in the tract of short and long term vasectomized mice. J Reprod Fertil 81:377–384

Barratt CLR, Cohen J (1988) Quantitative effects of short- and long-term vasectomy on mouse spermatogenesis and sperm transport. Contraception 37:415–424

Barratt CLR, Cooke ID (1988) Sperm loss in the urine of sexually rested men. Int J Androl 11:201–207

Barratt CLR, Cooke ID (1991) Sperm transport in the human female reproductive tract – a dynamic interaction. Int J Androl 14:394–411

Barratt CLR et al. (1989) The hypo-osmotic swelling test and the sperm mucus penetration test in determining fertilization of the human oocyte. Hum Reprod 4:430–434

Barratt CLR, Bolton AE, Cooke ID (1990) Functional significance of white blood cells in the male and female reproductive tract. Hum Reprod 5:639–648

Barratt CLR, Kessopoulou E, Thompson LA, Tomlinson MT (1992) The functional significance of leucocytes in human reproduction. Reprod Med Rev 1:115–129

Barratt CLR, McCann CT, Hornby DP, Andrews PD (1993) Recombinant human ZP3 expressed in Chinese hamster ovary cells (CHO) is a potent inducer of the acrosome reaction. Hum Reprod (Suppl) 8:407

Birkhead TR, Moller AP (1992) Sperm competition in birds: evolutionary causes and consequences. Academic Press, London

Black DL (1974) Neural control of oviduct musculature. In: AD Johnson, CW Foley (eds) The oviduct and its functions. Academic Press, New York, pp 65–118

Blackmore PF, Beebe SJ, Danforth DR, Alexander N (1990) Progesterone and 17-hydroxyprogesterone. Novel stimulators of calcium influx in human sperm. J Biol Chem 256:1376–1380

Boice ML, Geisert RD, Blair RM, Verhage HG (1990) Identification and characterization of bovine oviductal glycoproteins synthesized at estrus. Biol Reprod 43:457–465

Bongso A, Ng S-C, Fong C-Y, Ratnam S (1991) Cocultures: a new lead in embryo quality improvement for assisted reproduction. Fertil Steril 56:179–190

Buhi WC, Van Wert JW, Alvarez IM, Dones-Smith MM, Bernhish MA (1989a) Synthesis and secretion of proteins by post-partum human oviductal tissue in culture. Fertil Steril 51:75–80

Buhi WC, Vallet JL, Bazer FW (1989b) Do novo synthesis and release of polypeptides from cyclic and early pregnancy porcine oviductal tissue in explant culture. J Exp Zool 252:79–88

Burkman LJ, Overstreet JW, Katz DF (1984) A possible role for potassium and pyruvate in the modulation of sperm motility in the rabbit oviductal isthmus. J Reprod Fertil 71:75–80

Calvo L et al. (1989) Follicular fluid-induced acrosome reaction distinguishes a subgroup of men with unexplained infertility not identified by semen analysis. Fertil Steril 52:1048–1054

Cohen J (1991) The case for and against sperm selection. In: Baccetti B (ed) Comparative sper-

matology 20 years after. IV International Congress on Spermatology. Sienna, Italy (Serono Symposia)
Coll JC, Miller RL (1991) The nature of sperm chemo-attractants in corals and starfish. In: Baccetti B (ed) Comparative spermatology 20 years after. IV International Congress on Spermatology. Sienna, Italy (Serono Symposia)
Cornwall GA, Tulsiani DRP, Orgebin-Crist M-C (1991) Inhibition of the mouse sperm surface – D-mannosidase inhibits sperm-egg binding in vitro. Biol Reprod 44:913–921
Critoph FN, Dennis KJ (1978) Ciliary activity in the human oviduct. Br J Obs Gynae 84:216–218
Croxatto HB, Ortiz ME, Diaz S, Hess R, Balmaceda J, Croxatto HD (1978) Studies on the duration of egg transport by the human oviduct. Am J Obstet Gynecol 132:629–634
Dean J (1991) The zona pellucida genes encode essential proteins for mammalian fertilisation and early embryogenesis. Proc Soc Exp Biol Med 162:141–146
De Jonge CJ, Rawlings RG, Zaneveld LJD (1988) Induction of the acrosome reaction by the human oocytes. Fertil Steril 50:949–953
De Jonge CJ, Han H-L, Mack SR, Zaneveld LJD (1991a) Effect of phorbol diesters, synthetic diacylglycerols and a protein kinase C inhibitor on the human sperm acrosome reaction. J Androl 12:62–70
De Jonge CJ, Han H-L, Lawrie H, Mack SR, Zaneveld LJD (1991b) Modulation of the human sperm acrosome reaction by effectors of the adenylate cyclase/cyclic AMP second-messenger pathway. J Exp Zoology 258:113–125
De Jonge CJ, Barratt CLR, Radwanska E, Cooke ID (1993) The acrosome reaction inducing effect of human follicular fluid and oviductal fluid. J Androl 14:359–365
Ehrenwald E, Parks JE, Foote RH (1988) Cholesterol efflux from bovine sperm, I. Induction of the acrosome reaction with lysophosphatidylcholine after reducing sperm cholesterol. Gam Res 20:145–157
Ehrenwald E, Foote RH, Parks JE (1990) Bovine oviductal fluid components and their potential role in sperm cholesterol efflux. Mol Reprod Dev 25:195–204
Ellington JE, Schlafer DH, Foote RH (1991) Ultrastructural features of bull sperm cocultured with bovine uterine tube epithelial cells. J Androl (Suppl, Abs 11)
Fazleabas AT, Verhage HG (1986) The detection of oviduct-specific proteins in the baboon (*Papio anubis*). Biol Reprod 35:455–462
Florman HM, Babcock F (1989) Progress toward understanding the molecular basis of capacitation. Elem Fertil 105–132
Fraser LR, Harrison RAP, Herod JE (1990) Characterisation of a decapacitation factor associated with epididymal mouse spermatozoa. J Reprod Fertil 89:135–148
Frederichs CM, Ashton SH (1982) Effect of vasoactive intestinal polypeptide (VIP) on the in vitro and in vivo motility of the rabbit reproductive tract. Fertil Steril 37:845–850
Guerin J-F, Ouhibi N, Regnier-Vigouroux G (1991) Movement characteristics and hyperactivation of human sperm on different epithelial cell monolayers. Int J Androl 14:412–422
Harper MJK (1982) Sperm and egg transport. In: Austin CR, Short RV (eds) Germ cells and fertilisation, 2nd edn. Cambridge University Press, London, pp 102–127
Harrison RAP, Roldan ERS (1990) Phosphoinositides and their products in the mammalian sperm acrosome reaction. J Rep Fertil (Suppl) 42:51–67
Hunter RHF (1987) Human fertilisation in vivo with special reference to progression, storage and release of competent spermatozoa. Hum Reprod 2:329–332
Hunter RHF, Wilmut I (1984) Sperm transport in the cow: peri-ovulatory redistribution of viable cells within the oviduct. Reprod Nut Develop 24:597–608
Jansen RPS (1980) Cyclic changes in the human fallopian tube isthmus and their functional importance. Am J Obstet Gynecol 136:292–308
Jansen RPS (1984) Endocrine response in the fallopian tube. Endocr Rev 5:525–549
Jones R (1990) Identification and functions of mammalian sperm-egg recognition molecules during fertilization. J Reprod Fertil (Suppl) 42:89–105
Katz DF, Morales P, Samueld SJ, Overstreet JW (1990) Mechanisms of filtration of morphologically abnormal human sperm by cervical mucus. Fertil Steril 54:513–516
Kenemans P, Hafez ESE (1984) Clinical application of scanning electron microscopy in human reproduction. Scanning Electron Microscopy 1984/I:215–242
Kim SJ, Cho DJ, Chang KW, Song CH (1991) Effects of utero-tubal flush on sperm motility and survival in vitro. 47th meeting of the American Fertility Society. Orlando, Florida, Abstract P-164
Kim-Bjorklund T, Landgren B-M, Hamberger L, Johannisson E (1991) Comparative mor-

phometric study of the endometrium, the fallopian tube and the corpus luteum during the post ovulatory phase in normally menstruating women. Fertil Steril 56:842–850
Kopf GS (1990) Zona pellucida mediated signal transduction in mammalian spermatozoa. J Reprod Fert (Suppl) 42:33–49
Lambert H, Overstreet JW, Morales P, Hanson JW, Yanagimachi R (1985) Sperm capacitation in the human female reproductive tract. Fertil Steril 43:325–327
Lenton EA et al. (1988) The endocrine environment of the human oocyte. J Reprod Fertil 82:827–841
Lippes J, Wagh PV (1989) Human oviductal fluid (hOF) proteins. IV. Evidence for hOF proteins binding to human sperm. Fertil Steril 51:89–94
Lundberg JM, Hedlund B, Bartfai T (1982) Vasoactive intestinal polypeptide enhances muscarinic ligand binding in cat submandibular salivary gland. Nature 295:147–149
Maathuis JB, Aitken RJ (1978) Cyclic variation in concentrations of protein and hexose in human uterine flushings collected by improved techniques. J Reprod Fertil 52:289–295
Mbizvo MT, Burkman LJ, Alexander NJ (1990) Human follicular fluid stimulates hyperactivated motility in human sperm. Fertil Steril 54:708–712
McNutt TL, Killian GJ (1991) Influences of bovine follicular and oviduct fluids on sperm capacitation in vitro. J Androl 12:244–252
Menghi G, Scocco P, Materazzi G (1990) Changes in vasoactive intestinal polypeptide (VIP) levels in the rabbit oviduct at different hormonal stages. An immunohistochemical study. J Anat 171:139–146
Miller DJ, Ax RL (1990) Carbohydrates and fertilization in animals. Review article. Mol Reprod Develop 26:184–198
Miller DJ, Mecek MB, Shur BD (1992) Complementarity between surface 1,4 galactosyl transferase and egg coat ZP3 mediates sperm egg binding. Nature 357:589–593
Miller EG, Kurzrok R (1932) Biochemical studies of human semen. III Factors affecting migration of sperm through the cervix. Am J Obstet Gynecol 24:19–26
Moore HDM (1990) Development of sperm-egg recognition processes in mammals. J Reprod Fertil 42:71–78
Mortimer D, Camenzind AR (1989) The role of follicular fluid in inducing the acrosome reaction of human spermatozoa incubated in vitro. Hum Reprod 4:169–174
Mukherjee AB, Lippes J (1972) Effect of human follicular and tubal fluids on human, mouse and rat spermatozoa in vitro. Can J Genet Cytol 14:167–174
Nagai T, Moor RM (1990) Effect of oviduct cells on the incidence of polyspermy in pig eggs fertilized in vitro. Mol Reprod Dev 26:377–382
Oliphant G, Reynolds AB, Thomas TS (1985) Sperm surface components involved in the control of the acrosome reaction. Am J Anat 174:269–283
Parrish JJ, Susko-Parrish JL, Handrow RR, Sims MM, First NL (1989) Capacitation of bovine spermatozoa by oviduct fluid. Biol Reprod 40:1020–1025
Pollard JW et al. (1991) Fertilizing capacity of bovine sperm may be maintained by binding to oviduct epithelium cells. Biol Reprod 44:102–107
Pollow K, Inthraphuvasak J, Manz B, Grill H-J, Pollow V (1981) A comparison of cytoplasmic and nuclear oestradiol and progesterone receptors in human fallopian tube and endometrial tissue. Fertil Steril 36:615–622
Ramsewak SS, Barratt CLR, Li T-C, Gooch H, Cooke ID (1990) Peritoneal sperm recovery can be consistently demonstrated in women with unexplained infertility. Fertil Steril 53:1106–1108
Ravnik SE, Zarutski PW, Muller (1992) Purification and characterisation of a human follicular fluid lipid transfer protein that stimulates human sperm capacitation. Biology of Reproduction 47:1126–1133
Robberecht P et al. (1981) Presence of vasoactive intestinal polypeptide receptors to adenylate cyclase in rat lung membranes. Biochem Biophys Acta 678:76–82
Roldan ERS, Harrison RAP (1989) Molecular mechanisms leading to exocytosis during the sperm acrosome reaction. In: Bavister BD, Cummins J, Roldan ERS (eds) Fertilisation in mammals. Serono Symposia, USA
Rubenstein BB, Strauss H, Lazarus ML, Hankin H (1951) Sperm survival in women. Motile sperm in the fundus and tubes of surgical cases. Fertil Steril 2:15–19
Saling PM (1989) Mammalian sperm interaction with extracellular matrices of the egg. In: SR Milligan (ed) Oxford Review of Reproductive Biology II. Oxford University Press, Oxford
Saling PM (1991) How the egg regulates sperm function during gamete interaction: facts and fantasies. Biol Reprod 44:246–251

Settlage DSF, Motoshina M, Tredway DR (1973) Sperm transport from the external cervical os to the fallopian tubes in women: a time and quantitative study. Fertil Steril 24:655–661

Siiteri JE, Dandekar P, Meizel S (1988) Human sperm acrosome reaction – initiating activity associated with the human cumulus oophorus and mural granulosa cells. J Exp Zool 246:71–80

Sjöberg J, Wahlstrom T, Grudzinskas JG, Sinosich MJ (1986) Demonstration of pregnancy-associated plasma protein-A (PAPP-A)-like material in the fallopian tube. Fertil Steril 45:517–521

Smith TT, Yanagimachi R (1987) Distribution and number of spermatozoa in the oviduct of the golden hamster after natural mating and artificial insemination. Biol Reprod 37:225–234

Smith TT, Yanagimachi R (1989) Capacitation status of hamster spermatozoa in the oviduct at various times after mating. J Reprod Fertil 86:225–261

Smith TT, Yanagimachi R (1990) The viability of hamster spermatozoa store in the isthmus of the oviduct: the importance of sperm-epithelium contact for sperm survival. Biol Reprod 42:450–457

Smith TT, Yanagimachi R (1991) Attachment and release of spermatozoa from the caudal isthmus of the hamster oviduct. J Reprod Fertil 91:567–573

Suarez SS, Redfern K, Raynor P, Martin F, Phillips DM (1991) Attachment of boar sperm to mucosal explants of oviduct in vitro: possible role in formation of sperm reservoir. Biol Reprod 44:998–1004

Sullivan R, Duchesne C, Fahmy N, Morin N, Dionne P (1990) Protein synthesis and acrosome reaction-inducing activity of human cumulus cells. Hum Reprod 5:830–834

Sutton R, Wallace ALC, Engel H, Nancarrow CD (1984) Binding of sheep oviductal fluid proteins to spermatozoa. In: Lindsay D, Pierce D (eds) Reproduction in sheep. Australian Academy of Sciences, Australia, pp 140–143

Tesarik J, Pilka L, Drahorad J, Cechova D, Veselsky V (1988) The role of cumulus cell-secreted proteins in the development of human sperm fertilizing ability: implication in IVF. Hum Reprod 3:129–132

Tesarik J, Otras CM, Testart J (1990) Effect of the human cumulus oophorus on movement characteristics of human capacitated spermatozoa. J Reprod Fertil 88:665–625

Thomas P (1991) The effect of human follicular fluid on polyphosphoinositide metabolism in human sperm. In: Bacetti B (ed) Comparative spermatology 20 years after. IV International Congress on Spermatology. Sienna, Italy (Serono Symposia), pp 1075–1078

Thomas P, Meizel S (1988) An influx of calcium is required for initiation of the human sperm acrosome reaction induced by follicular fluid. Gamete Res 20:397–411

Thomas P, Meizel S (1989) Phosphatidylinositol 4, 5-bisphosphate hydrolysis in human sperm stimulated with follicular fluid or progesterone is dependant upon $Ca^{2+}$ influx. Biochem J 264:539–546

Thompson LA, Tomlinson MJ, Barratt CLR, Bolton AE, Cooke ID (1991) Positive immunoselection – a method of isolating leucocytes from leucocytic reacted cervical mucus samples. Am J Reprod Immunol 26:58–61

Thompson LA, Barratt CLR, Bolton AE, Cooke ID (1992) The leucocytic reaction of the human uterine cervix. Am J Reprod Immunol 28:85–89

Thompson LA, Barratt CLR, Thornton S, Bolton AE, Cooke ID (1993) The effects of clomosphere citrate and cyclofenil on cervical mucus volume and receptivity over the periovulatory period. Fertil Steril 59:125–129

Tuffrey M, Alexander F, Inman C, Ward ME (1990) Correlation of infertility with tubal morphology and function in mice with salpingitis induced by a human genital-tract isolate of *Chlamydia trachomatis*. J Reprod Fert 88:295–305

Verdugo P, Blandau RJ, Tam PY, Halbert SS (1976) Stochastic elements in the development of deterministic models of ovum transport. In: Harper MJK et al. (eds) Ovum transport and fertility regulation. Scriptor, Copenhagen, pp 126–137

Verhage HG, Bareither ML, Jaffe RC, Akbar M (1979) Cyclic changes in ciliation, secretion and cell height of the oviductal epithelium in women. Am J Anat 156:505–522

Verhage HG, Akbar M, Jaffe RC (1980) Cyclic changes in cytosol progesterone receptor of human fallopian tube. J Clin Endocrinol Metab 51:776–780

Verhage HG, Fazleabas AT, Donnelly K (1988) The in vitro synthesis and release of proteins by the human oviduct. Endocrinology 122:1639–1645

Wassarman PM (1992) Mouse gamete adhesion molecules. Biol Reprod 46:186–191

Wetzels AM, Bastiaans BA, Goverde HJM, Jansen HJG, Rolland R (1991) Vero cells stimulate human sperm motility in vitro. Fertil Steril 56:535–539

Williams M et al. (1992) Recovery of artificially inseminated spermatozoa from the oviduct of a woman undergoing total abdominal hysterectomy. Hum Reprod 7:506–509
Williams M et al. (1993) Uterine flushing: a method to recover spermatozoa and leucocytes. Hum Reprod 8:925–928
Williams M et al. (1993) Sperm numbers and distribution within the human fallopian tube around ovulation. Hum Reprod 8: 2019–2026
Zaneveld LJD, De Jonge CJ, Anderson RA, Mack SR (1991) Opinion: human sperm capacitation and the acrosome reaction. Hum Reprod 6:1265–1274
Zhu JJ, Barratt CLR, Cooke ID (1992) Effect of human cervical mucus on human sperm motion and hyperactivation in vitro. Hum Reprod 7:1402–1406
Zhu JJ, Barratt CLR, Lippes J, Pacey AA, Cooke ID (1994a) Human oviductal fluid prolongs sperm survival. Fertil Steril (in press)
Zhu JJ, Barratt CLR, Lippes J, Pacey AA, Cooke ID (1994b) The sequential effects of human cervical mucus, oviductal fluid and follicular fluid on sperm function. Fertil Steril (in press)
Zinaman MJ, Kiel ME, Albertson BD, Overstreet JW, Simon JA (1988) Effects of periovulatory follicular, peritoneal and uterine fluid on sperm motion characteristics and acrosomal status. 44th Annual meeting of the American Fertility Society, Atlanta, Georgia, Abstract 060
Zinaman MJ et al. (1989) The physiology of sperm recovered from the human cervix: acrosomal status and response to inducers of the acrosome reaction. Biol Reprod 41:790–797

# Section II
# Tubal Endoscopy

# Chapter 7
# Transcervical Tubal Endoscopy: Falloposcopy

J.F. Kerin

## Introduction

Rapid advances in the miniaturisation of fibre-optic and cannulation devices for use in small hollow organ systems have occurred in the past decade. Many of these devices have been pioneered in the cardiovascular. neuro-vascular and urological fields. During the past 5 years great interest has developed for their use in the female reproductive system. Until recently, the only section of the human female genital tract that had not been explored by endoscopy was the oviduct (Kerin et al. 1990a) extending from the utero-tubal ostium to the ampullary-isthmic junction. This narrowest and most medial segment is vulnerable to pathogenic organisms responsible for pelvic inflammatory disease. Oviductal disease is a major cause of infertility and ectopic pregnancy.

Until now, investigators have had to rely on the more indirect methods of hysterosalpingography (HSG) and hydrochromotubation under laparoscopic observation for assessing oviductal patency, stricture formation, dilatation, or obstruction. More recently, fluoroscopic oviductal catheterisation (Platia and Krudy 1985; Thurmond et al. 1987), hysteroscopic directed cannulation (Sulak et al. 1987; Novy et al. 1988), transcervical balloon tuboplasty, (Confino et al. 1986), and laparoscopic directed salpingoscopic techniques (Mohri et al. 1970; Hershlag et al. 1991) have yielded improved diagnostic and therapeutic approaches to oviductal disease. Until recently, it was considered impossible to pass probes atraumatically along the intramural segment of the human oviduct because of its tortuosity and small calibre (Sweeney 1962). These difficulties have been largely overcome through the development of flexible, delicate, self-seeking, guide wire-coaxial catheter systems, and linear eversion catheter techniques that were initially used for coronary angioplasty

(Grundfest et al. 1985) and peripheral vascular embolectomy (Fogarty et al. 1984). These systems have been miniaturised and used for microendoscopic procedures within the oviduct (Kerin et al. 1990b).

A description of a falloposcope and the technique for its introduction into the oviduct for both diagnostic and therapeutic purposes has been published in detail elsewhere (Kerin et al. 1990b). A falloposcopic classification and scoring system has been developed to characterise and quantify the site, type, and severity of oviductal disease and to correlate scores with endotuboplasty results and pregnancy outcome.

In this chapter falloposcopy is defined as microendoscopy of the oviductal lumen from the utero-tubal ostium to the fimbria by a non-incisional transvaginal approach (Kerin et al. 1990a,b,c).

## Initial Difficulties and Misconceptions about Retrograde Oviductal Cannulation Attempts

In 1954, Lisa studied the gross anatomy of the intramural oviduct from 300 hysterectomy specimens and noted that it averaged 2 cm in length and from 0.2 to 0.4 mm in diameter (Lisa et al. 1954). In 1963 Sweeney studied the course of the intramural oviduct in 100 post-hysterectomy uterine specimens (Sweeney 1963). He noted that the intramural oviductal length ranged from 1 to 3.5 cm and that its course through the uterine wall was variable in both calibre and direction. In 69% of cases the intramural oviduct was tortuous, in 23% straight, and in 8% curved. He concluded that it was not possible to pass probes from the uterine cavity along the oviduct lumen and that such attempts would cause damage. This sentiment was conveyed in a critical editorial by De Cherney as late as 1987 where he cautioned over-enthusiastic investigators about the complex, narrow and tortuous nature of the intramural oviduct and of the harm which might be done by retrograde cannulation procedures (De Cherney 1987).

## Cannulation Differences of the Ex Vivo and In Vivo Oviduct

Unlike a blood vessel the tubal lumen is collapsed and is therefore a potential space. Its primary longitudinal and secondary epithelial folds provide great surface area to the collapsed lumen which contains mucus-like secretions throughout most of the menstrual cycle. The tubes are paired organs which vary from 7 to 14 cm in length and are enclosed in the mesosalpingeal borders of the broad ligament. The smooth muscle wall becomes thinner in relation to both distance from the uterine horn and increases in diameter. Furthermore, the tubes may take a gentle C-shaped curve to a more tortuous path as they proceed from the uterine horn, antero-lateral and then posterior to the ovary. These variations in tubal configuration may be further distorted by uterine fibroids, peritubal adhesions, infection, ectopic pregnancy, intra-tubal disease, space-occupying tumours in the broad ligament, ovary and adjacent pelvic structures. An appreciation of the course and structure of the tubal lumen is essential for successful cannulation procedures. Our in vivo observations (Kerin et al. 1990a) show that the dimensions and path of the intramural lumen bears little resemblance to observations made ex vivo as described by Lisa et al. (1954), Hernstein and Neustadt (1924) and Sweeney (1963). It was pointed out by Corfman (1990) that observations of in vivo studies such as those of Rubin (1928), Rubin and Bendeick (1928) and Kerin et al. (1990a) indicate that the intramural tube is straight or gently curved. The tortuous course in non-living ex-vivo specimens may be an artefact secondary to myometrial contraction. In addition, the intramural lumen diameter of 0.2–0.4 mm, described by Lisa et al. (1954) in ex-vivo specimens is probably also the result of collapse and contraction. Falloposcopic studies indicate that the intramural tube is 0.8–1.2 mm in diameter and can accommodate a cannula of 1–1.2 mm without damage (Kerin et al. 1990a). The healthy elastic tubal wall can tolerate minor distension provided the cannula is flexible, smooth-walled and advanced with a coaxial (Kerin et al. 1990a) or a linear eversion system (Bauer et al. 1993). It is also important to understand that, like the ovary and endometrium, the tube is a dynamic organ which undergoes important cyclical changes. The first technique for placing the falloposcope into the oviduct used a coaxial delivery system (Kerin et al. 1990a,b,c). The alternative non-hysteroscopic technique involves the use of a miniaturised linear eversion catheter delivery system. Each system will be described in detail and the advantages outlined. However, it must be emphasised that the technique of falloposcopy is in its formative stages and these techniques are constantly being refined and upgraded. Conclusions drawn at this stage should be regarded as preliminary.

## Description of a Falloposcope and Miniature Hysteroscope System

Initial evaluations were made on women undergoing hysterectomy and salpingectomy. Prototype falloposcopes were developed by Olympus (Olympus PF-5X; Olympus Corp., Lake Success, NY), Intramed (Intramed Laboratories, San Diego, CA) Medical Dynamics (Medical Dynamics, Inc., Englewood, CO), Advanced Interventional Systems (AIS, Costa Mesa, CA) and Imagyn (Imagyn Medical Inc., San Clement, CA). The result is falloposcopes measuring 1.0–1.5 m in length, 0.5 mm in outside diameter (OD), and containing an atraumatic leading end and sufficient flexibility to minimise the risk of perforation or damage to the endosalpinx and myosalpinx.

Falloposcopes with optical qualities adequate for defining endotubal surface anatomy contain 1800–2200 imaging fibres with a centre-to-centre cross-sectional fibre distance of 4 μm, a distal lens of 0.3-mm diameter, a depth of field from 1 mm to infinity, two-point discrimination down to 10 μm, 8–50 times magnification, an angle of end-on field of view in air of 72°, in water of 54°, and 8–12 illuminating fibre bundles each of 100–130 μm in diameter. A 300-W xenon light source provides illumination through a flexible cable attached to the falloposcope at its proximal end. A 35–70 mm video coupler relays images from the falloposcope to a light-sensitive colour microchip video camera. During the procedure, the real time images are displayed on a high-resolution colour monitor and are recorded permanently on tape using a high quality video cassette recorder. Still photographs are obtained from the video tape using a computer graphics freeze-frame technique and a colour video printer for production of hard-copy prints.

Small flexible hysteroscopes have also been evaluated for guiding the falloposcope into the ostium of the fallopian tube under direct vision (Olympus Corp., Lake Success, NY; Intramed Laboratories, San Diego, CA). The 25–30-cm working fibre of these hysteroscopes is semirigid and the distal 5 cm is flexible and steerable about a tight radius of 1.5 cm with a range of movement from neutral (straight) to 90°. The focus and steering is operated from the proximal end, next to the eye-piece. The working channel of these hysteroscopes ranges from 1.6 to 2.2 mm in diameter, and is adequate to accommodate the cannulation and falloposcope instrumentation. The small OD (3.3–4.5 mm) of these hysteroscopes and their flexibility permit them to be introduced through the cervical canal without prior dilatation. The firm seal created between the hysteroscope and endocervical canal is important for producing adequate distension of the uterine cavity and tubal ostium: this allow good visualisation; facilitates easy passage of the falloposcope and associated guide wires and cannulas into the tube under direct vision; and is economical of the fluid distension medium, because of minimal leak back into the vagina.

## Technique Using a Coaxial Falloposcopy Delivery System

A hysteroscope is gently introduced through the cervical canal and into the uterine cavity. The uterine cavity is irrigated with lactate–Ringers solution at a rate of 10 to 40 ml per minute, using a gravity fed system. Under video monitoring, the distal tip of the hysteroscope is directed to within 3 mm of one of the tubal ostia so that a direct long axis view of the intramural tubal lumen is obtained. The coaxial technique involves the passage into the fallopian tube of small, “floppy”, steerable, tapered guide wires made of stainless steel or coated with Teflon (Target Therapeutics, Fremont, CA; Cook OB/GYN, Spencer, IN; Glidewire, Medi-Tech Incorporated, Watertown, MA) under video hysteroscopic monitoring. These flexible guide wires range from 0.3 to 0.8 mm OD and can negotiate the natural curvatures of the tubal lumen atraumatically. When the wire has passed to a point of resistance, or 15 cm beyond the utero-tubal ostium, flexible Teflon cannulas of 1.2–1.3 mm OD with polished leading ends (Target Therapeutics: Cook OB/GYN) are introduced over the guide wire and through the tubal ostium under direct hysteroscopic vision to a point of resistance or for approximately 15 cm to the region of the fimbrial segment of the fallopian tube and into the peritoneal cavity. The guide wire is then withdrawn while the Teflon cannula is kept in place and the falloposcope introduced into it. The cannula provides protection to the entire length of the falloposcope and serves as a conduit for fluid irrigation of the distal end of the falloposcope to permit a lens–fluid–epithelial interface for image facilitation. Direct apposition of the endothelium into the lens otherwise results in a “white out reflection”. By lifting the endothelium off the lens, the falloposcope can be advanced under direct vision, thus preventing epithelial damage. Furthermore, if the falloposcope meets with an obstruction or tubal distortion, this limited hydrotubation facilitates negotiation along a narrow intramural, isthmic, or ampullary segment, through strictures or intraluminal adhesions. Once the leading end of the falloposcope has passed beyond the fimbria the light is insufficient to illuminate the peritoneal cavity. However, when the falloposcope lens is within millimetres of bowel, mesentery or ovary, transient views of these organs are obtained (Kerin et al. 1990a). With laparoscopic peritoneal illumination, enough light is present for a tunnel view of intraperitoneal structures through the falloposcope. Better inspection of the tubal epithelium is obtained by withdrawal of the falloposcope towards the uterine ostium with continuous irrigation. This eliminates the "antegrade white out reflection" associated with advancing the falloposcope lens against a curvature of the tube. Dual video monitoring can be used for continuous hysteroscopic and falloposcopic recordings. A fluid-tight irrigation system has been achieved by using a Tuohy-Borst type Y adapter (Cook OB/GYN; Rotating Hemostatic Valve; Advanced Cardiovascular Systems; Temecula, CA) connection for introduction of the falloposcope and fluid via the proximal end of the hysteroscope operating channel. The instrumentation, normal falloposcopic appearance and dimensions of the intramural, isthmic, ampullary and fimbrial tube have been described in detail (Kerin et al. 1990a).

## Development of a Linear Eversion Catheter (LEC) Falloposcopy Delivery System

The coaxial technique is the commonest method of introducing the falloposcope. A promising refinement in catheter technology has been the development of a miniaturised linear eversion catheter system for the introduction of the falloposcope with or without a hysteroscope (Imagyn Medical Inc.). Unlike most coaxial catheter systems where guide wires and catheters need to be pushed along the tubal lumen, the linear eversion catheter system is rolled out along the tube using hydraulic pressure. A diagram of the LEC system is shown in Fig. 7.1.

This linear eversion catheter system has been approved by the Food and Drug Administration (FDA) for the construction of an instrument that is flexible enough to conform to the fallopian tube but retains sufficient radial integrity to maintain an open lumen under pressure. This open lumen facilitates irrigation and the free movement of the falloposcope or an embryo/gamete cannula. Once the tubal ostium is visualised and coaxial alignment is achieved, the LEC is advanced into the tube. The actual LEC consists of a long miniature tubular balloon with an outside diameter of 1.2 mm which is inverted on itself. Hydraulic pressure at the proximal end causes the inner lumen to roll outside itself to become its under lumen, thereby advancing along the tube. Furthermore, any cannula system in the inverted balloon lumen, such as a falloposcope, irrigation system or gamete transfer catheter, will be carried forward (Fig. 7.2).

The advantages of the LEC system are fourfold. Firstly, the LEC and its balloon automatically keep the falloposcope coaxially aligned along the tubal lumen. Secondly, the unrolling action eliminates any sheer forces between the balloon element and the inner walls of the tube. Thirdly, the forward progression concentrates energy at the tip, making it self guiding.

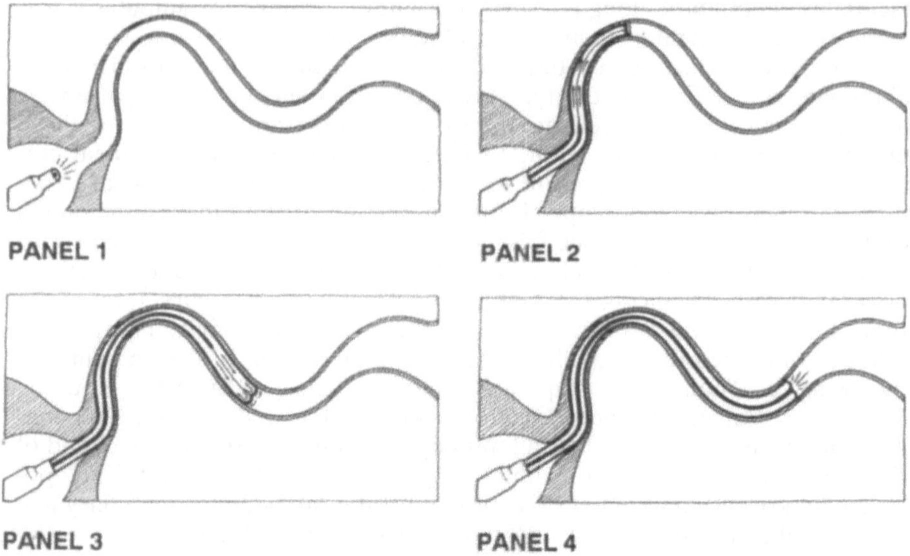


**Fig. 7.1.** Panel 1 displays the relationship of a precurved transuterine guiding catheter and falloposcope for end-on viewing of the tubal ostium. Panel 2 displays a close-up diagramatic view of the construction of the LEC delivery system showing the relationship between the outer transuterine catheter tip, balloon, scope and irrigation channel. Panel 3 displays the LEC delivery system carrying the falloposcope advanced through the intramural and isthmic segments of the tubal lumen. Panel 4 displays the LEC delivery system everted into the ampulla with the falloposcope flush with the balloon's end for optimal viewing. (With kind permission from Imagyn Medical, Inc.)

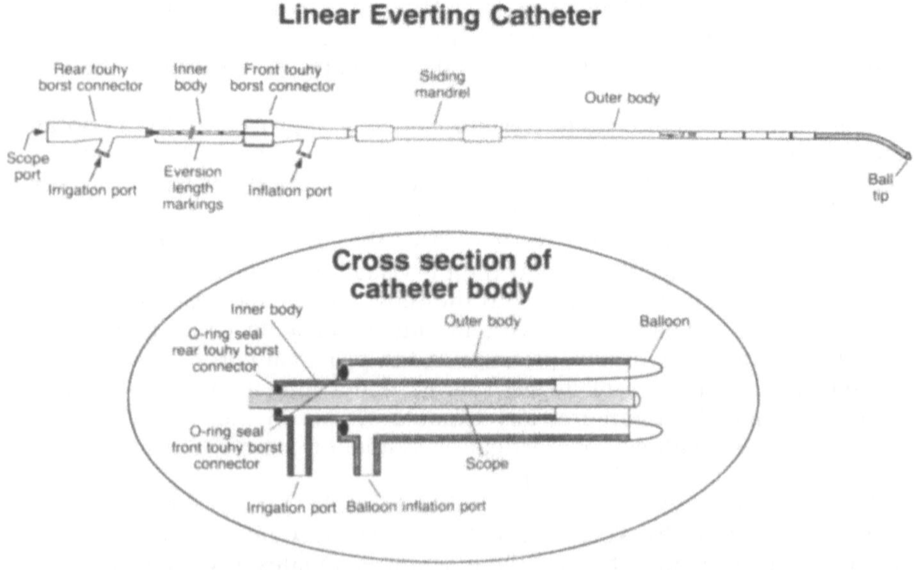


**Fig. 7.2.** A line diagram showing the relationships of the component parts which make up the falloposcope-LEC delivery system. (With kind permission from Imagyn Medical, Inc.)

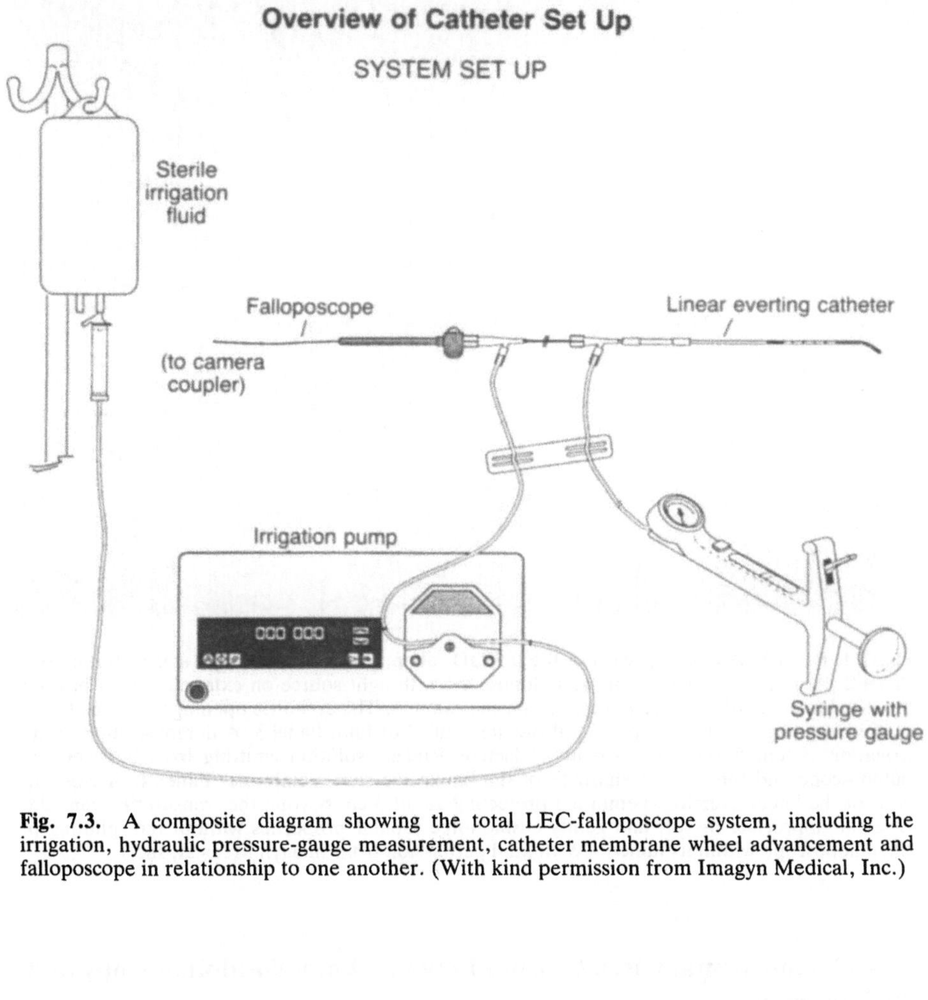


**Fig. 7.3.** A composite diagram showing the total LEC-falloposcope system, including the irrigation, hydraulic pressure-gauge measurement, catheter membrane wheel advancement and falloposcope in relationship to one another. (With kind permission from Imagyn Medical, Inc.)

Fourthly, the LEC system can be delivered via the transvaginal route to the utero-tubal ostium using either a hysteroscopic or non-hysteroscopic approach (Bauer et al. 1993). A composite diagram of the total LEC system including the irrigation, hydraulic pressure, catheter membrane advancement and falloposcope system is outlined in Fig. 7.3.

Using LEC systems, falloposcopy or tubal cannulation procedures can be performed in the non-anaesthetised woman with little or no sedation. This may make the system an attractive method for placing gametes or embryos at a known position in the oviductal lumen under direct visual monitoring. As the balloon catheter rolls out, it advances the falloposcope automatically, but the scope can still be adjusted independently for optimal visualisation and prevention of epithelial trauma, particularly during antegrade manoeuvres. This system is illustrated in Fig. 7.4.

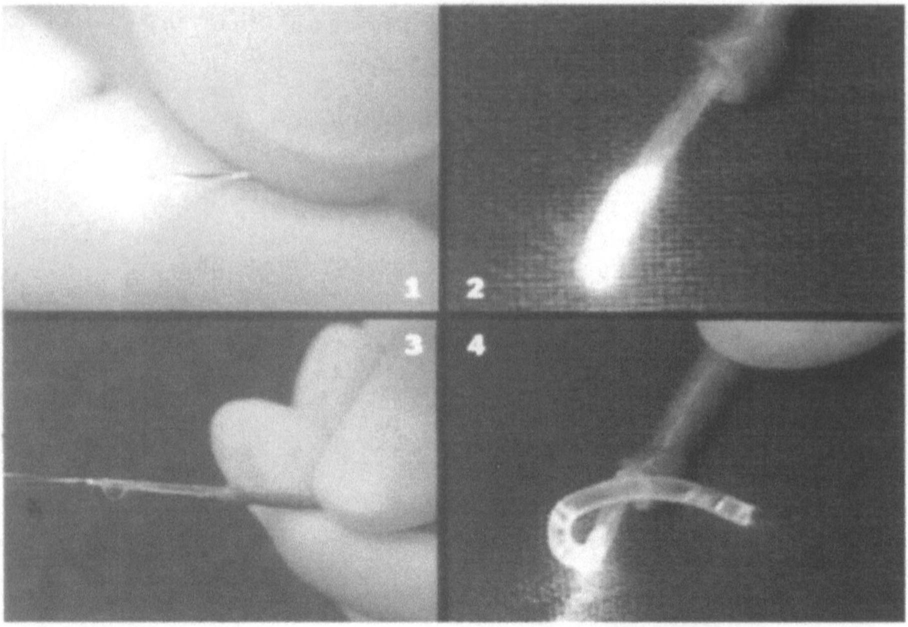


**Fig. 7.4.** Panel 1. A close-up view of the 0.5 OD falloposcope with the light source turned on. Panel 2. A more distant view of the falloposcope with light source on extending 2 cm beyond the distal opening of the precurved transuterine cannula. The eccentric opening tip of the transuterine cannula fits into the opening of the utero-tubal ostium. Panel 3. A demonstration of the irrigation system displaying a stream of lactate–Ringers solution emitting from between the falloposcope and the inner membrane of the linear eversion membrane. Panel 4. A close-up view of the linear eversion membrane projecting about 3 cm beyond the transuterine cannula. One can appreciate its soft and gently cushion-like tubular properties without the splinting of the falloposcope within its lumen. (With kind permission from Imagyn Medical, Inc.)

## The Complementary Relationship Between Ampullosalpingoscopy and Falloposcopy

Until the development of the falloposcope the only endoscopic means for assessing the oviductal lumen was ampullosalpingoscopy (Cornier et al. 1984; Brosens et al. 1987). These laparoscopic-assisted techniques could only explore the oviductal mucosa down to the ampullary-isthmic junction, but were valuable for studying epithelial integrity in relation to the likelihood of conception (Shapiro et al. 1988; Marana et al. 1990). To correlate salpingoscopic changes with pathological processes, abnormal areas of oviductal epthelium detected salpingoscopically underwent biopsy. With severe disease there was good concordance between salpingoscopic and histological diagnoses. However, moderate pathological changes documented by light microscopy and transmission electron microscopy were frequently not diagnosed salpingoscopically, even with magnification (Hershlag et al. 1991). Thus, current investigative tools may underdiagnose subtle tubal damage.

Salpingoscopy provides an additional tool for examination of the oviductal epithelium distal to the ampullary isthmic junction (Hamou and Taylor 1982; Mencaglia et al. 1986). The falloposcope can complement the salpingoscope by assessing the medial third of the oviduct using a transvaginal approach (Kerin et al. 1992).

## A Classification and Scoring System for the Falloposcopic Assessment of Oviduct Disease

A classification and scoring system for determining the localisation, nature, and extent of tubal lumen disease has been developed for objective evaluation of endoscopic findings (Kerin et al. 1992). Degree of patency, degree of adhesion formation, amount of dilatation, and abnormal intraluminal contents are scored as: 1 (normal), 2 (mild to moderate disease), and 3 (severe disease) for each of the four segments of both tubes. A score of 20 or less for each tube is normal; a score between 20 and 30, is mild to moderate endotubal disease; and a score of 30, is severe endotubal disease (Fig. 7.5).

The classification and scoring table is divided into sections: history, scoring chart, a diagram of the tubes, uterus, and ovaries, a treatment summary, pregnancy prognosis, and a recommendation for future treatment. If the tube is normal (score 20 or less), no further procedures are performed. Falloposcopic characterisation of each segment of the fallopian tube has been described by Kerin et al. (1990a). If the tubes contained debris or adhesions, simple cannulation and "aqua-dissection" are performed (Kerin et al. 1990b,c,d, 1992). If the tube contains polypoid structures, thicker adhesions, or short segmental strictures, the passage of flexible wires with outside diameters up to 0.8 mm (Cook OB/GYN, Spencer, IN; Target Therapeutics, Fremont, CA) can be used (Kerin et al. 1990b,c). With thick intraluminal adhesions and rigid structures or obstructions, small "Stealth" balloon catheters (Target Therapeutics, Fremont, CA) with OD of 1.0 mm in the deflated and up to 2.5 mm in the inflated state are used (Kerin et al. 1990b,c). Such procedures are performed under laparoscopic monitoring to monitor excessive tubal distortion, partial or complete perforation, or bleeding. These techniques have been described in detail (Kerin et al. 1990b). Before any procedure, the nature, site, and extent of the lesion was classified and scored. The lesion was falloposcopically reassessed immediately after the tuboplasty procedure to note improvement or tubal damage. Improvement was considered to be significant if a stenosis, adhesion, or obstruction has been visibly enlarged or broken down with an improved flow of fluid through the tube. Examples of falloposcopic images ranging from normal to abnormal observations are illustrated in Fig. 7.6 and Fig. 7.7. The patients in this study were given an intravenous antibiotic at the commencement of the falloposcopy procedure and reviewed at 1 week and then at 3-month intervals for at least 12 months. Patients with tubal patency were followed for 1 year to see if pregnancy occurred.

Patient's Name ______ Date ______ Phone # ______
Age ______ G ______ P ______ SAB ______ TAB ______ Ectopic ______ Infertile: Yes ______ No ______
Other Significant History (i.e. surgery, infection, etc.) ______

HSG ______ Sonography ______ Photography ______ Laparoscopy ______ Laparotomy ______
Cycle Details ______
Semen Details ______

| SITE of DISEASE | RIGHT TUBE INTRAMURAL | RIGHT TUBE ISTHMIC | RIGHT TUBE AMPULLARY | RIGHT TUBE FIMBRIAL | LEFT TUBE INTRAMURAL | LEFT TUBE ISTHMIC | LEFT TUBE AMPULLARY | LEFT TUBE FIMBRIAL |
|---|---|---|---|---|---|---|---|---|
| PATENCY<br>Patency — 1<br>Stenosis — 2<br>Fibrotic obstruction — 3 | | | | | | | | |
| EPITHELIUM<br>Normal — 1<br>Pale, Atropic — 2<br>Flat, featureless — 3 | | | | | | | | |
| VASCULARITY<br>Normal — 1<br>Intermediate — 2<br>Poor pallor — 3 | | | | | | | | |
| ADHESIONS<br>None — 1<br>Thin, weblike — 2<br>Thick — 3 | | | | | | | | |
| DILITATION<br>None — 1<br>Minimal — 2<br>Hydrosalpinx — 3 | | | | | | | | |
| * OTHER — 2–3 | | | | | | | | |
| CUMULATIVE SCORE | | | | | | | | |
| TOTAL SCORE | RIGHT TUBE = | | | (NORMAL = 20) | LEFT TUBE = | | | (NORMAL = 20) |

**A cumulative score for each tube of: 20 = Normal Tubal Lumen; > 20 but < 30 = Moderate Endotubal Disease; > 30 = Severe Endotubal Disease.**
*** Mucus Plugs or Tubal Debris, Endotubal Polyps, Endometriosis, Salpingitis Isthmica Nodosa, Inflammatory, Infectious, Neoplastic conditions and absent tubal segments are each assigned a score of 2 to 3 depending on the significance of the lesion.**

**Treatment (Specify R & L Tube Surgical Procedures).**

Nothing ______
Aquadissection ______
Guidewire Cannulation ______
Wire Dilitation ______
Direct Balloon Tuboplasty ______
Other ______

Prognosis for Conception:

______ Excellent (> 75%)
______ Good (50-75%)
______ Fair (25-50%)
______ Poor (< 25%)

Recommended Followup Treatment: ______

Surgeons ______

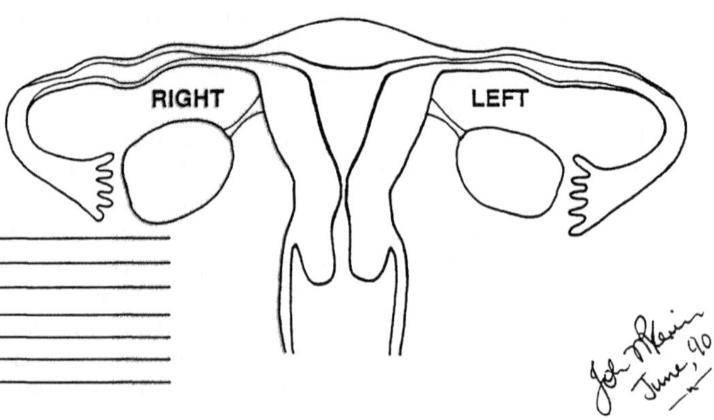


**Fig. 7.5.** Falloposcopic classification, scoring and localisation of tubal lumen disease.

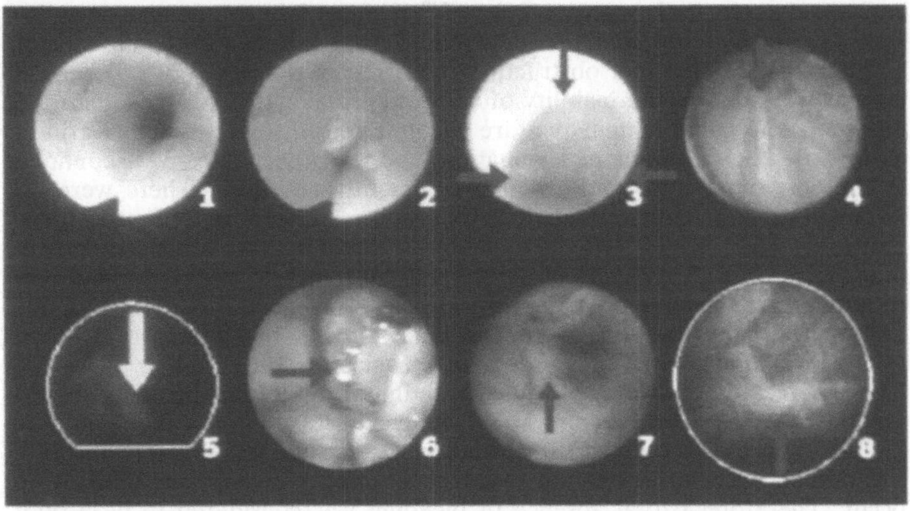


**Fig. 7.6. Examples of falloposcopic images, ranging from normal to abnormal observations.**

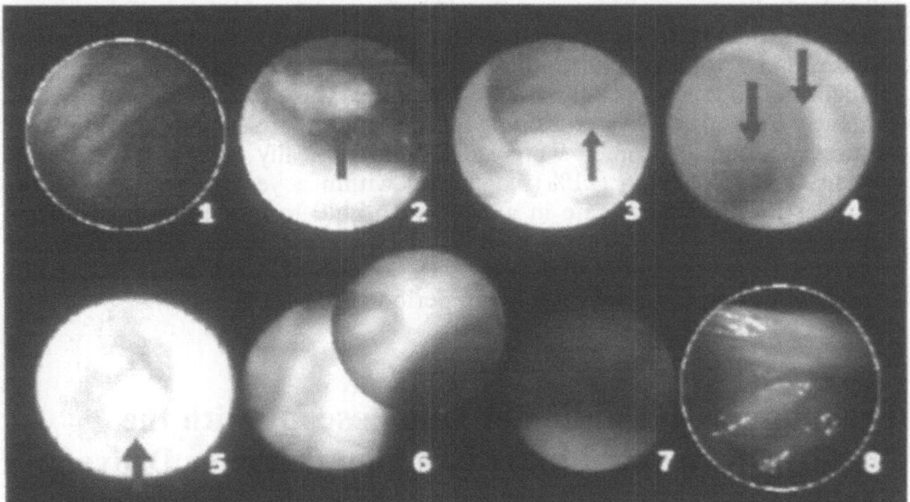


**Fig. 7.7.** Further examples of falloposcopic images, ranging from normal to abnormal observations.

## Clinical Results after Falloposcopy Procedures with the Coaxial Delivery System

Seventy-five women with a provisional diagnosis of oviductal endotubal disease had a total of 121 tubes available for falloposcopy. Falloposcopy was performed successfully within 112 tubes. Technical failures, defined as an inability to advance the falloposcope within the tubal lumen in the absence of a detectable intraluminal obstruction, occurred in 9 cases (7%). Technical failures were due to the inability of current coaxial systems to negotiate the more tortuous tubal lumens that are encountered in some women (Kerin et al. 1990a). The falloposcopic evaluations and pregnancy rates were confined to the 66 women who underwent a successful procedure. There were no intraoperative or post-operative complications related to the procedure. However, when flexible wire cannulation or direct balloon tuboplasty procedures were used, 5 instances of partial and 1 instance of complete tubal perforation were observed laparoscopically just proximal to an obstructive lesion. These perforations were the same size as the dilator or balloon (<1 mm in diameter). They were not associated with bleeding as viewed laparoscopically, but were associated with minor, endotubal bleeding viewed falloposcopically. This bleeding spontaneously resolved in less than 1 min on 2 of the 5 occasions on which it was noted. If the tube was severely fibrosed, the normal vascular epithelium was absent, and bleeding was unlikely to occur. Therefore a total absence of bleeding was considered to be a poor prognostic sign. In all instances, there was major intratubal disease, and the perforation did not further compromise the tubal status. There was no pyrexia, inflammation, or infection associated with either diagnostic or operative falloposcopy.

Sixty of the 112 tubes examined falloposcopically (54%) had evidence of disease, and a total of 119 lesions were detected (average 2 per tube). The incidence of falloposcopically disease-free tubes was 46%, despite suggestive evidence from prior hysterosalpingograms and hydrochromotubation procedures. Of the 28 women who had falloposcopically normal tubes (falloposcopy score = 20) 6 (21%) conceived within a year of the procedure. However the pregnancy rate in women with mild to moderate disease (falloposcopy score 21 to 30) was poor (2/22 (9%) in 1 year). None of the 16 women with severe endotubal disease (falloposcopy score greater than 30) conceived during the 1-year follow-up period (Kerin et al. 1992).

## Preliminary Evaluation of Falloposcopy with the Non-hysteroscopic Linear Eversion Catheter Delivery System

The LEC delivery system is designed to deliver a 0.5-mm OD falloposcope into the lumen of the fallopian tube using the transvaginal approach, without the need for hysteroscopic guidance. As a result the LEC falloposcope delivery system offers a number of advantages. The everting balloon principle minimises shear forces between the balloon element and the inner walls of the tube. The catheter automatically advances the falloposcope while allowing independent movement of the endoscope to optimise visualisation and prevent trauma. The forward progression concentrates energy at the tip, making the system self guiding. It can also mobilise debris, lyse fine intra-

**Table 7.1.** Multicentre (4) evaluation of the non-hysteroscopic linear eversion catheter delivery system

| | Successful eversion (per tube) | Successful imaging (per tube) | Lesions found (per tube) | Management modification (per patient) |
|---|---|---|---|---|
| Procedures | 34/36 | 32/36 | 20/32 | 13/19 |
| Percentage | 94 | 89 | 63 | 68 |

luminal adhesions and dilate selected stenoses. Finally, the linear everting catheter system can be delivered via the transvaginal route without hysteroscopy or cervical dilation, minimising the need for anaesthesia or sedation (Bauer et al. 1993). The system is potentially attractive for placing gametes or embryos at a known postion in the tubal lumen.

The balloon of the linear everting catheter system is quite distinct from the conventional "balloon catheters" used for tuboplasty procedures. The linear everting catheter balloon unrolls or everts to achieve linear progression, whereas conventional balloons expand radially, without advancing in a forward direction.

Studies to assess the clinical efficacy and safety of the LEC system are in progress in North America and the United Kingdom, Europe and Australia. Preliminary studies indicate that the LEC delivery system can reliably access the tubal lumen. Furthermore, useful diagnostic information can be obtained (Sweeney 1963). Studies in 5 institutions of 45 falloposcopy procedures using the LEC system, showed successful delivery and imaging in 89% of procedures. Lesions were found in 63% and were significant enough to alter management in 68% (Table 7.1).

Falloposcopy assisted in selection of candidates for IVF versus endotuboplasty or conventional microsurgery. Furthermore, falloposcopy can assess tubal mucosa and patency prior to transvaginal intra-tubal transfer procedures (Kerin et al. 1992).

# Conclusion

The falloposcope has now been refined to the point at which it has become a safe, reliable and useful diagnostic tool. It provides direct transvaginal, non-incisional visual access to the entire length of the tubal lumen. An objective classification and scoring system has been devised for diagnostic and prognostic purposes.

Neither the coaxial nor the LEC techniques have been associated with complications in a total of 148 procedures. However, the safety margins are narrow, and great care and acquired skill are required to negotiate the tortuous and delicate tubal lumen. Tactile sensitivity in passing guide wires etc is essential. If the slightest resistance is detected, force should never be applied. Technical failures become more rare with experience. For example, only two technical failures occurred in the last 70 procedures of our series.

The LEC system is particularly effective for negotiating the more tortuous tubes.

Falloposcopy demonstrated normal tubes in 46% of cases previously diagnosed as abnormal by HSG. Factors contributing to these differences include spasm of the ostium during cannulation. Intraluminal debris, particularly in the isthmus, has been identified with the falloposcope. Such debris may be a readily treatable cause of proximal tubal obstruction using salpingography, fallopian tube cannulation, or transcervical balloon tuboplasty. The falloposcope may displace debris into the folds of the ampullary tube or into the peritoneal cavity. Thus falloposcopy may be therapeutic. This may explain why the diagnosis of proximal tubal obstruction is more common after HSG and chromohydrotubation in which the head of hydrostatic pressure diminishes by the time it reaches the tube and is therefore less likely to dislodge intraluminal debris. Pregnancy rates may increase after HSG, perhaps because of mobilisation of loose debris. Falloposcopy can identify non-obstructive tubal disease that may be missed by HSG and laparoscopy.

In summary, improvements in falloposcopes and delivery systems will almost certainly establish their diagnostic and therapeutic roles; first, as a valuable, accurate and objective diagnostic procedure; second, as a therapeutic modality for treating minimal intraluminal disease such as debris or adhesions; third, they provide an accurate means for placing gametes and embryos into the oviduct.

# References


Bauer O et al. (1993) Transcervical access and intra-luminal imaging of the fallopian access technology. Human Reprod (in press)

Brosens IA, Boeckx W, Delattin PH, Puttemans P, Vasquez G (1987) Salpingoscopy: a new pre-operative diagnostic tool in tubal infertility? Br J Obstet Gynaecol 94:722–728

Confino E, Friberg J, Gleicher N (1986) Transcervical balloon tuboplasty. Fertil Steril 46:963–966

Corfman RS (1990) Falloposcopy: frontiers realised . . . a fantastic voyage revisited. Fertil Steril 54:574–576

Cornier E, Feintuch MJ, Boucara L (1984) La fibrotuboscopie ampullaire. J Gynecol Obstet Biol Reprod (Paris) 13:49–56

De Cherney AH (1987) Anything you can do I can do better . . . or differently! Fertil Steril 48:374–376

Fogarty TJ, Kinney TB, Finn JC (1984) Current status of dilatation catheters and guiding systems. Am J Cardiol 53:97–100

Grundfest WS et al. (1985) Pulsed ultraviolet lasers and the potential for safe laser angioplasty. Ann Surg 150:220–226

Hamou JE, Taylor PJ (1982) Panoramic contact and microcolpohysteroscopy in gynecologic practice. Curr Prob Obstet Gynecol 4:2

Hernstein A, Neustadt B (1924) Intramural portion of the fallopian tube. Ztschr Geburtsh u Gynak 88:431–437

Herschlag A et al. (1991) Salpingoscopy: light microscopic and electron microscopic correlations. Obstet Gynecol 77:399

Kerin J et al. (1990a) Falloposcopy: a microendoscopic technique for visual exploration of the human fallopian tube from the uterotubal ostium to the fimbria using a transvaginal approach. Fertil Steril 54:390–400

Kerin J, Daykhovsky L, Grundfest W, Surrey E (1990b) Falloposcopy: a microendoscopic transvaginal technique for diagnosing and treating endotubal disease incorporating guide-wire cannulation and direct balloon tuboplasty. J Reprod Med 35:606–612

Kerin J, Surrey E, Daykhovsky L, Grundfest W (1990c) Development and application of a falloposcope for transvaginal endoscopy of the fallopian tube. J Laparoendoscopic Surg 1:47–56

Kerin J, Surrey ES, Williams DB, Daykhovsky L, Grundfest WS (1990d) Falloposcopic observations of endotubal mucous plugs as a cause of reversible obstruction and their histological characterisation. J Laparoendoscopic Surg 1:97–101

Kerin JF et al. (1992) Falloposcopic classification and treatment of fallopian tube lumen disease. Fertil Steril (in press)

Lisa JR, Gioia JD, Rubin IC (1954) Observation of the interstitial portion of the fallopian tube. Obstet Gynecol 99:159–160

Marana R et al. (1990) Perilaparoscopic salpingoscopy in the the evaluation of tubal factor in fertile women. Int J Fertil 35:211

Mencaglia L, Hamou J, Perino A, Cosmi E (1986) Transcervical and retrograde salopingoscopy: evaluation of the fallopian tube in infertile patients. In: Siegler AM (ed) The fallopian tube: basic studies and clinical contributions. Futura 35:377

Mohri T, Mohri L, Yamadori F (1970) Tubaloscope: flexible glass fibre endoscope for intratubal observations. Endoscopy 2:226–229

Novy MJ, Thurmond AS, Patton P, Uchida BT, Rösch J (1988) Diagnosis of cornual obstruction by transcervical fallopian tube cannulation. Fertil Steril 50:434–440

Platia MP, Krudy AG (1985) Transvaginal fluoroscopic recanalisation of a proximally occluded oviduct. Fertil Steril 44:704–706

Rubin IC (1928) Observations on the intramural and isthmic portions of the fallopian tubes with special reference to so called "isthmospasm". Surg Gynecol Obstet 46:87–94

Rubin IC, Bendeick AJ (1928) Metrosalpingography with the aid of iodized oil. Am J Roentgenol 19:348–352

Shapiro BS, Diamond MP, De Cherney AH (1988) Salpingoscopy: an adjunctive technique for evaluation of the fallopian tube. Fertil Steril 49:1076

Sulak PJ, Letterie GS, Hayslip CC, Coddington CC, Klein TA (1987) Hysteroscopic cannulation and lavage in the treatment of proximal tubal occlusion. Fertil Steril 48:493–495

Sweeney WJ III (1963) The interstitial portion of the uterine tube – its gross anatomy, course and length. Ostet Gynecol 19:3–5

Thurmond AS, Novy MJ, Uchida BT, Rösch J (1987) Fallopian tube obstruction: selective salpingography and recanalisation. Radiology 63:511–514

Chapter 8

# Transabdominal Tubal Endoscopy

O. Djahanbakhch and S.D. Maguiness

## Introduction

The function of the fallopian tube is most commonly assessed by determining patency, observing a normal external appearance at endoscopy and internal appearance at hysterosalpingography. The recent development of small-diameter flexible and rigid endoscopes has facilitated the direct visualisation of the mucosal folds within the lumen. However, the information obtained by tubal endoscopy is still of only limited value in clinical practice. One reason is that most studies are based only on abnormal cases. Another is that there is limited information about variation in the appearance of the tubal lumen during the normal menstrual cycle, or in relation to age or drug therapy.

This chapter critically reviews all the transabdominal approaches which have been used to determine normal tubal function.

## Fallopian Tube Assessment at Laparotomy

### External Appearance

The gross external appearance of the fallopian tube at laparotomy has been classified by Boer-Meisel et al. (1986) and Winston and Margara (1991). Istre and Guttorm (1988) have suggested that women with fimbriae of normal appearance before tubal surgery had a higher subsequent pregnancy rate compared to those with atrophic fimbriae. They reported a good correlation between the macroscopic and microscopic appearance of the fimbriae. Boer-

Meisel et al. (1986) examined the microscopic appearance of the fimbrial mucosa during laparotomy, with an operating microscope. They reported a 77% pregnancy rate in women who have had tubal surgery for hydrosalpinges, provided the microscopic appearance of the tubal mucosa was normal.

Microbiopsies can be taken from the mucosa of the fimbriae (Brosens and Vasquez 1976; Vasquez et al. 1980, 1983) and from other sites in the tubal lumen during tubal surgery (Marchini et al. 1988). The percentage of ciliated cells correlates with the ability of the tube to transport the ovum, and is therefore a useful prognostic index for fertility (Brosens and Vasquez 1976). However, these findings were not confirmed by either Marchini et al. (1988) or Winston and Margara (1991).

Cytological examination of fluid from hydrosalpinges obtained at laparotomy has been reported to correlate with the morphological state of the tubal lumen when opened (Albrich et al. 1984), and may therefore be of value in assessing whether reparative surgery should be attempted.

### Internal Appearance

Henry-Suchet et al. (1981, 1983) reported the first endoscopic visualisation of the tubal lumen at laparotomy. The procedure was performed using a 4-mm hysteroscope in a 5-mm sheath, and was named "Tuboscopy". The endoscope was inserted into the fimbrial end of the tube, or via a surgical incision if the tube was blocked. Ringers–lactate solution flowed between the scope and sheath into the tube, distending the lumen thus facilitating visualisation as far as the isthmic-ampullary junction.

Henry-Suchet et al. (1985) then reported the prognostic value of this procedure for tuboplasties. Lesions observed during tuboscopy differed from those suspected at hysterosalpingogram in 50% of cases. The only women who became pregnant within 2 years had at least one tube which appeared normal at tuboscopy. Mencaglia et al. (1986), using a microhysteroscope and carbon-dioxide distension of the tube, reported a series of 27 women having tubal surgery for subfertility. Of the 12 women who had normal tubal folds and vascularity, 6 became pregnant after surgery.

## Laparoscopy

### External Appearance

As at laparotomy, the gross external appearance of the fallopian tube and fimbrial mucosa can be easily assessed. Fallopian tubes which are patent but with swellings and kinks were termed "tortuous" by Leeton and Selwood (1978). This finding was bilateral in 95% of women and was associated with a pregnancy rate of 90.5 % within 2 years of hydrotubation. Diagnostic laparoscopy has been extensively studied and has become an integral part of the investigation of subfertile women. It appears to increase the accuracy of over-all pelvic assessment (Israel and March 1976). Significant findings at laparoscopy have been reported in 38.7% of women attending a subfertility

**Table 8.1.** Cumulative results of the studies reviewed by Maguiness et al. (1992) comparing hysterosalpingography (HSG) and laparoscopy to determine the appearance of the fallopian tube. There is agreement between the appearance of the fallopian tubes at HSG and laparoscopy in 73.9% (59.5 + 14.4) and disagreement in 26.1% (17.4 + 8.7). Total number of cases = 2122. Information in this table comes from Duignan et al. 1972, Swolin and Rosenkrantz 1972, Maathuis et al. 1972, Kierse and Vandervellen 1973, Hutchins 1977, Taylor 1977, Gomel 1977, El-Minawi et al. 1978, Servy and Tzingounis 1978, Philipsen and Hansen 1981 and Blackwell 1989

| | | Appearance at hysterosalpingogram | |
|---|---|---|---|
| | | Normal | Abnormal |
| Laparoscopic appearance | Normal | 1263 (59.5%) | 184 (8.7%) |
| | Abnormal | 370 (17.4%) | 305 (14.4%) |

clinic (Templeton and Kerr 1977), and in 60% of women with unexplained subfertility (Peterson and Behrman 1970). Paavonen et al. (1984) reported peritubal adhesions in 31% of cases of primary subfertility at laparoscopy. Pregnancy has been reported to occur in 38% of women if laparoscopy was normal, compared to 31% if pathology involved one tube and 17% if both were involved (Stadler et al. 1984).

Studies comparing findings at laparoscopy with hysterosalpingography have been reviewed by Maguiness et al. (1992). The superior performance of laparoscopy in identifying tubal adhesions (Swolin and Rosencrantz 1972) is clearly demonstrated by the number of cases of tubal pathology diagnosed in women with an apparently normal hysterosalpingogram (17.4%), as Table 8.1 illustrates.

Overall, there is total agreement between the two methods in 73.9% of cases and disagreement in 26.1%. If it is assumed that laparoscopy gives a correct diagnosis with respect to tubal appearance, these figures suggest that the sensitivity of hysterosalpingography is only 45% ( 305/675 ) with respect to the diagnosis of tubal pathology. However hysterosalpingography is almost as specific in detecting the nature of an abnormality as laparoscopy (1263/1447 = 87.3%).

The disadvantages of laparoscopy are that it is usually performed under a general anaesthetic and does not give information about the uterine cavity. However, because of the additional information obtained about the pelvic organs (Table 8.2), this procedure has superseded the hysterosalpingogram

**Table 8.2.** Information relevant to fertility, other than tubal appearance or patency, obtained at hysterosalpingogram or endoscopy (n = 1865) reviewed by Maguiness et al. (1992). Information in this table comes from Duignan et al. 1972, Kierse and Vandervellen 1973, Moghissi and Sim 1975, Gabos 1976, Hutchins 1977, Taylor 1977, El-Minawi et al. 1978, Servy and Tzingounis 1978, Philipsen and Hansen 1981 and Rice et al. 1986

| | | Endoscopy | Hysterosalpingogram |
|---|---|---|---|
| Uterus | Congenital | 3 | 18 |
| | Synechiae/polyps | 0 | 43 |
| | Myoma | 49 | 8 |
| | "Filling defects" | 0 | 2 |
| Pelvis | Endometriosis | 223 | 0 |
| | Ovaries: Polycystic/cysts | 72 | 0 |

as the primary method of assessing the fallopian tubes (Templeton and Kerr 1977).

## Internal Appearance

The tubal mucosa was first visualised at laparoscopy by Cornier (1985, 1986) using a 3.5-mm flexible bronchoscope which was passed, via the operating channel of the laparoscope, into the tubal lumen as far as the isthmic-ampullary junction. A saline infusion, in which the mucosal folds float, was used to enhance visualisation. Flexible endoscopes are expensive and give an image of poorer quality than a rigid endoscope; however they are still used. Brosens et al. (1987) used a dedicated 3-mm-diameter rigid tuboscope to assess the ampulla and infundibulum of the tube. This rigid tuboscope was modified to allow easier insertion and visualisation of the tubal mucosa (Brosens et al. 1987). The 2.8-mm-diameter endoscope extends 40 mm beyond the end of a 3-mm-diameter sheath, down which an obturator can be passed to aid insertion into the tubal lumen. Atraumatic grasping forceps are applied just behind the fimbria to hold the fallopian tube against the sheath. The obturator is withdrawn, the endoscope inserted and an infusion of distending fluid commenced. This opens up the potential space of the tubal lumen and facilitates visualisation of the mucosal folds which float in the distending medium. In a normal fallopian tube, major and minor mucosal folds can be seen around the whole circumference of the lumen. The complexity of the mucosal folding and the vessels within the folds increases towards the fimbriated end (Fig. 8.1).

To visualise the fimbria they can be floated in lactate–Ringers solution in the Pouch of Douglas and examined with the laparoscope (Nezhat et al. 1990). Classifications of lesions identified at salpingoscopy have been proposed by Brosens and Puttemans (1989) and Kerin (see Hershlag et al. 1991).

Brosens et al. (1987) reported that tuboscopy in 7 of 27 subfertile women with a normal hysterosalpingogram, revealed abnormalities of the folds such as adhesions (Fig. 8.2), agglutination, inflammatory vascular patterns, and, in one woman, a circular stricture. A control group of women with normal fertility had no abnormalities of the tubal mucosa.

Subsequently Brosens and Puttemans (1989) have reported a group of subfertile women with a normal laparoscopy and hysterosalpingogram; 5% of these women had lesions of the tubal mucosa at salpingoscopy. Shapiro et al. (1988) have also described the use of both flexible and rigid tuboscopes, noting that 23.5% of women had salpingoscopic findings different from those which would have been expected from the pelvic appearance at laparoscopy.

In women with endometriosis, Nezhat et al. (1990) found no association with intratubal disease, while Shapiro et al. (1988) reported abnormal intratubal findings in 4 of 6 women studied. These studies used women undergoing sterilisation or diagnostic laparoscopy as control groups.

Puttemans et al. (1987) reported that 53% of women with a hydrosalpinx had mucosal lesions at salpingoscopy which were not diagnosed by hysterosalpingogram or laparoscopy. De Bruyne et al. (1989) performed a prospective trial to evaluate the value of salpingoscopy in the assessment of

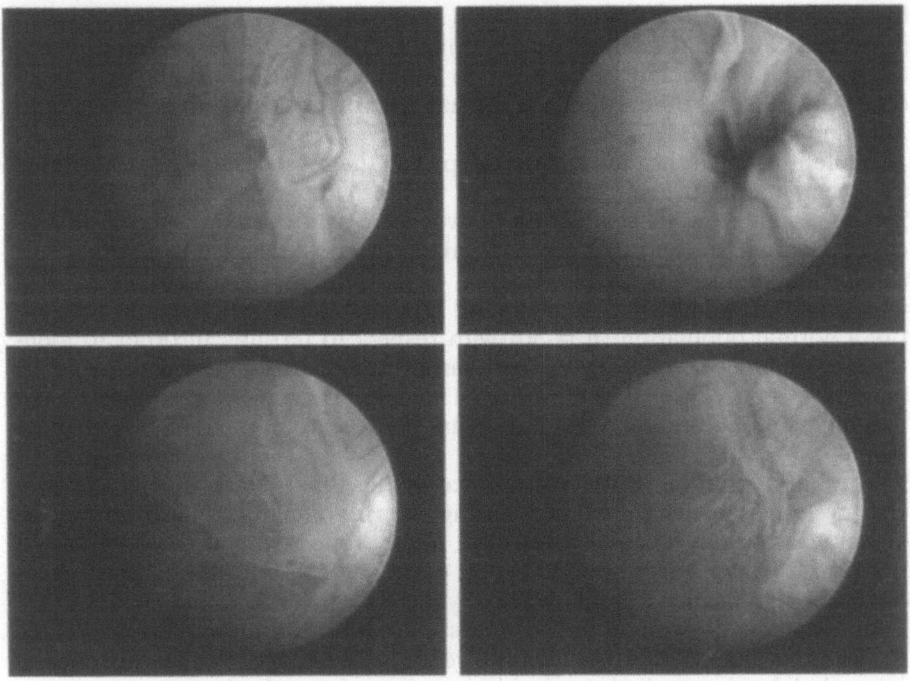

**Fig. 8.1.** Normal appearance of the tubal lumen at endoscopy.

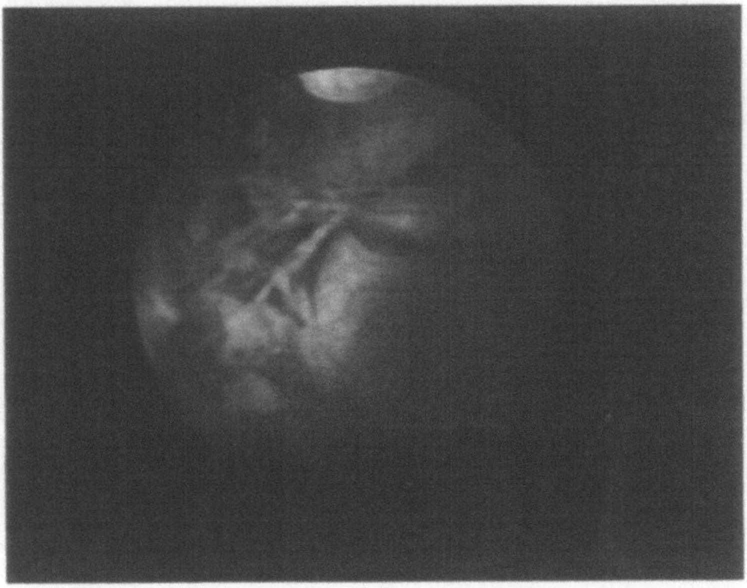

**Fig. 8.2.** Adhesions between mucosal folds seen at salpingoscopy.

hydrosalpinges. They reported a 59%, pregnancy rate when there were no intratubal adhesions. Salpingoscopy may also prove to be of value in the assessment of fallopian tubes prior to tubal surgery, as lesions have been observed at sites other than the actual site of occlusion (Maguiness and Djahanbakhch 1991).

While it is apparent that salpingoscopy can diagnose lesions not detectable by other methods even the use of contact magnification (×80, Storz 26001A) yields a poor correlation between the salpingoscopic and histological appearance of the tubal mucosa unless the tubal damage is severe (Hershlag et al. 1991).

A prospective study (Maguiness and Djahanbakhch 1992) set out to identify a normal population (n = 30) with respect to fertility, in order to identify any changes in relation to the ovarian cycle, or lesions which could be perceived as a cause of subfertility. The salpingoscopic appearance of the ampulla and fimbria of both fallopian tubes was normal in 20 of these women.

The only variation in the appearance of the tubal lumen during the ovarian cycle was seen in 3 women during the pre-ovulatory phase: the blood vessel walls in the mucosal folds were highly reflective and the edge of the mucosal folds appeared rounded (Fig. 8.3). The cause of these appearances and their significance is unknown.

In 10 of the 30 women in the series there were intratubal lesions (Table 8.3). In this small series there was no relationship between the occurrence of intratubal lesions and obstetric history, time from the last pregnancy, or contraceptive usage.

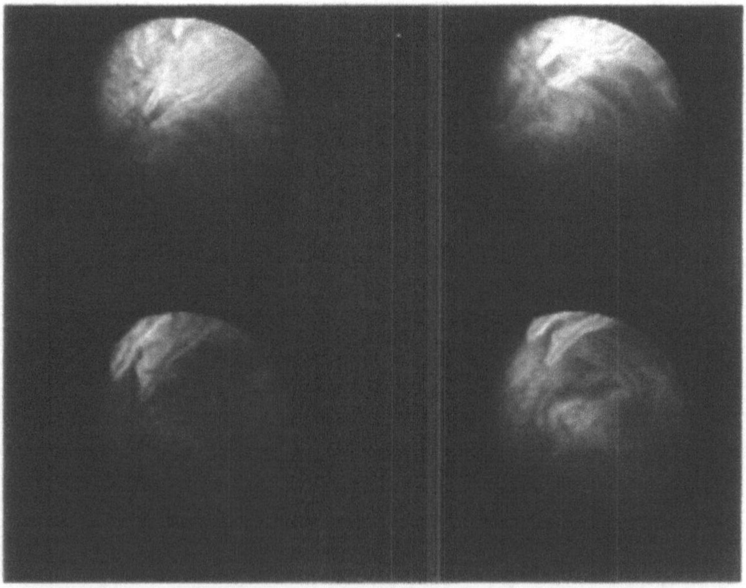

**Fig.8.3.** Highly reflective blood vessel walls in the mucosa of the fallopian tube seen at salpingoscopy in women in the periovulatory phase of the ovarian cycle.

**Table 8.3.** Salpingoscopic findings in a population of fertile women undergoing sterilisation (n = 30; Maguiness and Djahanbakhch 1992)

| | | Unilateral | Bilateral | Total |
|---|---|---|---|---|
| Normal | | | 20 | 20 |
| Abnormal[a] | Intratubal adhesions | 2 | | 2 |
| | Fronds | | 4 | 4 |
| | Abnormal mucosal folds | 1 | 2 | 3 |
| | Blood vessels with an irregular lumen | | 2 | 2 |
| | Black "spots" | 1 | 2 | 3 |

[a] Some women had more than one abnormal finding.

The presence of intraluminal adhesions in apparently normal women is consistent with similar findings in 2 women amongst a control group of 10 in a study of transcervical falloposcopy by Kerin et al. (1990). The black "spots" seen in the mucosal folds may be similar to the haemorrhagic spots described by Brosens and Puttemans (1989); however there was no associated increase in fold vascularity to suggest an inflammatory process. The irregularity of blood-vessel diameter has not been previously reported and is of unknown significance.

In earlier studies some of these observations may be considered to be pathological thus causing subfertility. Women undergoing sterilisation, diagnostic laparoscopy or laparotomy have been used as control groups for studies of salpingoscopy (Henry-Suchet et al. 1985; Brosens et al. 1987; Nezhat et al. 1990). The reproductive and gynaecological characteristics of these control groups are never described in detail. In contrast to this, we observed "abnormalities" in the fallopian tube of women with a normal reproductive career, no history of abdominal pathology and a normal pelvic appearance at laparoscopy; earlier studies may have described these as pathological.

## Conclusion

Direct visualisation of the fallopian tube is of benefit in the selection of patients for gamete intrafallopian transfer, in-vitro fertilisation or tubal surgery. While it would appear that salpingoscopy is of value in the assessment of a hydrosalpinx prior to reconstructive surgery, its use in the assessment of subfertility will only become apparent following further and larger prospective studies of normal women.

## References

Albrich W, Peters-Welte A, Gotz A, Hammer C (1984) The cytology of tubal secretion of salpingostomies by microsurgical technique. In: Harrison RF, Bonnar J, Thompson W (eds)

Diagnosis and management of tubouterine factors in infertility. MTP Press Ltd, Lancaster, pp 189–191
Blackwell RE (1989) The infertility workup and diagnosis. J Reprod Med 34:81–85
Boer-Meisel ME, te Velde ER, Habbema JDF, Kardaun JWPF (1986) Predicting the pregnancy outcome in patients treated for hydrosalpinges: a prospective study. Fertil Steril 45:23–29
Brosens IA, Puttemans PJ (1989) Double-optic laparoscopy. In: Sutton C (ed) Ballière's Clinical Obstetrics and Gynaecology, Vol 3, pp 595–608
Brosens IA, Vasquez G (1976) Fimbrial microbiopsy. J Reprod Med 16:171–178
Brosens I, Boeckx W, Delattin Ph, Puttemans P, Vasquez G (1987) Salpingoscopy: a new preoperative diagnostic tool in tubal infertility? Br J Obstet Gynaecol 94:768–773
Cornier E (1985) L'ampulloscopie per-coelioscopique. J Gynecol Obstet Biol Reprod 14:459–466
Cornier E (1986) Ampullosalpingoscopy. In: Siegler AM (ed) The fallopian tube: basic studies and clinical contributions. Futura Publishing Company, Mount Kisco, New York, pp 383–389
De Bruyne F, Puttemans P, Boeckx W, Brosens IA (1989) The clinical value of salpingoscopy in tubal infertility. Fertil Steril 51:339–340
Duignan NM, Jordan JA, Coughlan BM (1972) One thousand consecutive cases of diagnostic laparoscopy. J Obstet Gynaecol Brit Commonw 79:1016–1024
El-Minawi MF, Abdel-Hadi M, Ibrahim AA, Wahby O (1978) Comparative evaluation of laparoscopy and hysterosalpingography in infertile patients. Obstet Gynecol 51:29–32
Gabos P (1976) A comparison of hysterosalpingography and endoscopy in evaluation of tubal function in infertile women. Fertil Steril 27:238–242
Gomel V (1977) Laparoscopy prior to reconstructive surgery for infertility. J Reprod Med 18:251–253
Henry-Suchet J, Tesquier L, Loffredo V (1981) Endoscopies tubaires: premiers resultats. Gynecologie 23:293–295
Henry-Suchet J, Tesquier L, Pez JP, Loffredo V (1983) Endoscopie tubaire ou tuboscopie: une exploration complementaire utile dans la chirurgie reparatrice des trompes. XXXIe assises franc. de gynec, Masson (ed), Paris
Henry-Suchet J, Loffredo V, Tesquier L, Pez JP (1985) Endoscopy of the tube (= Tuboscopy): its prognostic value for tuboplasties. Acta Europ Fertil 16:139–145
Hershlag A et al. (1991) Salpingoscopy: light microscopic and electron microscopic correlations. Obstet Gynecol 77:399–405
Hutchins CJ (1977) Laparoscopy and hysterosalpingogram in the assessment of tubal patency. Obstet Gynecol 49:325–327
Israel R, March CM (1976) Diagnostic laparoscopy: a prognostic aid in the surgical management of infertility. Am J Obstet Gynec 125:969–975
Istre O, Guttorm E (1988) The appearance of the fimbria as prognostic sign for successful fertility surgery. Nordisk Forening For Obstetrikk og Gynekologi XXVI Kongress, Abstr.
Kerin J et al. (1990) Falloposcopy: microendoscopy of the human fallopian tube from the utero-tubal junction to the fimbria using a trans cervico-uterine approach. Fertil Steril 54:390–400
Kierse MJNC, Vandervellen R (1973) A comparison of hysterosalpingography and laparoscopy in the investigation of infertility. Obstet Gynecol 41:685–688
Leeton J, Selwood T (1978) The tortuous tube: pregnancy rate following laparoscopy and hydrotubation. Aust NZ J Obstet Gynaecol 18:259–262
Maathuis JB, Horbach JGM, van Hall EV (1972) A comparison of the results of hysterosalpingography and laparoscopy in the diagnosis of fallopian tube dysfunction. Fertil Steril 23:428–431
Maguiness SD, Djahanbakhch O (1991) Tuboscopy in a previously sterilised patient. Br J Obstet Gynaecol 98:326–327
Maguiness SD, Djahanbakhch O (1992) Salpingoscopic findings in women undergoing sterilization. Hum Reprod 7:269–273
Maguiness SD, Djahanbakhch O, Grudzinskas JG (1992) Assessment of the fallopian tube. Obstet Gynec Survey 41:587–603
Marchini M et al. (1988) Ultrastructure of endosalpingeal biopsies in infertile patients: correlation with reproductive success. Int J Gynecol Obstet 27:239–245
Mencaglia L, Hamou J, Perino A, Cosmi E (1986) Transcervical and retrograde salpingoscopy: evaluation of the fallopian tube in infertile patients. In: Siegler AM (ed) The fallopian

tube: basic studies and clinical contributions. Futura Publishing Company, Mount Kisco, New York, pp 377–381
Moghissi KS, Sim GS (1975) Correlation between hysterosalpingography and pelvic endoscopy for the evaluation of tubal factor. Fertil Steril 26:1178–1181
Nezhat F, Winer WK, Nezhat C (1990) Fimbrioscopy and salpingoscopy in patients with minimal to moderate pelvic endometriosis. Obstet Gynecol 75:15–17
Paavonen J, Berg M, Lahtinen M, Heinonen PK (1984) Diagnostic laparoscopy in primary infertility. In: Harrison RF, Bonnar J, Thompson W (eds) Diagnosis and management of tubo-uterine factors in infertility. MTP Press Ltd, Lancaster, pp 167–170
Peterson EP, Behrman SJ (1970) Laparoscopy of the infertile patient. Obstet Gynecol 36:363–367
Philipsen T, Hansen BB (1981) Comparative study of hysterosalpingography and laparoscopy in infertile patients. Acta Obstet Gynecol Scand 60:149–151
Puttemans P, Brosens I, Delattin P, Vasquez G, Boeckx W (1987) Salpingoscopy versus hysterosalpingography in hydrosalpinges. Hum Reprod 2:535–540
Rice JP, London SN, Olive DL (1986) Reevaluation of hysterosalpingography in infertility investigation. Obstet Gynecol 67:718–721
Servy EJ, Tzingounis VA (1978) Tubal patency: hysterosalpingography compared with laparoscopy. South Med J 71:1511–1512
Shapiro BS, Diamond MP, DeCherney AH (1988) Salpingoscopy: an adjunctive technique for evaluation of the fallopian tube. Fertil Steril 49:1076–1079
Stadler C, Maassen G, Poehner G, Stauber M (1984) Laparoscopic findings in 801 sterile patients. In: Harrison RF, Bonnar J, Thompson W (eds) Diagnosis and management of tubo-uterine factors in infertility. MTP Press Ltd, Lancaster, pp 139–142
Swolin K, Rosencrantz M (1972) Laparoscopy vs. hysterosalpingography in sterility investigations. A comparative study. Fertil Steril 23:270–273
Taylor PJ (1977) Correlations in infertility: symptomatology, hysterosalpingography, laparoscopy, and hysteroscopy. J Reprod Med 18:339–342
Templeton AA, Kerr MG (1977) An assessment of laparoscopy as the primary investigation in the subfertile female. Br J Obstet Gynaecol 84:760–762
Vasquez G, Boeckx W, Winston RML, Brosens IA (1980) Human tubal mucosa and reconstructive microsurgery. In: Crosignani PG, Rubin BL (eds) Microsurgery in female infertility. Academic Press, London, pp 41–56
Vasquez G, Winston RML, Boeckx W, Gordts S, Brosens IA (1983) The epithelium of human hydrosalpinges: a light optical and scanning electron microscopic study. Br J Obstet Gynaecol 90:764–770
Winston RML, Margara RA (1991) Microsurgical salpingostomy is not an obsolete procedure. Br J Obstet Gynaecol 98:637–642

Chapter 9

# Transabdominal Salpingoscopy: The Significance of Mucosal Lesions in Infertility

I.A. Brosens

## Introduction

Tubal endoscopy or salpingoscopy is an additional tool to hysterosalpingography and laparoscopy in the exploration of tubal infertility. The rationale is based on the endoscopic identification of tubal lesions and the clinical significance of these lesions.

In this chapter the lesions of the tubal mucosa and their relationship with infertility will be discussed.

## Lesions of the Tubal Mucosa in Infertility

The use of microbiopsies for the clinical investigation of the fallopian tube in infertility was described by Brosens and Vasquez in 1976. A correlation was found between the ciliation of the tubal mucosa and the outcome of pregnancy. Subsequently research was focused on the microanatomical lesions of the fallopian tube in different conditions of tubal infertility (Vasquez et al. 1980, 1983).

### Tubal Phimosis

Deciliation of the fimbriae can be found in patients with tubal phimosis and appears to be associated with a poor fertility prognosis (Table 9.1).

**Table 9.1.** Deciliation and fertility outcome in fimbrial phimosis (27 patients)

| Ciliation | n | Intra-uterine pregnancy | Tubal pregnancy | Non-pregnant |
|---|---|---|---|---|
| Normal | 10 | 7 (70%) | 0 (0%) | 3 (30%) |
| Deciliation | 17 | 2 (12%) | 2 (12%) | 13 (76%) |

**Table 9.2.** Tubal lesions and fertility outcome in hydrosalpinx (50 patients)

| Mucosal lesions | Intra-uterine pregnancy (15) | Tubal pregnancy (3) | Non-pregnancy (32) |
|---|---|---|---|
| Flattening | 13 | 3 | 32 |
| Deciliation | 11 | 3 | 28 |
| Inflammation | 4 | 3 | 19 |
| Adhesions | 4 | 3 | 22 |

## Hydrosalpinx

In hydrosalpinx flattening of the mucosal folds, adhesions between folds, fibrosis of folds, desquamation and deciliation of the epithelium and abnormal ciliary structures can be found. In addition, inflammatory changes and fibrosis are seen.

In a prospective study ampullary micro-biopsies were obtained in 50 patients at the time of salpingostomy and were correlated with the pregnancy outcome after salpingostomy (Table 9.2). No pregnancies occurred in thick-walled hydrosalpinges. In thin-walled hydrosalpinges pregnancy was more likely to occur in the absence of adhesions and inflammatory changes. Deciliation is seen in most hydrosalpinges, but there is no correlation between the degree of deciliation and the outcome of pregnancy. On the contrary, the deciliation is usually more pronounced in the thin-walled than in the thick-walled hydrosalpinx. Experimental work by Karbowski et al. (1988) has shown that ciliation can regenerate in mechanical hydrosalpinges after salpingostomy.

## Proximal Tubal Block

The underlying pathology in proximal tubal block includes fibrosis, chronic infection, salpingitis isthmica nodosa, cornual polyps and endometriosis and can be associated with more extensive, even ampullary lesions. Several investigators have found a poor fertility prognosis in lesions characterised by inflammatory changes and in salpingitis isthmica nodosa. These findings were also confirmed in our follow-up (Table 9.3).

## Pelvic Endometriosis

In severe endometriosis the fimbriae and ampulla can be involved in adhesions. Agglutination of the folds or compression of the infundibulum give

**Table 9.3.** Fertility outcome in proximal tubal pathology (37 patients)

| | n | Intra-uterine pregnancy | Tubal pregnancy | Non-pregnancy |
|---|---|---|---|---|
| Fibrosis | 13 | 8 (61%) | 3 (23%) | 2 (16%) |
| Chronic infection | 11 | 1 (9%) | 3 (27%) | 7 (64%) |
| Salpingitis isthmica nodosa | 6 | 2 (33%) | 0 (0%) | 4 (67%) |
| Cornual polyps | 4 | 1 (25%) | 0 (0%) | 3 (75%) |
| Endometriosis | 3 | 0 (0%) | 0 (0%) | 3 (100%) |
| Total | 37 | 12 (32%) | 6 (16%) | 19 (52%) |

rise to phimosis, a stenotic ostium or even a hydrosalpinx. When fimbrioplasty is performed the removal of adhesions usually reveals a normal mucosa and a patent infundibulum. In a series of 32 patients with pelvic endometriosis in whom a fimbrioplasty was performed as part of reconstructive surgery the percentage of ciliated cells ranged from 38.3% to 79.2% (mean 57.2% ± 8.5%) except for one hydrosalpinx which had 26.3% ciliated cells. In 25 patients the folds were uniformly ciliated, the cilia having a normal aspect. However in 7 patients agglutinated and irregularly orientated cilia and/or areas with marked deciliation were observed. When extensive bridges were present in the fimbriae (3 patients) the percentage of ciliated cells was low and coexisted with round-cell infiltration. The difference of the overall cilia population although lower than in normal fertile woman, was not statistically significant.

### Tubal Tuberculosis

In some patients the fallopian tube is patent. The fimbrial ostium is usually stenotic and the ampullary folds show flattening, adhesions, deciliation ranging from patchy to an almost complete absence of cilia and abnormally thin cilia.

In most patients the fallopian tube is completely changed into a thick fibrous hydrosalpinx. The folds show atrophy, desquamation and deciliation, as in pelvic inflammatory disease (PID), but the marked adenomatous patterns, the generalised pleiomorphism of individual cells together with pronounced deciliation are seldom so conspicuous in non-tuberculous chronic salpingitis.

## Technique of Salpingoscopy

There is no doubt that the rigid salpingoscope as developed by Brosens et al. (1987) allows excellent visualisation of the mucosa of the infundibulum and ampulla (Fig. 9.1). The view is clear, bright and wide. Both the anatomical structure of the mucosa and the fine vascular network of the folds can be investigated. The rigid scope is less expensive than the flexible. The salp-

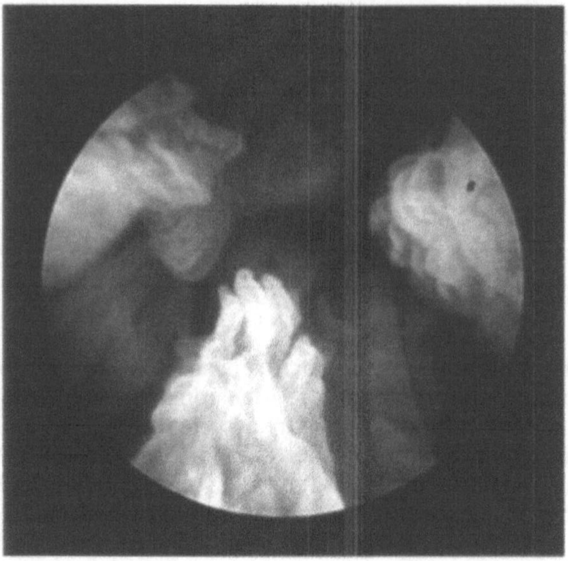

**Fig. 9.1.** View of the mucosal fold system in the ampulla.

ingoscope consists of an outer sheath with a connection for a saline drip, an obturator and a 2.8-mm endoscope (Fig. 9.2). As in hysteroscopy the distension of the cavity by a saline drip allows full inspection of the folds. This is optimally achieved by clamping the tube with a round-ended atraumatic forceps around the sheath of the scope at the level of the infundibulum. Air bubbles should be allowed to escape as they may create artefacts by

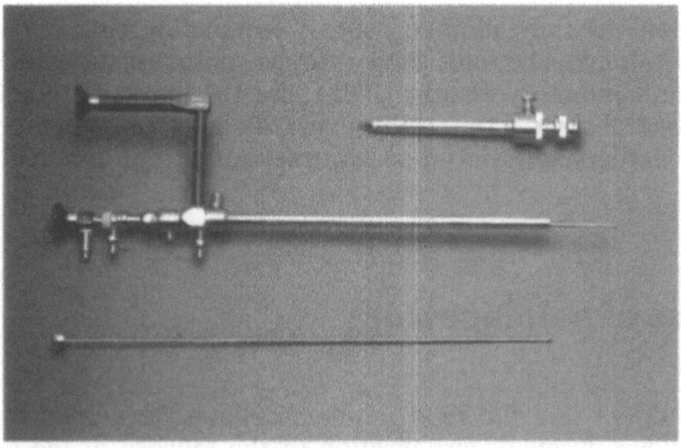

**Fig. 9.2.** The salpingoscope consists of a sheath with a connection for a saline drip, an obturator for cannulating the tube and a 2.8-mm endoscope.

compressing the folds to the wall giving the false impression of a foldless tube.

Complications rarely occur when the salpingoscope is manoeuvred with care. Manipulation of the tube by grasping forceps can produce some serosal bleeding. Only flushing with saline is necessary. Perforation of the tubal mucosa can occur if the telescope is advanced blindly and the saline drip can produce oedematous swelling of the mesosalpinx. Oedematous swelling of the mesosalpinx can also occur in diseased tubes with desquamation of the mucosa.

## Findings

### *Normal Structure*

In the ampulla there are four to five major longitudinal folds with several accessory folds arising from them on each side. Between the major folds there are four or five minor folds. These folds have a delicate structure with a fine vascular network. At the level of the isthmo-ampullary junction, the major folds level off to four or five small, rounded folds which continue into the narrow, isthmic segment. At first the fluid in the ampullary segment may be turbid with flocculent material, particularly when salpingoscopy is performed around the time of menstruation or following hysteroscopy. It is interesting to note that the lateral wall of the folds is densely ciliated, while the top of the folds is deciliated. This could explain counter-current movements in the ampullary segment. The egg is likely to be transported in the ampulla between two opposing major folds.

### *The Tortuous Tube*

In the so-called convoluted or tortuous tube the lumen is very distensible, the folds are flattened and separated and the wall is extremely thin and transparent. Cannulation of the ampulla can be difficult as the infundibulum may be stenotic and the tortuosity prevents the tube from longitudinal stretching. This abnormality has been explained by herniation of the tubal mucosa or aplasia of the myosalpinx. It can involve segments or the entire ampulla. Hysterosalpingography or injection of methylene blue into this tube may create the impression of a hydrosalpinx, because of the extensive dilatation and stenotic infundibulum. However, tortuous tubes are unlikely to be a cause of infertility as they are found in patients with proven fertility.

### *Vascular Abnormalities*

Cyclic vascular changes have recently been described by Maguiness and Djahanbakhch (1992). Vascular abnormalities such as small venectasias can be seen in the folds. Their significance is not known. A marked vascularisation and haemorrhagic spots are suggestive of chronic inflammation.

**Table 9.4.** Salpingoscopy: classification of the ampullary lesions in hydrosalpinges

| | |
|---|---|
| Grade 1 | Normal fold pattern |
| Grade 2 | Separation and flattening of folds |
| Grade 3 | Focal lesions, e.g. small adhesions |
| Grade 4 | Adhesive or destructive lesions over the entire ampulla |
| Grade 5 | Fibrosis and complete loss of folds |

### *Lesions*

Filmy adhesions between the ampullary folds are avascular and adhere between otherwise normal folds. These adhesions can occur focally or extensively in the ampulla. Severe adhesions are thick and vascularised and the fold structure is distorted. They usually extend over the entire length of the ampullary segment. A complete loss of the mucosal folds by fibrosis makes the tube appear as a rigid, hollow channel with some remnants of folds. A classification for these lesions has been proposed in hydrosalpinges by De Bruyne et al. (1989) (Table 9.4).

## Clinical Value

Salpingoscopy allows detailed examination of the tubal mucosa and is a logical extension of the endoscopic examination of the female genital tract. In patients with pelvic adhesions but with patent fallopian tubes salpingoscopy allows the detection of mucosal adhesions. The presence of minor mucosal adhesions is not incompatible with normal fertility (Maguiness and Djahanbakhch 1992). In the presence of a tubocornual block salpingoscopy is the only technique to evaluate the quality of the mucosa of the ampullary segment. In hydrosalpinx, hysdrosalpingography (HSG) and laparoscopy are frequently inadequate. Puttemans et al. (1987) demonstrated at salpingoscopy mucosal lesions that were not detected at HSG or laparoscopy in 52% of patients. On the other hand, adhesions were absent in 43% of patients who were suspected of having a defective fold pattern on HSG (Table 9.5). A prospective study of salpingostomy showed a 59% pregnancy rate in patients when salpingoscopy showed absence of intratubal adhesions (De Bruyne et al. 1989).

Salpingoscopy is apparently superior to HSG and laparoscopy in the exploration of the tubal mucosa. Therefore it could be useful in the selection of patients for gamete intrafallopian transfer (GIFT) by excluding unsuspected tubal lesions.

Salpingoscopy can also be useful in patients with ectopic pregnancy. The salpingoscope can be introduced into the fallopian tube with an unruptured tubal pregnancy to evaluate the presence and extent of lesions and to locate the ectopic pregnancy. In addition it is particularly important to evaluate the quality of the contralateral fallopian tube. The laparoscopic appearance of a tube is *no* guarantee of an intact mucosa. Prospective studies are in progress to assess the value of salpingoscopy in the estimation of the risk of recurrent ectopic pregnancy.

**Table 9.5.** Correlation between findings at hysterosalpingography (HSG) and salpingoscopy in hydrosalpinges (Puttemans et al. 1987)

| Information from HSG | Salpingoscopy | | | | | Total | Conformity |
|---|---|---|---|---|---|---|---|
| | Folds preserved | | Abnormal fold pattern | | | | |
| | Grade 1 | Grade 2 | Grade 3 | Grade 4 | Grade 5 | | |
| Normal fold pattern | 5 | 6 | 7 | 2 | 3 | 23 | 48% |
| Abnormal or defective fold pattern | 3 | 6 | 3 | 4 | 5 | 21 | 57% |
| No visualisation | 1 | 1 | 0 | 4 | 1 | 7 | 0% |
| Total | 9 | 13 | 10 | 10 | 9 | 51 | |

Conclusion: HSG was false negative in 52%, false positive in 43% and of no use in 14%.

**Table 9.6.** Laparoscopy vs salpingoscopy (Gordon, personal communication)

| Laparoscopy | | Salpingoscopy | |
|---|---|---|---|
| | n | Normal | Abnormal |
| Normal tubes | 160 | 157 (98%) | 3[a] (2%) |
| Damaged tubes | 67 | 37 (55%) | 30 (45%) |

[a] One patient with history of ectopic pregnancy in the contralateral tube

In non-selected patients with normal findings at laparoscopy unsuspected lesions of the tubal mucosa are detected in not more than 3% (Table 9.6) (Gordon, personal communication).

# Summary

Salpingoscopy allows detailed visualisation of the mucosal pattern of the tubal ampulla as far as the isthmo-ampullary junction. With experience, it takes 10 minutes to perform salpingoscopy on both sides. Transabdominal salpingoscopy is an extension of laparoscopy and should be performed in all cases when tubal disease is suspected. Comparative studies proved the technique to be superior to HSG. In conditions like a tubocornual block, transabdominal salpingoscopy is the only technique to provide information on the ampullary mucosa. Salpingoscopic inspection of a phimosis or a hydrosalpinx can be performed quite easily and the findings are important in the management and selection between surgical repair, GIFT or in-vitro fertilisation. Salpingoscopy may also prove to be a useful tool in the estimation of the risk of recurrent ectopic pregnancy.

# References

Boer-Meisel ME, Te Velde ER, Habbema JDF, Kardaun JWPF (1986) Predicting the pregnancy outcome in patients treated for hydrosalpinges: a prospective study. Fertil Steril 45:23–29

Brosens I, Vasquez G (1976) Fimbrial microbiopsy. J Repr Med 16:171–178

Brosens I, Boeckx W, Delattin Ph, Puttemans P, Vasquez G (1987) Salpingoscopy: a new preoperative diagnostic tool in tubal infertility? Br J Obstet Gynaec 94:722–728

Cornier E (1985) l'Ampulloscopie per-coelioscopique. J Gynéc Obstét Biol Reprod 14:459–466

De Bruyne F, Puttemans P, Boeckx W, Brosens IA (1989) The clinical value of salpingoscopy in tubal infertility. Fertil Steril 51:339–340

Henry-Suchet J, Loffredo V, Tesquier L, Pez J (1985) Endoscopy of the tube (= tuboscopy): its prognostic value for tuboplasties. Acta Eur Fertil 16:139–145

Karbowski B, Vasquez G, Boeckx W, Brosens I, Schneider HPG (1988) An experimental study of tubo-ovarian function following restoration of patency in hydrosalpinges. Eur J Obstet Gynaec 28:305–315

Maguiness SD, Djahanbakhch O (1992) Salpingoscopic findings in women undergoing sterilization. Hum Reprod 7:269–273

Puttemans P, Brosens I, Delattin Ph, Vasquez G, Boeckx W (1987) Salpingoscopy versus hysterosalpingography in hydrosalpinges. Hum Reprod 2:535–540

Vasquez G, Boeckx W, Winston RML, Brosens IA (1980) Human tubal mucosa and reconstructive microsurgery. In: Crosignani PG, Rubin BL (eds) Microsurgery in Female Infertility. Academic Press, London, pp 41–56

Vasquez G, Winston RML, Boeckx W, Gordts S, Brosens IA (1983) The epithelium of human hydrosalpinges: a light optical and scanning electron microscopic study. Br J Obstet Gynaec 90:764–770

Section III

# Diagnosis and Treatment of Tubal Disease

Chapter 10

# Proximal Tubal Disease: Diagnosis and Endoscopic Treatment

N. Gleicher

## Introduction

Under normal circumstances the physiology and natural history of specific organ systems is well understood *before* their respective medical conditions are treated. However, because of difficulty with access, our understanding of tubal physiology and pathology has lagged behind knowledge of other pelvic organs. While the concept of transvaginal tubal catheterisation is probably over 100 years old, only in recent years has technology been developed that permits a transvaginal, transcervical approach to the oviducts.

The biggest break-throughs have taken place in conjunction with the treatment of proximally occluded oviducts. Until a transvaginal catheter approach was attempted in the mid-eighties (Platia and Krudy 1985; Confino et al. 1986; Thurmond et al. 1987), proximal tubal occlusion was universally treated with microsurgery, which almost always included excision of the affected tubal segment. While initial attempts at tubal catheterisation were greeted with scepticism (De Cherney 1987), the approach is now considered as established. Eighty percent to 90% success in tubal recanalisation and approximately 50% pregnancy rates (in the absence of distal tubal disease) have been reported by at least two groups of investigators with considerable experience (Thurmond and Rösch 1990; Confino et al. 1990). Moreover, procedural complication rates as well as tubal pregnancies are exceedingly rare.

In properly selected cases of tubal disease the inexpensive and ambulatory tubal catheterisation has thus quite rapidly replaced the more costly and invasive tubal microsurgery. Moreover, a very short procedure under para-cervical block or, at most, mild sedation, has taken the place of segmental tubal resection, a major surgical procedure under general anaesthesia. Tubal catheterisation procedures have also given us considerable new insights into the pathophysiology of proximal tubal occlusion.

## Diagnosis

Sulak et al. (1987a) reported that a percentage of cases of proximal tubal occlusions were *not* the result of inherent tubal disease but rather the consequence of intraluminal plaque formation. Their observation explained why tubal surgeons were often unable to detect pathology in tubal segments that were resected for proximal occlusion. The experience with tubal catheterisation procedures took this observation a step further. In accordance with Sulak's findings, proximally recanalised oviducts often appear completely normal on contrast studies. Therefore, segmental resection of affected fallopian tubes, converts a normal oviduct into a "scarred" one.

Unfortunately, this has proved an oversimplification. A normal opacification pattern with contrast medium does *not* necessarily reflect completely normal tubal status. For example, normal opacification can occur in the presence of highly increased tubal perfusion pressures. In fact Confino et al. (1992) demonstrated that tubal catheterisation procedures can reduce tubal perfusion pressures dramatically, though not necessarily to normal levels. Moreover, different tubal catheterisation procedures affect tubal perfusion pressures to varying degrees. For example, selective salpingography (SS), a highly effective method for re-establishing tubal patency in milder cases of proximal tubal occlusion (see below), reduces perfusion pressures less than does transcervical balloon tuboplasty (Confino et al. 1992). Whether this is responsible for the differences in pregnancy rates with different treatment methods remains to be established. Recently data from our Centre, suggest that the pressure required to perfuse oviducts correlates with tubal function as defined by opacification patterns (Gleicher et al. 1992d). It is tempting to speculate that it can also be predictive of the potential of any particular oviduct to allow pregnancy.

To evaluate tubal perfusion pressures we have used a contrast injection system for hysterosalpingography (HSG) and SS. A standardised volume of contrast medium is injected per unit time into each patient. Except for obvious anatomical differences between patients, the resulting pressure curves must reflect the compliance of the vessel receiving the contrast medium. Our early studies revealed that evaluation of perfusion pressures during HSG was of limited value since those pressures reflect only the outlet of least resistance from the system. An HSG is, therefore, unable to detect differences in resistance between two oviducts, unless there is delayed filling on one side. Moreover, uterine pathology, such as myomas or septae, can also affect the symmetrical distribution of contrast medium and thus affect the interpretation of perfusion pressure measurements. In contrast, perfusion pressure evaluations during SS are highly reliable and probably predictive of tubal reproductive capacity. Experienced tubal surgeons know that "stiff" oviducts have poor pregnancy potential. It is exactly those "stiff" tubes that de-

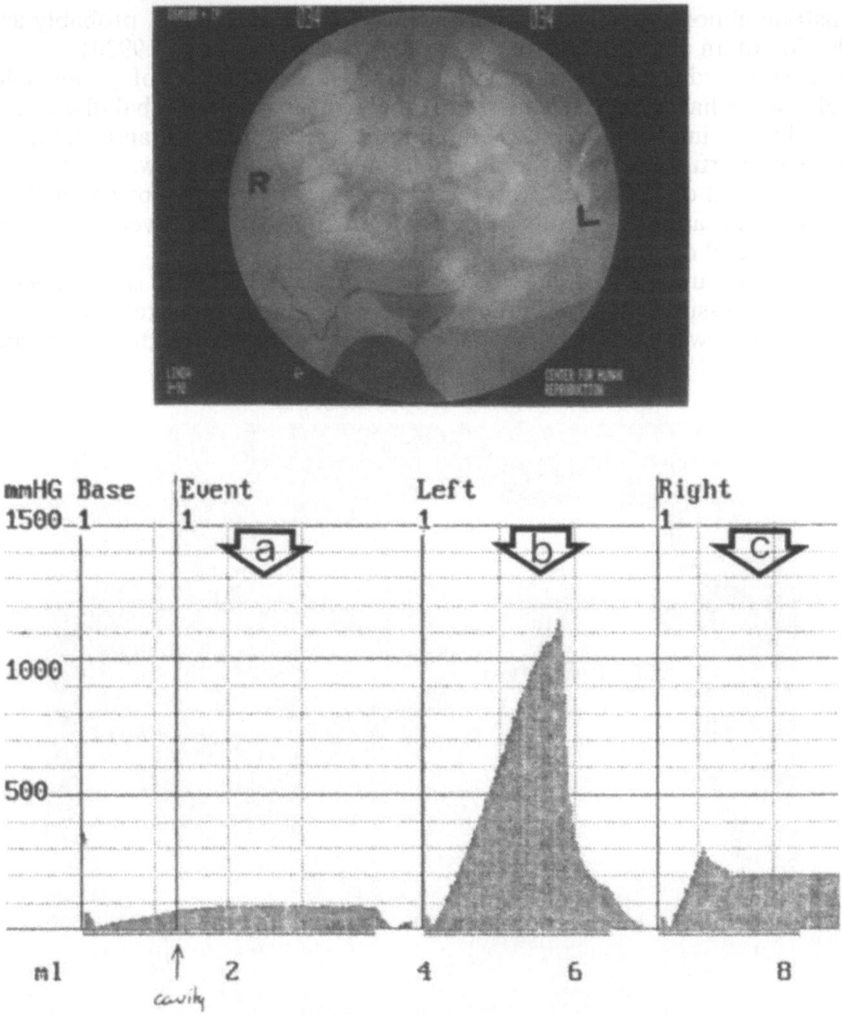


**Fig. 10.1.** The tubal opacification pattern alone here could result in a misleading diagnosis in this patient. The HSG revealed in real time an apparently normal bilateral tubal opacification pattern. Review of the study from digital memory revealed, however, a clear delay in left in comparison to right tubal opacification (upper panel). We therefore performed bilateral selective salpinography which demonstrates evidence of initial cornual obstruction on the left, only overcome at exceedingly high perfusion pressure, while the normal right oviduct shows normal pressure measurements (lower panel) **a**. HSG; **b**. left SS; note abnormal opening pressure of 1150 mm Hg which reduces to normal flow levels of less than 200 mm Hg once the initial obstruction is overcome. **c**. right SS with a normal pressure perfusion curve.

Normal SS pressures are approximately twice the level of normal HSG pressures, which is a reflection of vessel size into which contrast medium is injected since infusion speed and delivery system diameter are identical for both procedures.

monstrate abnormally elevated perfusion pressures during SS, probably as a reflection of an abnormal fibrotic myosalpinx (Gleicher et al. 1992d).

The standard gynaeco-radiological diagnostic evaluation of patients for tubal disease has to be re-evaluated. If there is suspicion of tubal disease, an HSG alone is inadequate. At a minimum, a concomitant SS, and preferably a pressure perfusion study, should be obtained. Fig. 10.1 shows a case study in which tubal opacification studies alone would have been grossly misleading. Only the addition of tubal perfusion pressure studies revealed the real extent of tubal disease.

We are still unable to define in detail the prognostic clinical significance of perfusion pressures. In a preliminary study we reported that tubal perfusion pressures below 350 mm Hg may be normal since they correlate with normal

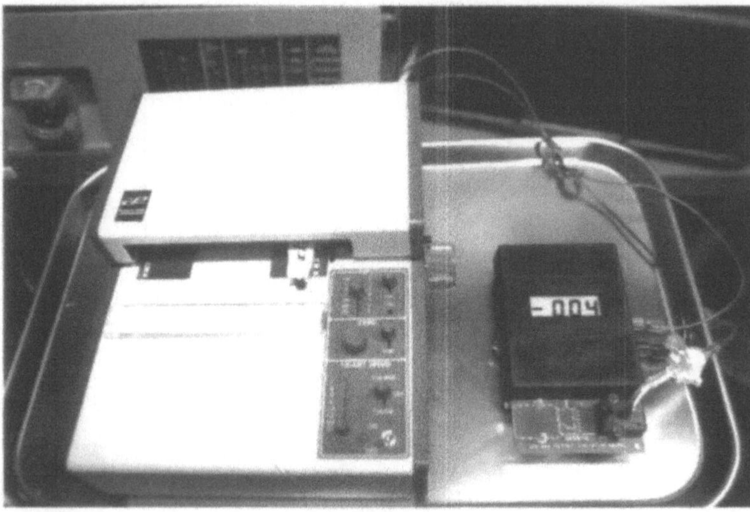

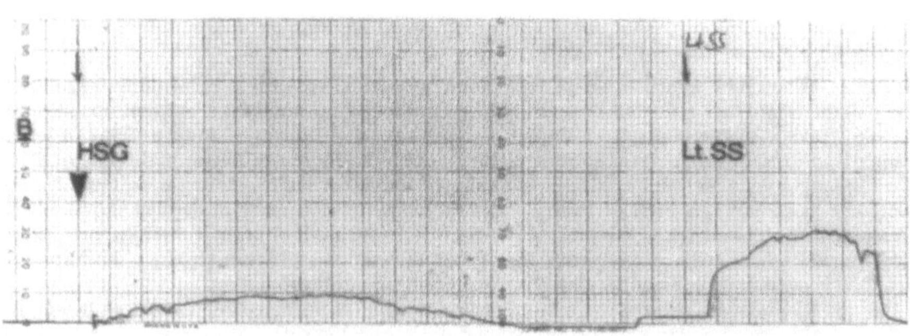


**Fig. 10.2.** **a**. Experimental device used at The Center for Human Reproduction in Chicago to assess opening pressures during HSG and SS. **b**. Example of normal pressure recordings during HSG and left SS in a patient undergoing a re-evaluation after a transabdominal myomectomy and left tuboplasty. Pressures are recorded on tracing paper. HSG, hysterosalpingogram; Lt SS, left selective salpingography. (From Gleicher N (ed) (1992) Tubal Catheterization Procedures, Wiley-Liss, with permission.)

opacification patterns (Gleicher et al. 1992d). Since normal opacification patterns can, however, be obtained in the presence of tubal disease, a cut-off at 350 mm Hg may be excessive and might include patients with significant tubal disease. Our clinical impression is that the truly normal oviduct perfuses at less than 150 mm Hg. This has also been suggested by a Japanese study (Kaseki et al. 1991) and the study by Confino et al. (1992). Unfortunately, in that study we utilised a rather primitive hand-held manometer to assess pressure values ("The Wizard", Bard Reproductive Systems Haverhill, Massachusetts). From there we graduated to an assembled injection and digital pressure measurement device, which also provided a print-out (Fig. 10.2; this was the device utilised in the previously noted study (Gleicher et al. 1992d). Since calibration of this system had to be performed manually, considerable variations in pressure measurements between cases were unavoidable. We have since further advanced to a fully computerised system (Fig. 10.3), which was provided to us as a custom device by Bard Reproductive Systems, Haverhill, Massachusetts, and which should be able to

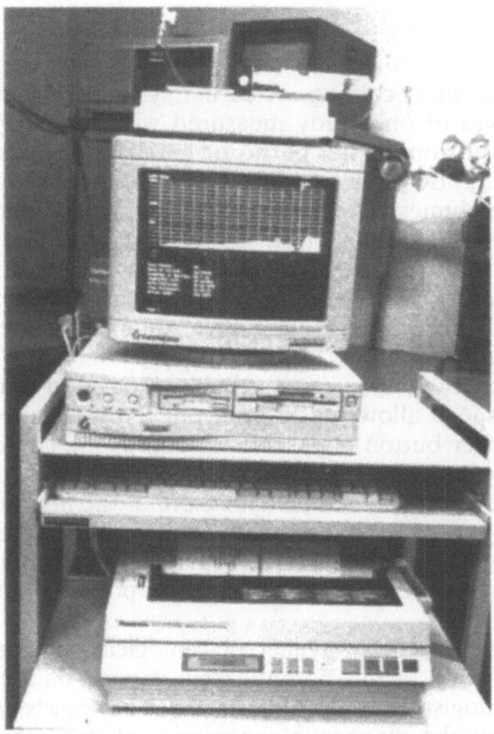

**Fig. 10.3.** Advanced computerised perfusion pressure measuring device, provided to us as a custom device by Bard Reproductive Systems, Haverhill, Massachusetts. The infusion pump is seen on top of the screen, which demonstrates the perfusion pressure curve of a HSG, followed by the beginning of a pressure curve during left SS. Both curves demonstrate normal pressures. The numbers on the $x$-axis are indicative of amount of contrast medium injected and therefore allow uterine cavity volume assessments. An outline printer is shown on the lower shelf, as a hard copy of the screen picture is being generated for the medical record.

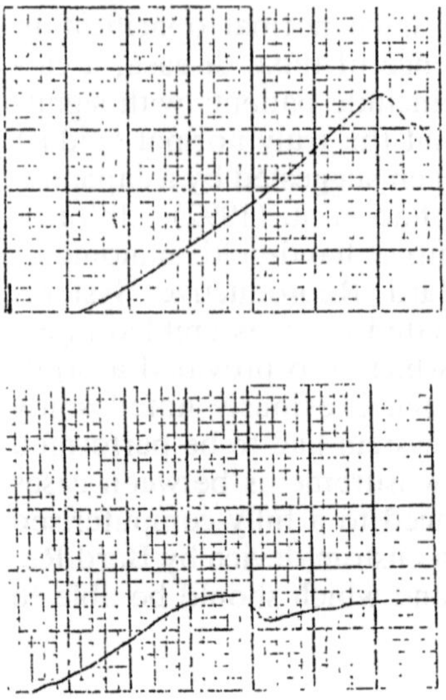

**Fig. 10.4.** Perfusion pressure curve during SS demonstrates a clearly elevated pressure profile (upper panel). After tubal catheterisation by wire guide tubal perfusion pressures are clearly reduced (lower panel).

overcome fully the short-comings of earlier systems. Fig. 10.4 demonstrates the pressure curves of one study measured with this new device. The improvement in detail from earlier perfusion curves is obvious.

This new system also allows for the first time the accurate determination of uterine cavity volumes. The literature is surprisingly sparse on this clinical parameter. For example Sher et al. (1989) suggested that cavity depth can serve as an important predictor of IVF success. If so, volume may be an even better indicator. Cavity volume may also correlate with pregnancy success in women with Müllerian anomalies, though we are unaware of any actual volume studies in support of this concept.

Endometrial cavity volume can easily be assessed in our system since the preset injection speed allows us to print out the injected volume at regular invervals. A marker button is pushed as soon as the contrast enters one or both of the fallopian tubes. That moment is thus marked. The amount of previously injected contrast is then a measure of the uterine cavity volume.

In preliminary work, we have found cavity volume especially valuable in the evaluation of uteri with distorted cavities due to myomas. Long-term follow-up studies on the relevance of fertility potential and pregnancy outcome are in progress.

The diagnostic potential of gynaeco-radiological procedures is expanding. The proper utilisation of this potential will depend on a co-operative effort between gynaecologists and radiologists. Gynaecologists can be expected to be sceptical about the diagnostic capabilities of fluoroscopically controlled procedures since most of them do not have direct access to X-ray machines and are generally unfamiliar with this medium. Radiologists, who have the instrumentation and experience, lack, however, the integrated knowledge of infertility therapy and usually do not have direct access to the infertile patient. Consequently, only a co-operative approach will lead to a further expansion in gynaeco-radiology.

# Treatment

The treatment of tubal disease by non-surgical means is very new. The modern era of transvaginal, transcervical tubal catheterisation procedures began in the mid-eighties when Platia and Krudy (1985), Thurmond et al. (1987) and Confino et al. (1986) reported their first attempts. Their efforts received considerable support from the work of Sulak et al. (1987a), who demonstrated that many cases of proximal tubal occlusion were not due to tubal disease per se, but were caused by intraluminal plaques, which were amenable to dislocation by transvaginal catheter procedures.

Despite this pathophysiological explanation of early successes, the profession's initial response towards a transvaginal approach was highly sceptical. Such scepticism was also reflected in the literature (De Cherney 1987) after some small pilot studies were published (Platia and Krudy 1985; Confino et al. 1986; Thurmond et al. 1987; Sulak et al. 1987b).

Most of the scepticism was based on anatomical considerations. The intramural portion of the oviduct was felt to be too narrow to allow the passage of a catheter system which could provide useful information for pre-treatment assessment. Moreover, the tortuosity of the first half of the fallopian tube was also felt to represent a major impediment to successful catheterisation (De Cherney 1987). Lastly, such an approach had to overcome the basic resistance that meets any innovation which attempts to replace an established and widely practised procedure with a simpler, less invasive and more cost-effective approach.

Early studies established that the fallopian tube could be catheterised with relative ease (Platia and Krudy 1985; Confino et al. 1986; Thurmond et al. 1987; Confino et al. 1988). Gynaecologists almost instantly embraced the approach and today tubal catheterisation procedures are widely performed.

Despite rapid acceptance of the transvaginal approach towards the fallopian tube, there is nevertheless concern about the generalised use of the technique. Even today, only limited data are available on the therapeutic effectiveness of various tubal catheterisation procedures. The number of prospective and well-controlled studies, utilising a large enough sample size, is small. Moreover, much of the prospectively accumulated data utilised a fluoroscopically controlled approach towards tubal catheterisation (Thurmond and Rösch 1990; Confino et al. 1990). In contrast, most tubal catheterisation procedures performed today are done during hysteroscopy. Our own experience (Confino et al. 1988) and the data of other investigators strongly suggest that outcome data are not comparable under those two circumstances.

The proliferation of tubal catheterisation procedures has also resulted in the description of a wide variety of tubal catheterisation systems. While the use of a multitude of different catheters may be a desirable end-point of a procedural development process, it complicates the interpretation of outcome data. Moreover, the use of different technologies prohibits extrapolation of results from one study to another.

The various treatments will be described with special emphasis on the guidance system (for example, fluoroscopy vs hysteroscopy), specific treatment options (for example, selective salpingography vs tubal catheterisation) and catheter technology (for example, wire guide catheterisation vs balloon tuboplasty).

## High Pressure Perfusion versus Tubal Catheterisation

Most published experience refers to proximal tubal occlusion. Proximal tubal occlusion represents around 20% of all tubal disease (Musich and Behrman 1983) and can occur as an isolated lesion (*unipolar disease*) or in conjunction with distal disease (*bipolar tubal disease*). The differentiation between those two forms is important because pregnancy rates after successful proximal recanalisation are close to 50% with unipolar and barely 10% with bipolar disease (Gleicher et al. 1993). Moreover, the risk of tubal pregnancy is significantly higher with bipolar disease (Zbella 1992).

The diagnosis of proximal tubal occlusion is complicated by an apparently high incidence of so-called "tubal spasm", which might result in the false-positive diagnosis of proximal tubal occlusion. The concept of tubal spasm was initially based on the observation that proximal tubal occlusion might appear to be intermittent: one hysterosalpingogram (HSG) may show it, while the next will not. Hysteroscopic observations of the tubal ostia confirmed that the normal rhythmic peristalsis of the ostia can be interrupted by prolonged periods of spasm.

As a consequence, the literature abounds with techniques to differentiate between tubal spasm and true proximal occlusion, with tubal spasm being considered as a *normal* physiological variation.

We have concluded that tubal spasm is probably *never* a normal physiological state. We are convinced that a normal tubal ostium will *always* be patent to contrast medium as long as the gynaeco-radiological procedure is performed correctly. We have reached this opinion based on a number of observations: 1) Patients referred to our centre with the diagnosis of tubal spasm almost uniformly demonstrate elevated tubal perfusion pressures during selective salpingography (SS). 2) Patients who entered the Multicenter Balloon Tuboplasty (TBT) study (Confino et al. 1990; Gleicher et al. 1993) were prescreened with at least one HSG and one laparoscopy. Nevertheless, approximately 10% of patients with alleged bilateral proximal tubal occlusion by those two tests, were found to have at least one patent tube on HSG performed as the initial step of the TBT procedure. These patients were then excluded from the full TBT procedure but were still followed up. Their pregnancy rates were dismal (below 10%) and significantly lower than pregnancy rates in patients treated either with SS or TBT (Gleicher et al. 1993). These observations thus strongly suggest that patients with intermittent tubal patency during HSG have a significant degree of tubal disease that warrants treatment. What form that treatment should take is still undetermined. Some of our preliminary data suggest that the reduction of perfusion pressures through tubal catheterisation procedures may be helpful. Fig. 10.4 demonstrates tubal perfusion pressure curves before and after a wire guide catheterisation of an abnormal oviduct. As can be seen, the "rotor rootering" of the fallopian tube reduced a significantly elevated perfusion pressure to a normal level below 100 mm Hg.

Once proximal occlusion is confirmed a variety of non-surgical treatment options exist, all based on transvaginal catheter techniques.

### *Selective Salpingography (SS)*

The simplest technique is *therapeutic* selective salpingography. This is not only a diagnostic procedure of great importance, but can also have considerable therapeutic benefits (Gleicher et al. 1992a; Gleicher et al. 1991; Capitanio et al. 1991). In the Multicenter TBT Study some 10% of patients, who were confirmed as occluded by HSG, achieved at least unilateral tubal patency by SS. These patients, in contrast to those who were patent after HSG, achieved pregnancy rates comparable to TBT patients, though with a time delay of approximately 1 year (Gleicher et al. 1993). It is tempting to conclude that SS results in similar pregnancy rates to tubal catheterisation procedures (Capitanio et al. 1991). Obviously such a conclusion is wrong since only SS failures advanced to TBT in the Multicenter TBT Study and other published SS experiences described patient populations that were not as stringently prescreened for tubal occlusion as patients from the Multicenter TBT Study.

The only definite conclusion about published data on SS and tubal catheterisation procedures is that the literature does not contain a single report of randomisation between the two. SS may represent a valid first choice of therapy in any randomly chosen patient population with proximal tubal occlusion. Our own data suggest that SS alone will be successful in over 90% of such cases (Gleicher et al. 1991). What remains to be established is whether pregnancy rates are truly similar to those achieved with tubal catheterisation procedures and whether pregnancy occurs within similar time periods.

Selective salpingography is less successful in recanalising tubal obstruction if patients have been repeatedly prescreened, as in the Multicenter TBT Study. If tubal obstruction has been confirmed by at least two independent evaluations, SS will be successful in only around 10% of cases (Confino et al. 1990). This suggests that SS will be successful in milder cases, while the more impacted lesions require tubal catheterisation procedures. Consequently, one has to be careful in equating data in the literature that refers to SS procedures as well as tubal catheterisation techniques. However, SS is a valid first choice in the patient who presents with proximal tubal occlusion. In the tubal catheterisation system used at our Centre (Bard Reproductive Systems, Haverhill, Massachusetts), the selective salpingography catheter is also the delivery system for the TBT catheter. Consequently, the SS catheter is placed first and an attempt at SS is made. Only if SS is unsuccessful is a TBT catheter advanced, and a TBT procedure carried out (Fig. 10.5).

This approach seems logical and cost-effective and is probably the current standard of care. We are, however, increasingly concerned that this approach may have to change. Our concern is based on a number of observations: Confino et al. (1992) have found that the tubal perfusion pressure after successful SS is still significantly higher than after successful TBT. The difference was apparent not only immediately following the re-

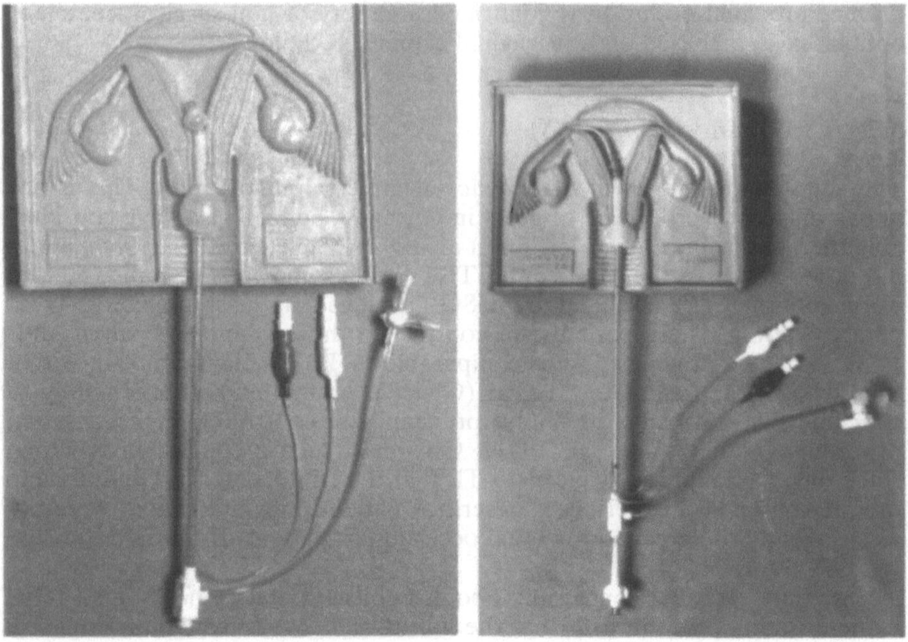

a b

**Fig. 10.5.** The Bard[R] transcervical balloon tuboplasty system in a uterine model. Note the double-balloon HSG catheter situated in the cervix. **a**. The interior balloon prevents not only the backflow of contrast but also expulsion of the catheter when high pressures are exerted. The exterior balloon "fixes" the HSG catheter in place and prevents its forward movement into the cavity. **b**. The SS catheter is placed through the HSG catheter into the uterine cornua. (From Gleicher N (ed) (1992) Tubal Catheterization Procedures, Wiley-Liss, with permission.)

spective procedures but was maintained at 6-month follow-up. This observation again suggests that the achievement of tubal patency is not an ideal endpoint for successful treatment. Moreover, in the Multicenter TBT Study, SS patients lagged significantly behind TBT patients in the time to conception, even though they comprised milder cases of tubal impaction (Gleicher et al. 1993). Therefore, pregnancy results after SS can probably be improved further if SS is followed by a tubal catheterisation procedure, even though patency has already been achieved.

## *Tubal Catheterisation Procedures*

Tubal catheterisation procedures take four different approaches. These are *wire guide cannulations* alone, *coaxial catheter systems* on a guide wire, a *linear everting catheter* system and *balloon tuboplasty*. *Wire guide cannulation* alone can be successful in many cases that have failed SS, but the pregnancy rates are disappointing. In 30 patients treated in this way we achieved no clinical pregnancy and only one tubal gestation. Even though this patient group comprises women with very severe tubal disease, pregnancy rates were significantly lower than in women with bipolar tubal disease who had undergone TBT (Gleicher et al. 1993). We no longer recommend wire guide cannulation as the sole therapy for proximal tubal occlusion.

*Coaxial catheter systems* were introduced by the Oregon group. In a number of studies they demonstrated that this system achieves tubal patency rates in over 80% of patients and pregnancy rates in a range of 25% to almost 50%, dependent on patient selection (Thurmond et al. 1987; Thurmond and Rösch 1990). The authors are describing their technique elsewhere in this volume (see Chap. 11).

The *linear everting catheter* represents an interesting concept. This uses a flexible membrane which, under hydraulic pressure, gently unrolls forward through the tube. The system is in clinical trial and is produced by Imagyn Medical, a California based company. Whether it can overcome tubal obstruction has not so far been reported. At present it is primarily used as a delivery system for transvaginal GIFT, ZIFT or PROST and for tuboscopy instrumentation.

The *Transcervical Balloon Tuboplasty (TBT) System* (Bard Reproductive Systems, Haverhill, Massachusetts) was co-developed with our group and is the catheterisation system most familiar to us. We believe that this system has a number of advantages over competing catheters.

The first advantage is that it allows a stepwise approach towards the new infertility patient. The Bard TBT System consists of a *cervical cannula* (also called *HSG catheter*) which is introduced into the cervix (Fig. 10.5). This can be done with no anaesthesia, a paracervical block or, on rare occasions, under mild sedation. Most tubal catheterisation procedures at our centre are performed under only paracervical block. The double balloon design of the cervical cannula creates a fixed platform for all subsequent catheters, which are passed through the lumen of the cannula. As soon as the cannula is in place, we introduce an SS (or secondary) catheter, but do *not* advance it *into* the uterus at this time. After flushing this catheter with contrast it is only advanced towards the cranial opening of the cannula and serves as the injection catheter for the HSG procedure. While an HSG can be performed by directly injecting through one of two portals of the cannula, we prefer to use the SS catheter as our injection portal in order to standardise the delivery system between HSG and SS. This then allows us to compare perfusion pressures between amounts per unit time of contrast medium delivered through a catheter of equal diameter.

We use a fluoroscopy C-arm for our gynaeco-radiological procedures (General Electric Stenoscope, Milwaukee, Wisconsin), which allows for continuous digitalised documentation of the whole study and at any point can be replayed from memory on a frame-by-frame basis (Fig. 10.6). The system also provides for image enhancement, image enlargement and contrast modification. This multitude of options improves the diagnostic capacity of gynaeco-radiological procedures far beyond those of spot films. As a consequence, our need for diagnostic laparoscopies has been reduced by approximately 40% (Gleicher et al. 1992b).

Hysterosalpingography is performed in routine manner, with the usual attention to uterine cavity filling, symmetric opacification of oviducts, symmetric spillage and normal spill of contrast into the peritoneal cavity. In addition, however, we also obtain perfusion pressure measurements during this process. Unfortunately, perfusion pressures during HSG are of limited

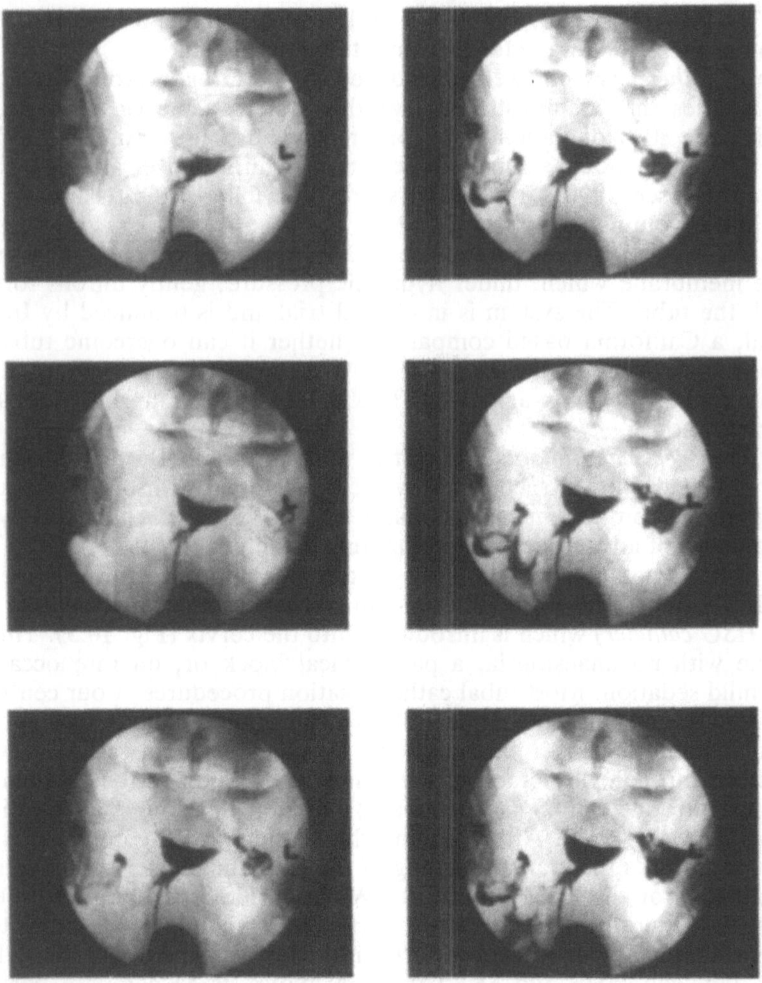


**Fig. 10.6.** Demonstration of memory. Individual frames can be recalled from memory. This allows a detailed review of dynamic changes, which often are only split seconds apart. Recall from memory also permits documentation on hard copy, as here demonstrated through an HSG study, which shows a normal uterine cavity partially filled in frame 10 and completely filled in frame 11. Frame 11 also demonstrates early left tubal opacification. Frame 13 demonstrates bilateral tubal opacification with early distal spill. Frame 15 demonstrates a normal spill on the right side and an apparent collection peritubally on the left side. This picture is confirmed in frames 17 and 19 and suggests left peritubal adhesions. Frames 10–19 are approximately 10 sec apart. Memory also allows one to revisit the frames between frames 10 and 19. (From Gleicher N (ed) (1992) Tubal Catheterization Procedures, Wiley-Liss, with permission.)

value since they only represent the uterine outlet of least resistance. If both tubes are asymmetrically affected by disease, the HSG pressure measurements can be very misleading. A similar error can be introduced by uterine cavity distortions (Gleicher et al. 1992d).

Upon completion of the HSG, the SS catheter is advanced into either the

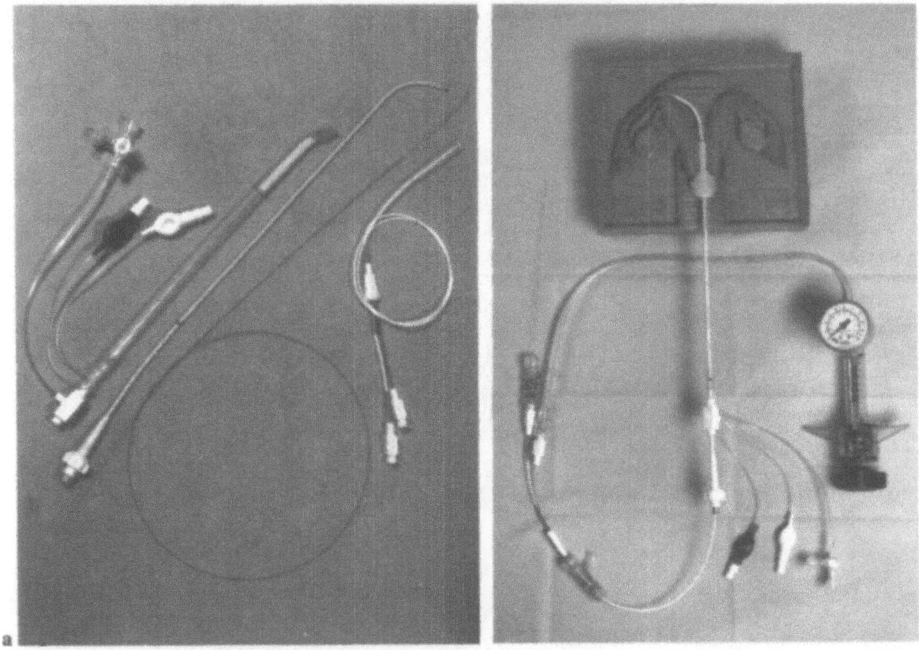

**Fig. 10.7.** TBT catheter system (Bard Reproductive Systems). **a**. System components separately shown from top to bottom: HSG catheter, SS catheter, wire guide, TBT catheter (inflation device, Wizard$^R$, not shown) **b**. The same system assembled within a uterine model inclusive of inflation device (Wizard$^R$) on the right. (From Gleicher N (ed) (1992) Tubal Catheterization Procedures, Wiley-Liss, with permission.)

right or left cornua and an SS is performed. Once again, the perfusion pressure is obtained concomitantly. The SS catheter is easily flipped to examine the contralateral side.

If SS confirms tubal occlusion, the TBT catheter, preloaded with a slightly protruding wire guide, is advanced through the SS catheter towards the tubal obstruction. When it is as close as possible to the site of obstruction, the balloon catheter is inflated (Fig. 10.7). This achieves two goals: first, the balloon stretches the tubal walls laterally, secondly, the balloon wedges the catheter. This, in turn, presents reflux of contrast which is now injected through the catheter forward into the oviduct, thus increasing the ejection force (Fig. 10.8).

The Multicenter TBT Study suggests that even the most recalcitrant of proximal tubal occlusions can be recanalised in 90% of patients, at least unilaterally. As noted earlier, with unipolar tubal disease, subsequent pregnancy rates will approach 50%, while complication rates are extremely low (Gleicher et al. 1993). Ectopic pregnancy rates are not increased over expected levels and are usually located away from the treatment site. This finding is compatible with the known increase in tubal pregnancy with bipolar tubal disease (Zbella 1992).

TBT is a very attractive and cost-effective primary treatment approach for the persistent proximal tubal occlusion. Whether TBT should also be per-

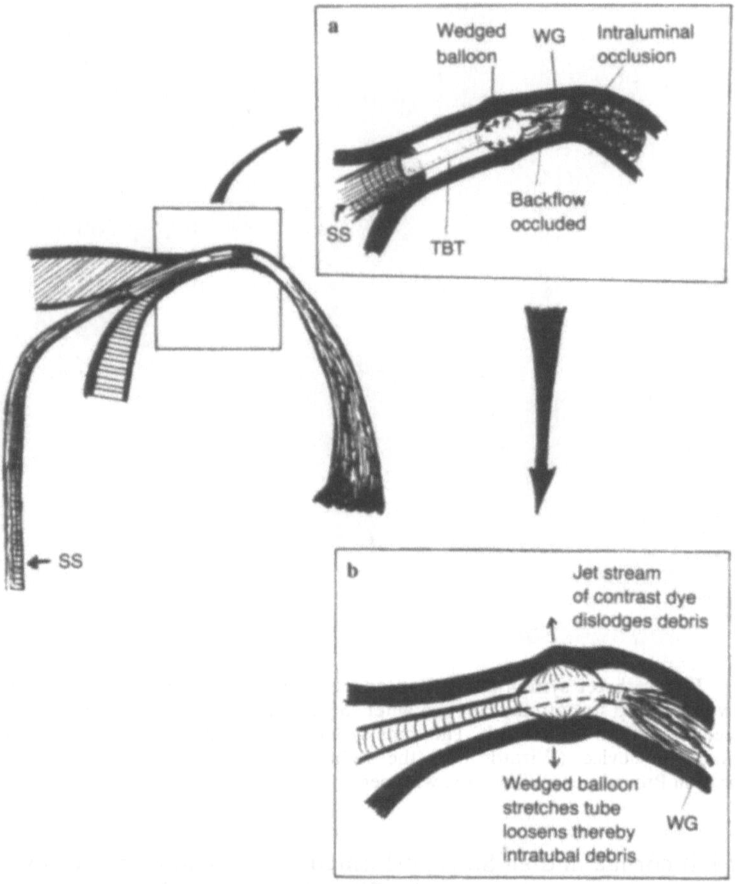


**Fig. 10.8.** Method of action of the TBT balloon catheter within the fallopian tube. **a**. The TBT catheter (TBT) is advanced through the guide catheter as close to the intraluminal occlusion as possible. The wire guide (WG), which protrudes slightly, leads the way. When in place, the TBT catheter is expanded, stretching the tubal walls laterally and occluding the tubal lumen ("wedging of catheter"). **b**. Wedged catheter prevents backflow of contrast medium which now is injected through the TBT catheter. Wedging of balloon "loosens" intratubal debris, which now is dislodged by a jet stream of contrast medium. (From Gleicher N (ed) (1992) Tubal Catheterization Procedures, Wiley-Liss, with permission.)

formed after successful SS if perfusion pressures remain high still needs to be determined. Our impression is that this approach improves pregnancy rates and/or shortens the conception time.

The TBT system is so far the *only* tubal catheterisation system that has undergone a *prospective multicentre* trial of a rigorously preselected patient population with *bilateral* tubal occlusion. It is also the only system that has been subject to review by the Food and Drug Administration.

## Fluoroscopic versus Hysteroscopic Guidance

Most tubal catheterisation procedures are performed during endoscopic procedures under hysteroscopic and/or laparoscopic guidance. This is unfortunate because there are no substantial studies in the literature to determine outcome data from such an approach. In contrast, there is considerable evidence in support of a fluoroscopic approach (Thurmond et al. 1987; Thurmond and Rösch 1990; Confino et al. 1990; Gleicher et al. 1993).

We began tubal catheterisation procedures via the hysteroscopic approach (Confino et al. 1988). During that initial pilot phase, it rapidly became apparent that a fluoroscopic approach has a number of significant advantages. First, it allows immediate integration of the tubal catheterisation procedure into the diagnostic work-up, following HSG and/or SS. Secondly, it reduces the need for expensive time in the operating theatre and for anaesthesia. Thirdly, it allows instant recognition of whether tubal patency has been achieved, while an exclusively hysteroscopic approach does not. While a concomitant laparoscopy will permit an instant diagnosis, even the combination of both these procedures will not give comparable information on the endotubal architecture once patency has been acheived. Finally, we have concluded that the fluoroscopically guided approach is quicker and simpler and will result in superior patency rates. This is confirmed by the very limited published literature comparing these approaches (Confino et al. 1988; Novy 1989; Patton et al. 1991). Overall, hysteroscopically controlled tubal recanalisation succeeds in approximately 60% of patients, while fluoroscopically controlled procedures uniformly achieve patency in approximately 90% of cases (Confino et al. 1988; Novy 1989; Patton et al. 1991; Hisao Osada, Nihon University, personal communication, Tokyo, Japan, March 1992).

It is unusual for a gynaecologist to promote a radiological approach; however, the conclusions reached at our Center are now based on nearly 500 procedures utilising a gynaeco-radiological approach. Our situation is unique in that we have our own fluoroscopy room. This obviously simplifies our approach, whereas most gynaecologists will be dependent on a co-operative effort with radiologists. We strongly recommend such a co-operative effort. Radiologists have become quite active in the area of tubal recanalisation treatment (Thurmond et al. 1987; Thurmond and Rösch 1990). They would clearly also benefit from the co-operation of gynaecologists which would ensure a more integrated approach to infertility treatment. Gynaecologists, in turn, would benefit from easy access to the newest fluoroscopic technology and would gain the opportunity to learn a new medium.

There are also some indications for a hysteroscopically guided approach. This makes sense during separately indicated endoscopic procedures. The various catheter technologies are applicable in either way. Moreover, a third approach, using sonographic guidance, has also been suggested (Confino et al. 1989; Stern et al. 1991). The latter has been proposed primarily out of concern for X-ray exposure to the ovaries, even though modern fluoroscopy equipment and limited exposure times are associated with an extremely low risk (Gleicher et al. 1992b).

# Diagnosis and Treatment of Ectopic Pregnancies

A special application of transvaginal tubal catheter technology is diagnosis and treatment of ectopic pregnancies. Even very small tubal pregnancies can be diagnosed with HSG and especially SS (Gleicher et al. 1992c). Other investigators have reported conservative treatment of tubal pregnancies utilising tubal catheterisation techniques (Risquez et al. 1990).

# Conclusion

Diagnosis and treatment of proximal tubal disease has changed radically over the last few years. Primarily as a result of various new catheterisation techniques, the transvaginal approach towards the fallopian tube has become routine. Considerable additional progress in this area can be expected as new techniques and instrumentation are being developed.

# References

Capitanio, GL et al. (1991) Transcervical selective salpingography: a diagnostic and therapeutic approach to cases of proximal tubal injection failure. Fertil Steril 55:1045–1050

Confino E, Friberg J, Gleicher N (1986) Transcervical balloon tuboplasty. Fertil Steril 46:963–966

Confino E, Friberg J, Gleicher N (1988) Preliminary experience with transcervical balloon tuboplasty (TBT). Am J Obstet Gynecol 159:370–375

Confino E, Tur-Kaspa I, Friberg J, Gleicher N (1989) Sonographic transcervical balloon tuboplasty. Presented at the 45th Annual Meeting of the American Fertility Society, San Francisco, California, November 13–16

Confino E et al. (1990) Transcervical balloon tuboplasty. JAMA 264:2079–2082

Confino E, Tur-Kaspa I, Gleicher N (1992) Sonographic balloon tuboplasty. Hum Reprod 7:1271–1274

De Cherney AH (1987) Anything you can do better . . . or differently! Fertil Steril 48:374–378

Gleicher N, Parrilli M, Redding L, Pratt D (1991) Hysterosalpingography (HSG) and selective salpingography (SS) as therapeutic procedures. Presented at the 47th Annual Meeting of the American Fertility Society, Orlando FL, October 19–24, 1991

Gleicher N, Pratt DE, Parralli M (1992a) Treatment of tubal disease by hysterosalpingography and selective salpingography. In: Gleicher N (ed) Tubal catheterization procedures. Wiley-Liss, New York, pp 55–69

Gleicher N, Pratt DE, Parrilli M (1992b) Diagnosis of tubal disease by hysterosalpingography and selective salpingography. In: Gleicher N (ed) Tubal catheterization procedures. Wiley-Liss, New York, pp 28–53

Gleicher N, Parrilli M, Pratt DE (1992c) Hysterosalpingography and selective salpingography in the differential diagnosis of chemical intrauterine versus tubal pregnancy. Fertil Steril 57:553–558

Gleicher N, Harlow L, Zilberstein M (1992d) The regulatory effect of antiphospholipid antibodies (APA) on signal transduction: a possible model for autoantibody induced reproductive failure. Fertil Steril 58:1136–1141

Gleicher N et al. (1993) The multicenter transcervical balloon tuboplasty study: conclusions and comparison to alternative technologies. Hum Reprod 8:1264–1271

Kaseki H, Akira S, Ienaga S, Araki T (1991) The measurement of intrafallopian pressure. Seventh World Congress on IVF and Assisted Procreation, Paris, France June 30–July 3 Human Reproduction (suppl) P236, pp 249–250
Musich JR, Behrman SJ (1983) Surgical management of tubal obstruction of the uterotubal junction. Fertil Steril 40:423–441
Novy MJ (1989) Combined hysteroscopic and microsurgical approach to intrauterine sequelae and cornual occlusion. Annual meeting of the American Fertility Society, San Francisco, Nov 13–16
Patton PE, Hickok LR, Wolf DP (1991) Succesful hysteroscopic cannulation and tubal transfer of cryopreserved embryos. Fertil Steril 55:640–641
Platia MP, Krudy AG (1985) Transcervical fluoroscopic recanalization of proximally occluded oviduct. Fertil Steril 44:704–706
Risquez F et al. (1990) Diagnosis and treatment of ectopic pregnancy by retrograde selective salpingography and intraluminal methotrexate injection: work in progress. Hum Reprod 5:759–762
Sher G, Vaught LK, Vaught WG, Knutzen VK (1989) The influence of age, uterine length, pre-post egg retrieval pressure estradiol drop, and the number of cleaved embryos transferred to the uterus, on outcome following in vitro fertilization and embryo transfer (IVF/ET). Sixth World Congress on In Vitro Fertilization and Alternate Assisted Reproduction, Jerusalem, Israel, April 2–7, Proceedings, Plenum, New York, p 70
Stern JJ, Peters AJ, Coulam CB (1991) Transcervical tuboplasty under ultrasonographic guidance: a pilot study. Fertil Steril 56:359–360
Sulak PJ et al. (1987a) Histology of proximal tubal occlusion. Fertil Steril 48:437–440
Sulak PJ, Letterie GS, Hayslip CC, Coddington CC, Klein TA (1987b) Hysteroscopic cannulation and lavage in the treatment of proximal tubal occlusion. Fertil Steril 48:493–495
Thurmond AS, Rösch J (1990) Nonsurgical fallopian tube recanalization for treatment of infertility. Radiology 174:371–374
Thurmond AS, Novy M, Uchida BT, Rösch J (1987) Fallopian tube obstruction: selective salpingography and recanalization. Radiology 163:511–515
Zbella EA (1992) Clinical approach to tubal disease. In: Gleicher N (ed) Tubal catheterization procedures. Wiley-Liss, New York, pp 15–25

Chapter 11

# Transcervical Tubal Cannulation in the Diagnosis and Treatment of Tubal Obstruction

A.S. Thurmond

## Introduction

The placement of small catheters directly in the proximal fallopian tube with selective injection of contrast agent allows us to overcome tubal "spasm" and improve visualisation of tubal anatomy. Probing of the proximal fallopian tube with a small guide wire is effective in dislodging debris or breaking up fine adhesions which cause tubal occlusion and result in infertility. In the past these patients would have needed laparotomy with tubal microsurgery, or in vitro fertilisation (Patton et al. 1986; Gillett and Herbison 1989).

## Indications

Patients with obstruction visualised by hysterosalpingography or laparoscopy in the interstitial or proximal isthmic portions of the tube (usually within 3 cm of the uterine cavity) are candidates for tubal cannulation. Obstruction in this region is often caused by amorphous debris or fine adhesions, and is amenable to catheter techniques (Sulak et al. 1987). Obstruction at the fimbriated portion of the tube tends to be caused by fibrosis and peritubal disease which are probably not amenable to simple catheter techniques.

Selective salpingography should be performed if the patient will benefit from visualisation of the entire tube on the side of the proximal obstruction, or if it is felt that the proximal tubal obstruction is a cause of infertility.

The procedure should not be performed if there is active vaginal bleeding, pelvic infection, or the possibility of early pregnancy. If there is an intrauterine mass which is blocking the cornual region on the side of the tubal obstruction, consideration should be given to surgical removal (often possible with hysteroscopy). This is because the mass may be the cause of the tubal obstruction; even if it is not the cause it may well interfere with effective catheterisation. Obstructions which are clearly at the site of a previous tubal reanastomosis are more difficult to recanalise, presumably because the cause is usually fibrosis. Occasionally recanalisation has been successful in these patients; however the success rate is lower than in patients who have blockage and no history of proximal tubal anastomosis.

# Technique

Fallopian tube catheterisation in patients with tubal disease is best performed using fluoroscopic guidance with injection of iodinated contrast media through the catheter. This allows the best visualisation of the fallopian tube for diagnostic purposes (Fig. 11.1). Fallopian tube catheterisation for proximal tubal obstruction has been performed using ultrasound guidance (Lisse and Sydow 1991; Stern et al. 1991). However, the inability to visualise the distal anatomy or to differentiate between perforation or successful recanalisation limits the use of ultrasound. Hysteroscopy/laparoscopy has been successfully used to guide catheters for proximal tubal recanalisation (Novy et al. 1988). This may be the preferred method if the patient also has pelvic adhesions which could be removed laparoscopically at the same time.

The procedure is performed during the follicular phase of the menstrual cycle at least 2 days after bleeding has stopped (to avoid flushing of blood into the fallopian tubes or peritoneal cavity), and before the patient has ovulated. The patient receives doxycycline 100 mg by mouth b.i.d. for 5 days starting 2 days before the procedure, or 200 mg by mouth just before the procedure followed by 100 mg by mouth b.i.d. for 5 days. Atropine and small doses of midazolam may be given intravenously before the procedure, and small doses of fentanyl citrate or other pain medication may be given during the procedure. For most patients intravenous medication is not necessary.

A hysterosalpingography (HSG) device is applied to the cervix e.g., a vacuum cup type device (Thurmond-Rosch Hysterocath; Cook, Inc., Bloomington, IN, or Cook OB/Gyn, Spencer, IN). This provides a sterile conduit through which catheters can be advanced, and allows traction on the uterus without a tenaculum (Thurmond et al. 1990). A conventional hysterosalpingogram is performed initially which allows localisation of the uterine cornua (Fig. 11.1a). Diluted water-soluble contrast medium (such as Conray 60 diluted 1:2 with saline) is used so as not to obscure visualisation of the catheters. A coaxial catheter system is used to engage the tubal ostium, and then to catheterise the proximal fallopian tube (Thurmond and Rösch 1990a). A 0.035-inch diameter-J guide wire, supported by a 9-F Teflon sheath and 5.5-F polyethylene catheter, is advanced into the uterine cornua (Fig. 11.1b,c). The 5.5-F catheter is advanced over the guide wire into the

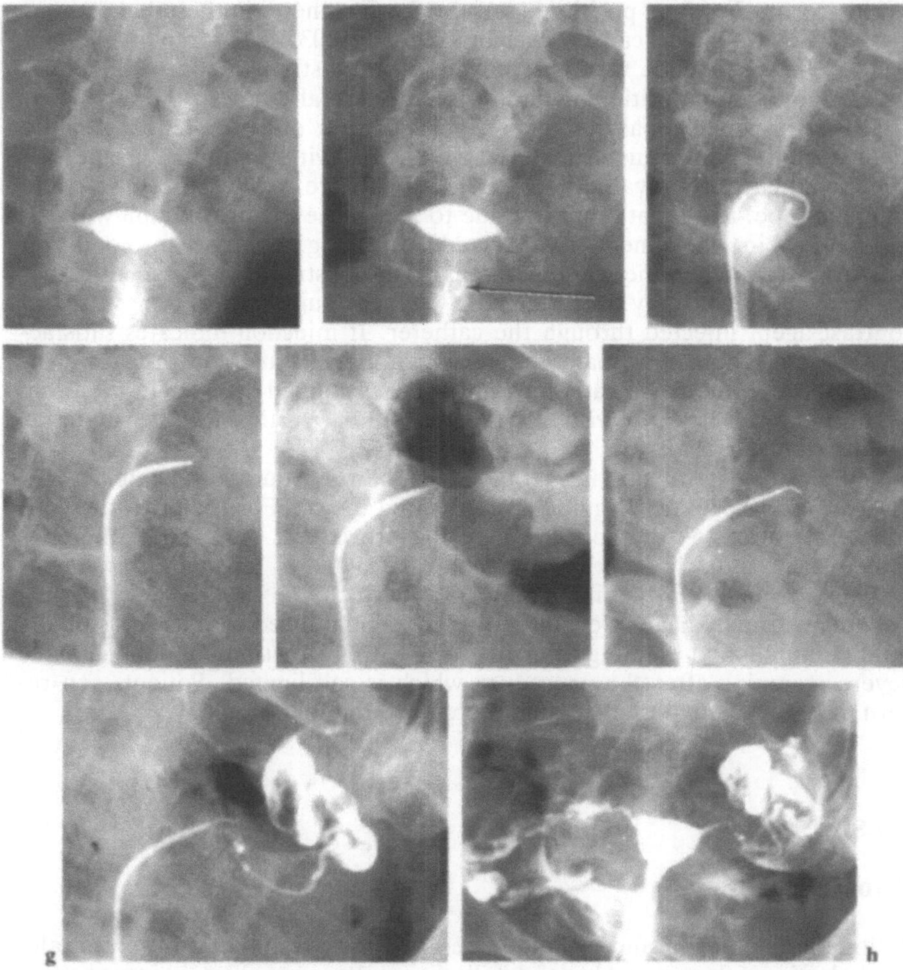


**Fig. 11.1a,b,c,d,e,f.** 28-year-old woman with 3 years of primary infertility. Prior to this examination she had one hysterosalpingogram (HSG) and 2 laparoscopies which documented bilateral proximal tubal obstruction. During the most recent laparoscopy she had bilateral fimbrioplasty performed. Bilateral catheter recanalisation of the proximal tubal obstructions was requested. **a.** Initial HSG confirms the bilateral proximal tubal obstruction. **b.** The 5.5-F catheter (not visible) and 0.035-inch J-guide wire (arrow) are coaxially advanced through the Hysterocath and endocervical canal. **c.** Using fluoroscopic guidance, the catheter and wire are advanced into the left uterine cornu. **d.** The catheter is wedged into the tubal ostium using a 0.035-inch straight guide wire (visible), and then the guide wire is removed. **e.** Full-strength contrast medium is directly injected into the left tube and obstruction approximately 2 mm from the tip of the catheter is confirmed. **f.** A .0015-inch guide wire and 3-F catheter are used gently to probe the obstruction. (Wire is visible, catheter tip is marked by a radiopaque bead.) **g.** Injection through the 5.5-F catheter shows that the tube is now widely patent, and there are some nodules in the isthmic portion of the tube at the site of the prior obstruction, consistent with salpingitis isthmica nodosa. **h.** Similar procedure was performed on the right side. Repeat HSG at the conclusion of the procedure demonstrates bilateral tubal patency.

uterine cornu. For final positioning of the 5.5-F catheter in the tubal ostium, the 0.035-inch J-guide can be exchanged for a 0.035-inch straight LT wire (Fig. 11.1d). The guide wire is removed, and full-strength contrast agent is injected to confirm positioning and to attempt visualisation of the tube (Fig. 11.1e). If proximal tubal obstruction persists after direct injection into the tubal ostium, a 0.015-inch diameter guide wire with platinum tip and 3-F Teflon catheter are advanced together through the 5.5-F catheter into the fallopian tube, and an attempt is made to recanalise the obstruction with to-and-fro probing movements of the guide wire (Fig. 11.1f) (Thurmond and Rösch 1990b). When the guide wire passes the obstruction, the small catheter is advanced coaxially over the guide wire, the guide wire is removed, and contrast agent injected through the catheter. If injection indicates satisfactory recanalisation, the small catheter is withdrawn, and contrast agent injected through the 5.5-F catheter (which has remained in place in the tubal ostium) in order better to visualise the entire tube, particularly the site of recanalisation (Fig. 11.1g).

If the contralateral side is also blocked, the procedure is repeated by reinserting the 0.035-inch J-guide and directing the 5.5-F catheter to the contralateral cornu. At the conclusion of the procedure, the 5.5-F catheter is drawn back into the uterus, and contrast agent is injected for a post-catheterisation hysterosalpingogram (Fig. 11.1h).

Patients usually have a few days of mild vaginal bleeding and occasionally mild cramping and bloating after the procedure. Occasionally patients have severe cramping after the procedure which is self-limited. Patients can return to normal activities including intercourse the following day.

# Results

## Tubal Visualisation

Using the equipment and technique described above, reported success rates for selective salpingography and fallopian tube recanalisation range from 75% to 92% (Thurmond 1991). Transcervical balloon tuboplasty, which uses different equipment but essentially the same technique, has also yielded high success rates (Confino et al. 1990). Approximately one-third of patients who undergo fallopian tube catheterisation for proximal tubal obstruction (unilateral or bilateral), have normal-appearing tubes following the procedure. Another one-third have normal tube; however the appearance of the peritoneal spill suggests peritubal adhesions. Of the remaining patients, 8% will have a small dilation at the site of the recanalisation; 8% will have frank salpingitis isthmica nodosa; and 8% will have a distal occlusion or hydrosalpinx. Approximately 10% will have unsuccessful attempts at recanalisation and will have persistent proximal tubal obstruction.

## Pregnancy Rates

We evaluated the therapeutic effect of fallopian tube recanalisation in 20 carefully selected patients in whom proximal tubal obstruction was thought to be the primary or sole cause of infertility (Thurmond and Rösch 1990b). All had bilateral proximal tubal obstruction by at least two HSGs and by laparoscopy, with no distal tubal disease identified by laparoscopy. The average duration of infertility was 4 years. Seven of the 20 women had additional infertility factors. All 20 patients had been recommended for tubal microsurgery or in vitro fertilisation, but underwent catheter recanalisation instead. Recanalisation of one or both tubes was successful in 19 women (95%). Fifty-eight percent of the women conceived by 1 year, without receiving any other therapy, and all pregnancies were intrauterine. Similar pregnancy rates have been reported by others (Confino et al. 1990; Platia et al. 1989).

### Reocclusion Rate

The tubal reocclusion rate is difficult to determine because in part it is time-dependent. In patients who do not conceive, some 50% of tubes reocclude by 6 months. If it is assumed that the tubes are patent in the patients who conceive, this gives an approximate reocclusion rate of 25% (Thurmond and Rösch 1990a; Confino et al. 1990; Kumpe et al. 1990). Repeat catheter recanalisation is technically possible and pregnancies have resulted after the second procedure.

## Complications

Perforation of a tube occurs in 5%–10% of cases (Thurmond 1991; Kumpe et al. 1990). The perforation rate has remained stable as we have gained more experience, and appears to be more related to the underlying pathology than to technical factors. Adverse consequences of perforation have not been reported and additional monitoring or treatment has not been necessary.

In patients with patent tubes following fallopian tube recanalisation, the reported ectopic pregnancy rate has varied between 0% and 13%. It appears that the risk of developing an ectopic pregnancy is increased in the presence of distal tubal disease. In our series all ectopic pregnancies were located in the ampulla of the tube, several centimetres distal to the site of the proximal catheterisation. The proportion of ectopic pregnancies is lower in studies in which patients with known concurrent distal disease were excluded (Thurmond and Rösch 1990a; Confino et al. 1990).

Pelvic infection following tubal catheterisation is a possibility. Using the prophylactic regimen described above the incidence of pelvic inflammation requiring treatment has been less than 0.5%. Patients should be warned of this complication, nonetheless, since occasionally even standard hysterosalpingography has resulted in severe, life-threatening pelvic infection.

Estimated radiation dose to the ovaries from the procedure is about 1 rad, which is within acceptable limits for a diagnostic procedure in women of child-bearing age (Kumpe et al. 1990; Hedgpeth et al. 1991).

As with all catheter procedures there is the possibility of bleeding, vasovagal reaction, or idiosyncratic reaction to contrast media. If the appropriate technique and standard precautions are used the incidence of these complications should be very low.

## Summary

Selective salpingography and fallopian tube recanalisation offer an improved method of diagnosis and treatment for proximal tubal obstruction. This procedure has an 85%–90% chance of opening the tube and allowing its visualisation. The risks and side effects are minimal. Selective salpingography and fallopian tube recanalisation should be the next step in evaluating a woman with proximal tubal obstruction by hysterosalpingogram or laparoscopy. The more expensive and more invasive techniques of tubal microsurgery or in vitro fertilisation should be reserved for the small number of patients in whom fallopian tube recanalisation is not successful.

## References

Confino E et al. (1990) Transcervical balloon tuboplasty. JAMA 264:2079–2082

Gillett WR, Herbison GP (1989) Tubocornual anastomosis: surgical considerations and coexistent infertility factors in determining the prognosis. Fertil Steril 51:241–246

Hedgpeth PL, Thurmond AS, Fry R, Schmidgall JR, Rösch J (1991) Ovarian radiation dose in radiologic fallopian tube recanalization. Radiology 180:121–122

Kumpe DA, Zwerdlinger SC, Rothbarth LJ, Durham JD, Albrecht BH (1990) Proximal fallopian tube occlusion: diagnosis and treatment with transcervical fallopian tube catheterization. Radiology 177:183–187

Lisse K, Sydow P (1991) Fallopian tube catheterization and recanalization under ultrasonic observation: a simplified technique to evaluate tubal patency and open proximally obstructed tubes. Fertil Steril 56:198–201

Novy MJ, Thurmond AS, Patton PE, Uchida BT, Rösch J (1988) Diagnosis of cornual obstruction by transcervical fallopian tube cannulation. Fertil Steril 50:434–440

Patton PE, Williams TJ, Coulam CB (1986) Microsurgical reconstruction of the proximal oviduct. Fertil Steril 47:35–39

Platia M, Chang R, Loriaux DL, Doppman JL (1989) Therapeutic potential of transvaginal recanalization for proximal fallopian tube obstruction. Paper #O-056, presented at the AFS annual meeting, San Francisco, CA, November 14

Stern JJ, Peters AJ, Coulam CB (1991) Transcervical tuboplasty under ultrasonographic guidance: a pilot study. Fertil Steril 56:359–360

Sulak PJ et al. (1987) Histology of proximal tubal occlusion. Fertil Steril 48:437–440

Thurmond AS (1991) Selective salpingography and fallopian tube recanalization. AJR 156:33–38

Thurmond AS, Rösch J (1990a) Nonsurgical fallopian tube recanalization for treatment of infertility. Radiology 174:371–374

Thurmond AS, Rösch J (1990b) Fallopian tubes: improved technique for catheterization. Radiology 174:572–573

Thurmond AS, Uchida BT, Rösch J (1990) Device for hysterosalpingography and fallopian tube catheterization. Radiology 174:571–572

Chapter 12

# Laser Technology: Endometriosis and Tubal Surgery

C. Sutton

## Introduction

The theoretical possibility of using laser energy in fertility surgery has existed ever since 1917, when Einstein published his quantum theory of radiation (Einstein 1917) but it was not until 1958 that Townes and Schavlow actually proposed the concept of stimulated emission of radiation to produce laser light (Schavlow and Townes 1958). Maiman (1960) created the first laser, a Ruby laser and for a long time this was an invention awaiting an application. In 1964 Patel, working for Bell Communications, developed the $CO_2$ laser (Patel et al. 1964) but the argon laser was the first to be introduced into medicine and was used initially in ophthalmology. Since then lasers have been used to a greater or lesser extent in virtually all specialities (Sutton and Hodgson 1992).

## Tissue Effects and Healing with the $CO_2$ Laser

In gynaecology the $CO_2$ laser was first used for the treatment of cervical intra-epithelial neoplasia because it had the advantage over cold-knife or diathermy conisation of rapid healing. When the cervix was examined 6 weeks after laser treatment it was difficult, with the naked eye, to differentiate between the area that had been treated and the surrounding normal tissue. The fact that all tissue debris is evacuated as smoke in the laser plume means that healing occurs with very little tissue oedema, and therefore less pain. There is minimal scarring, wound contracture and anatomical distortion (Allen et al. 1983). Thus, the $CO_2$ laser should be the ideal instrument for the delicate microsurgery required to restore fertility with the added advantage that the light energy can be passed down hollow metal tubes or silicone-quartz wave-guides for tissue vaporisation at laparoscopic surgery.

The first experimental studies of wound healing on the peritoneal surface were conducted by Bellina et al. (1984) on New Zealand white rabbits. He found that laser wounds healed better than those of electrocautery. The beam is strongly absorbed by water and since the majority of biological tissue volume is water, the penetration of the $CO_2$ laser is very superficial; 99.9% of the incident power is absorbed in the first 0.1 mm of soft tissue. This mode of action limits the zone of irreversible tissue damage to 70 $\mu$m (Baggish 1980), and even as little as 50 $\mu$m with the new generation of ultrapulse lasers (Coherent, Cambridge, UK) which deliver very high-pulse energy bursts of up to 250 mJ and average powers of 950 mW (Sutton and Hodgson 1993). Although there is some cellular damage up to 200 $\mu$m, healing from this area occurs rapidly and without scarring (Bellina 1978). Thus, using a $CO_2$ laser beam with a TEM oo mode and a spot size of 200 $\mu$m it is possible, given rapid speed of transit and high power density, for the surgeon to make a 350-$\mu$m incision (Kelly 1990). This is not possible with other techniques. Microcautery will make an incision of less than 1 mm, but the area of thermal necrosis (irreversible tissue damage) extends 1 mm deeper than the incision base and 1 mm lateral on either side, resulting in an incision that is 2–3 mm in width (Kelly 1990).

Some micro-surgeons attempt laser surgery without any training or real understanding of the interaction of laser light with human tissues. To use it in a comparable way to a microdiathermy needle will lead to poor results and disenchantment with the laser as a surgical tool. The surgeon must have a clear idea of the correct spot size, operating mode and speed of transit of the laser beam over the target tissue to achieve the power density necessary to vaporise tissue rather than to cause carbonisation and charring (Absten 1992; Reid 1992).

Bellina (1974) first introduced the $CO_2$ laser into tubal reconstructive surgery, aiming the laser beam by a micromanipulator through an operating microscope. The fine control thus achieved might enable the surgeon to produce clean, haemostatic incisions with minimal lateral damage and a decrease of adhesions and scarring. Sadly, this promise has not been realised. All that can now be claimed is that it makes certain cases technically easier. For example, in awkward access situations such as the posterior surface of an adherent ovary the laser light can be reflected off a gold-plated mirror (Kelly 1990).

There are many published retrospective studies (Winston 1980; Gomel and Swolin 1980; Mage and Bruhat 1983; Bellina et al. 1984; Kelly and Roberts 1983). The prospective study of Tulandi et al. (1984) and Tulandi and Vilos (1985) showed little advantage of the $CO_2$ laser over conventional electrocautery apart from a shorter surgery to conception interval at 1-year follow-up (Tulandi et al. 1984) although even that was not statistically different at 2 years (Tulandi and Vilos 1985).

Despite the initial enthusiasm for using a “no-touch” surgical technique the initial results, even in terms of adhesion formation, were disappointing (Diamond et al. 1987). A reduction in peritoneal mesothelial plasminogen activator activity (PAA) due to trauma tissue ischaemia is the likely mechanism of postsurgical adhesion formation (Buckman et al. 1976; Raftery 1981; Menzies and Ellis 1989). The biological interaction between lasers and living tissue minimises this trauma. Infection is less likely with laparoscopy than laparotomy; the ischaemia produced by surgical knots, which are used extensively in microsurgery, is avoided by the use of lasers. Although prospective studies have shown no difference in adhesion reformation between the laser and the microdiathermy needle (Tulandi 1987) animal experiments have clearly shown a marked reduction of adhesion formation, and less adhesion formation with laparoscopic adhesiolysis (Luciano et al. 1989). The ability to perform surgery laparoscopically is the most important feature; the laser merely provides the most convenient tool for this surgery.

## Laser Laparoscopic Tubal Surgery

The precise incisions yielded by the $CO_2$ laser make it an ideal instrument for the division of peri-tubal or peri-ovarian adhesions (Fig. 12.1). This is particularly true of a superpulse or ultrapulse mode which have the smallest spot size and high power density. However, great care must be taken to avoid opening the venous plexus between the tube and ovary. In this situation a back-stop should always be used.

Patients with adhesions following peritonitis, usually secondary to appendicitis, tend to have a normal endosalpinx with undamaged cilia and healthy mucosal folds. They have excellent pregnancy rates following laser salpingolysis. During the past 8 years we have treated 56 of these patients in Guildford and 34 (61.7%) have become pregnant, the majority within the subsequent 6 cycles. Donnez and Nisolle (1989) have reported a similar success rate; 108 (58%) viable pregnancies in 186 patients. In neither of these series were any ectopic pregnancies reported. Similar success rates have been re-

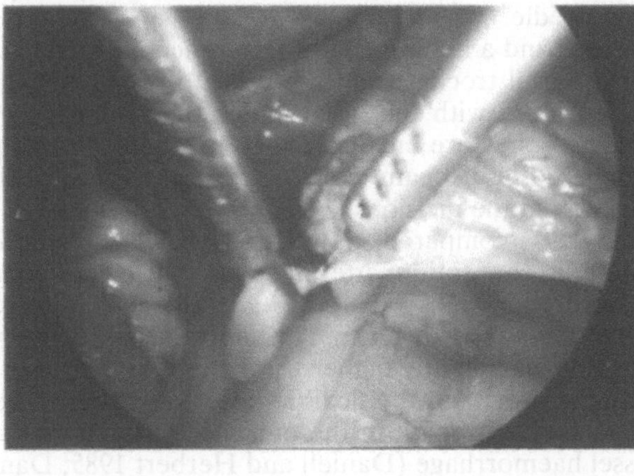

**Fig. 12.1.** Laparoscopic removal of fimbrial cyst with KTP fibre laser.

ported by laparoscopic procedures using scissors, with or without electrodissection, but these series have all reported ectopic pregnancy rates of 5%–8% (Gomel 1983; Bruhat et al. 1983; Reich 1987). Both methods are equally suitable for thin avascular lesions. However the $CO_2$ laser is more effective when the adhesions are dense and vascular since it allows more precise incision with minimal damage to adjacent tissue. Laser adhesiolysis is always more effective if traction is applied with atraumatic grasping forceps. Vaporisation is quicker and accompanied by less heat generation if a high power density, and a superpulse mode, is employed. It is imperative when operating in the vicinity of the fallopian tubes or bowel to use a back-stop, either on the laser probe as a "firing platform" or a titanium rod placed behind the adhesion to protect distal tissues from damage.

## Laparoscopic Laser Salpingostomy for Tubal Infertility

The commonest site of tubal occlusion is at the fimbrial end. The overall success rate of tubal surgery for hydrosalpinges, even when performed by microsurgical techniques, is poor, with a success rate in most series varying between 20% and 40% (Tulandi and Vilos 1985; Donnez and Casanas-Roux 1986; Singhal et al. 1991; Winston and Magara 1991). It is no longer justifiable to subject patients to major surgery when similar results can be obtained by laparoscopic salpingostomy (Gomel 1977; Daniell et al. 1986; Donnez and Nisolle 1989; Bruhat et al. 1989) or assisted conception techniques (Guzicks et al. 1986).

The procedure is as follows. The hydrosalpinx is distended with methylene blue dye instilled transcervically. A cruciate incision is made with a $CO_2$ or KTP/532 laser using a 300 $\mu$m fibre. An Nd:YAG laser with a fibertom tip (MBBS, Munich, Germany), artificial sapphire tips (SLT, Malvern, Penn, USA) or sculpted quartz tips (Sharplan, Tel Aviv, Israel) can also be used but the tissue damage produced is purely due to a thermal effect (Keckstein 1989, 1992) which could just as easily be produced by a microdiathermy needle.

Grasping forceps and a hook made of non-reflective metal are inserted via third and fourth portal trochars and are used to display the tissue edges as the incision is enlarged with the laser. Once the four flaps of the fimbrae have been prepared they are encouraged to evert like flower petals using a low power defocused laser beam over the serosal surface of the tube a few millimetres away from the incisions.

Daniell et al. (1991) compared the $CO_2$ and KTP lasers in a series of 120 patients attempting conception after laparoscopic neosalpingostomy. The tubal patency rate at 6 weeks was 83%. Overall there were 63 pregnancies (52%) of which 28% went to term, 12% aborted and 13% were ectopics. The pregnancy rate was slightly higher using the KTP/532 laser (31% against 25% with the $CO_2$ laser) and the flexible fibre was easier to use, generating less smoke. The ability to work in the presence of fluids was useful in stopping small vessel haemorrhage (Daniell and Herbert 1985; Daniell 1989).

## Laser Laparoscopic Treatment of Endometriosis

Since laparoscopy is essential to establish the diagnosis of pelvic endometriosis (Jansen and Russell 1986; Martin et al. 1989a) it is convenient for the patient if reduction of endometrial implants and restoration of normal tubo-ovarian anatomy can be achieved at the same time. The most precise way to vaporise ectopic endometrial tissue and to divide adhesions is to use a $CO_2$ laser transmitted down the central channel of the laparoscope (Donnez and Nisolle 1989) or, more safely, via a second portal probe (Daniell and Herbert 1985; Sutton 1985; Borten and Friedman 1986).

With the new generation of $CO_2$ lasers which incorporate an ultrapulse facility (Coherent Lasers, Palo Alto, California; Cambridge, UK) it is possible to limit the adjacent zone of irreversible tissue necrosis to as little as 50 $\mu$m. In skilled hands this accurate char-free tissue destruction allows endometriosis to be removed from potentially hazardous areas such as the bladder, bowel and ureter (Wilson 1988).

If laser technology is not available electrocautery is an alternative (Murphy et al. 1991) but may be less safe because of the difficulty in assessing the depth of tissue destruction. If electrosurgery is employed great care must be taken to avoid thermal or electrical conductance injuries to the bowel, bladder and ureter (Cheng 1976; DiNovo 1983; Baumann et al. 1988). However if recognised at the time it is now possible to repair such injuries laparoscopically (Reich and McGlynn 1990; Gomel and James 1991; Nezhat 1991).

## Laparoscopic Laser Surgery for Ovarian Endometriomas

In patients with more diffuse deposits and in those with ovarian endometriomas (chocolate cysts) and gross distortion of pelvic anatomy, a Potassium-Titanyl-Phosphate (KTP/532) visible light laser is more suitable (Laserscope, San Jose, California). This emerald-green visible light-laser can be transmitted down flexible silicone quartz fibres to allow laser energy to be delivered to otherwise inaccessible sites (Fig.12.2). It also has the advantage of working in the presence of blood and haemosiderin. Since the wave length of 532 nm is close to the absorption band for haemoglobin, it is selectively taken up by pigmented endometriotic tissue.

The argon laser produces a mixture of blue-green light of several wave lengths between 488 nm and 515 nm. It has tissue effects similar to the KTP laser with regard to photocoagulation but does not perform as well at laparoscopic surgery when cutting is required. This is because the end of the fibre burns off during the cutting procedure. Continuous measurements of the loss of laser power at the fibre tip during cutting show a nearly exponential decrease of power output with length of cut. After 50 cm only 10% of the laser power exits from the fibre tip. Correspondingly, the cutting efficiency is re-

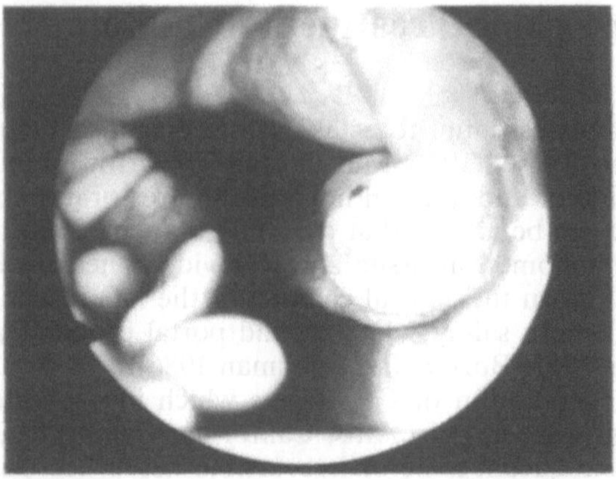

**Fig. 12.2.** Endometriosis of tube. Tube swollen and congested, but invariably patent.

duced to 30% but without any influence on the coagulation zone (Keckstein et al. 1988). This explains the disappointment felt by some surgeons when trying to use this laser for laparoscopic salpingolysis or salpingostomy. It is essentially a coagulating laser and is not as effective a surgical tool as the KTP laser. Moreover it requires special plumbing for water cooling and lacks the ability of the KTP laser to produce pure Nd:YAG energy by a simple switch mirror mechanism (Daniell 1992; Sutton and Hodgson 1992).

The argon and KTP/532 lasers are particularly suitable for the laparoscopic treatment of ovarian endometriomas (chocolate cysts) for which photocoagulation of the cyst lining is associated with a low recurrence rate (Brosens and Puttemans 1989; Marrs 1991). The thinnest part of the ovarian capsule overlying the endometrioma is fenestrated using a 300-$\mu$m fibre. The chocolate fluid is aspirated and irrigated until clear and the entire lining of the endometrioma can then be examined under the magnification gained by placing the tip of the laparoscope close to the endothelial surface. Several biopsies can be taken before photocoagulating the entire surface and sealing all blood vessels with the visible light laser at about 12 W.

We have used this technique in Guildford over the past 3 years. Most of our patients have been tertiary referrals with extensive fibrotic endometriosis, thick adhesions distorting the tubo-ovarian anatomy, complete obliteration of the cul-de-sac with the rectum densely adherent to the back of the uterus and large endometriomas between 4 cm and 12 cm in diameter. All 65 patients had an American Fertility Society (AFS) score of greater than 75. All had previously been on different types of drug therapy and many had undergone conventional conservative surgery by laparotomy. Ten of the 33 patients (30.3%) with infertility became pregnant within 5 months of the laser laparoscopy after a length of infertility ranging from 14 years to 2 years (mean 6.5 years). Of the 52 women with pelvic pain, 34 (65.4%) reported resolution or marked improvement in their symptoms following laser laparoscopic surgery.

Employing the same technique Daniell et al. (1991) have recently reported pain relief in 79.4% of 29 patients with pelvic pain due to large endometriomas and a crude pregnancy rate of 37.5% in 32 patients trying to conceive. This may be compared with the total lack of pregnancies in patients with severe endometriosis after laparoscopic removal of the fluid from the Pouch of Douglas and dye hydrotubation (Olive et al. 1985).

Although the Neodymium:YAG laser has been used by some surgeons (Corson 1992) this instrument produces an unacceptably large zone of tissue necrosis beneath the surface (Fisher 1987) making it less suitable for delicate fertility surgery and particularly intra-ovarian surgery. Attempts to minimise this laser tissue effect by the use of sapphire tips or sculpted quartz fibres rely on a purely thermal effect which can be achieved much more cheaply by electrodiathermy (Keckstein 1989, 1992).

The use of fibre-optic lasers facilitates these procedures by allowing rapid photocoagulation of the cyst wall. However, they can be resected laparoscopically by a combination of blunt traction with ovarian biopsy forceps and scissor dissection (Reich and McGlynn 1986).

Some authors advocate ovarian closure with sutures (Cook and Rock 1991) but this is illogical since the ischaemia produced by surgical knots will increase the likelihood of post-operative adhesion formation (Buckman et al. 1976; Raftery 1981; Menzies and Ellis 1989; Brumstead et al. 1990; Martin 1991; Macdonald and Sutton 1992).

## Laparoscopic Uterine Nerve Ablation and Pre-sacral Neurectomy

Jenkins et al. (1986) using laparoscopy observed that 30% of patients have deposits of endometriosis in the Pouch of Douglas and 15%–20% on the utero-sacral ligaments. The sensory parasympathetic fibres to the cervix and the sensory sympathetic fibres to the corpus traverse the cervical division of the Lee–Frankenhauser plexus which lies in, under and around the attachments of the utero-sacral ligament to the cervix. Sympathetic fibres can also be found in this area which reach the cervix with the uterine arteries. Cyclical bleeding around these fibres from deeply infiltrating endometriosis gives rise to intense dysmenorrhoea, and the deposits in the cul-de-sac give rise to deep dyspareunia. In many patients this is of such a severity that it constitutes an additional infertility factor.

It is unrealistic to expect conservative surgery to cure this disease (Sutton 1990). The aim of laser laparoscopy is restoration of normal tubo-ovarian anatomy and the amelioration of pain by vaporising deposits on the ovaries and utero-sacral ligaments, many of which infiltrate deeply (Martin et al. 1989b; Cornillie et al. 1986). This is best performed by laparoscopic uterine nerve ablation, destroying the parasympathetic component originating from the first to the third and fourth sacral nerves which reach the plexus by the pelvic nerves (nervi erigentes). These parasympathetic fibres in the anterior two-thirds of the utero-sacral ligaments and the small ganglia around the area where the ligaments attach to the cervix have been demonstrated in several studies on cadavers (Latarjet and Roget 1922; Davis 1936; Campbell 1950).

## Safety Precautions and Hazards

The intra-peritoneal use of lasers is potentially very dangerous, yet paradoxically they have enjoyed an excellent safety record largely because the surgeon has to be extremely careful to ensure that the aiming beam is exactly on the targetted tissue before he fires the laser. The surgeon must displace any loops of bowel out of the cul-de-sac and identify the ureter and the vessels running lateral to the utero-sacral ligament before activating the laser. A relatively high power density is used to vaporise a crater about 1 cm in diameter and sufficient depth is achieved when the nerve bundles no longer appear. Care should be taken not to vaporise too deeply because an artery courses deep in the ligament. It is essential to have haemostatic equipment in the form of endocoagulator, bipolar diathermy or endoscopic clips instantly available. If the utero-sacral ligaments are well formed a considerable amount of tissue is vaporised, generating a large amount of smoke which must be extracted while at the same time maintaining sufficient pneumo-peritoneum to continue the procedure.

This simple operation, easily performed with the $CO_2$ laser (Sutton 1989) or KTP laser (Daniell 1989) provides spectacular relief of dysmenorrhoea and deep dyspareunia particularly when the utero-sacral ligaments are infiltrated with endometriosis (Feste 1985; Sutton 1990) and is one of the few procedures in the endoscopic surgical literature that has been subjected to a randomised prospective double-blind trial (Lichten and Bombard 1987).

Another prospective study (Tjaden et al. 1990) has shown that pre-sacral neurectomy performed by laparotomy is effective in relieving mid-line dysmenorrhoea in patients with advanced endometriosis. A similar procedure can be performed laparoscopically using the $CO_2$ laser and hydrodissection to expose the pre-sacral nerve bundle which is then transected. This is very advanced and technically difficult laparoscopic surgery but in skilled hands gives excellent results (Nezhat et al. 1991). The retroperitoneal space in front of the sacral promontory is extremely vascular and the operation is facilitated by the Argon Beam Coagulator in which a unipolar diathermy current passes down a jet of argon gas. This displaces tissue debris and blood out of the surgical field thus allowing effective haemostasis (Daniell 1992a,b).

## Cytoreduction of Endometriosis and Infertility

The association between endometriosis and infertility is imperfectly understood. Even in the absence of anatomical distortion the visual diagnosis of the disease is more common in infertile women (Bancroft et al. 1989; West 1990; Halme et al. 1987; Thomas and Prentice 1992). Nevertheless, cytoreduction of peritoneal implants by lasers, restoration of normal tubo-ovarian anatomy by the division of adhesions and surgical treatment of ovarian endometriomas result in fecundity rates as high as 5.79% even in patients with Stage IV disease (Martin and Olive 1986). This is much superior to the results achieved with anti-endometriosis drugs (Siebel et al. 1982; Olive and Haney 1986). Expectant management alone results in no pregnancies at all in patients with severe disease (Olive et al. 1985). Furthermore there is evidence (Evers 1989) that the disease tends to recur within 2 cycles of cessation of drug therapy whereas in our series of 228 patients followed for 5 years recurrent disease was only present in 9.09% of women during the duration of the study. On second-look laparoscopy it was almost invariably in different locations (Sutton and Hill 1990). We are conducting a prospective double-blind randomised study comparing the results of laser laparoscopy with expectant management. Until such a study has been completed the role of laser laparoscopy in endometriosis-related infertility and pelvic pain remains unknown (Haney 1991).

# References


Absten GT (1992) The physics of light and lasers. In: Sutton CJG (ed) Lasers in gynaecology. Chapman and Hall, London, pp 1–23

Allen JM, Stein DS, Shingleton HM (1983) Regeneration of cervical epithelium after laser vaporisation. Obstet Gynecol 62:700

Baggish MS (1980) High power density carbon dioxide laser therapy for early cervical neoplasia. Am J Obstet Gynecol 136:117–125

Bancroft K, Vaughan Williams CA, Elstein M (1989) Minimal/mild endometriosis and infertility. A review. Br J Obstet Gynaecol 96:454–460

Baumann H, Jaeger P, Hugh A (1988) Ureteral injury after laparoscopic tubal sterilisation by bipolar electrocoagulation. Obstet Gynecol 71:483–485

Bellina JH (1974) Gynaecology and the laser. Contemp Ob Gyn 4:24–34

Bellina JH (1978) Carbon dioxide microsurgery in gynaecology. Int Adv Surg Onc 1:227–236

Bellina JH (1984) Microsurgery of the fallopian tube with the carbon dioxide laser: analysis of 230 cases with a 2 year follow-up. Lasers Surg Med 3:255–260

Bellina JH, Hemmings R, Voros IJ, Ross LF (1984) $CO_2$ laser and electrosurgical wound study with an animal model. A comparison of tissue damage and healing patterns in peritoneal tissue. Am J Obstet Gynecol 148:327

Borten M, Friedman EA (1986) Visual field obstruction in single puncture operative laparoscopy. J Reprod Med 31:1102–1105

Brosens IA, Puttemans PJ (1989) Double-optic laparoscopy: salpingoscopy, ovarian cystoscopy and endo-ovarian surgery with the argon laser. In: Sutton CJG (ed) Laparoscopic surgery. Bailliere's Clinical Obstet Gynaecol Vol 3, no 3, pp 595–608

Bruhat MA et al. (1983) Laparoscopy procedures to promote fertility. Ovariolysis and salpingolysis results of 93 selected cases. Acta Euro Fert 14:113–115

Brumstead JR, Deaton J, Lavigne E, Riddick DH (1990) Postoperative adhesion formation after ovarian wedge resection with and without ovarian reconstruction in the rabbit. Fertil Steril 53:723

Buckman RF, Woods M, Sargent L, Gervin AS (1976) A unifying pathogenic mechanism in the aetiology of intraperitoneal adhesions. J Surg Res 20:1–5

Campbell RM (1950) Anatomy and physiology of sacro-uterine ligaments. MJ Obstet Gynecol 59:1

Cheng VS (1976) Ureteral injury resulting from laparoscopic fulguration of endometriosis implants. Am J Obstet Gynecol 126:1045–1046
Cook AS, Rock JA (1991) The role of laparoscopy in the treatment of endometriosis. Fertil Steril 55:663–680
Cornillie FJ, Oosterlynck D, Lauweryns JM, Konincks PR (1976) Deeply infiltrating pelvic endometriosis: histology and clinical significance. Fertil Steril 53:978–983
Corson SL (1992) Nd:YAG laser laparoscopy. In: Sutton CJG (ed) Lasers in gynaecology, Chapman and Hall, London, pp 141–154
Daniell JF (1989) Fibreoptic laser laparoscopy. In: Sutton CJG (ed) Laparoscopic surgery. Bailliere's Clinical Obstetrics and Gynaecology. Vol 3, No 3, pp 545–562
Daniell JF (1992a) Advanced operative laser laparoscopy. In: Sutton CJG (ed) Lasers in Gynaecology. Chapman and Hall, London, pp 119–139
Daniell JF (1992b) The argon beam coagulator. In: Sutton CJG, Diamond M (eds) Endoscopy surgery for gynaecologists. WB Saunders, London
Daniell JF, Herbert CM (1985) A new second puncture probe for $CO_2$ laser laparoscopy. J Reprod Med 30:89–92
Daniell JP et al. (1986) Clinical results of terminal salpingostomy with the use of the $CO_2$ laser. Fertil Steril 45:175–178
Daniell JP, Kurtz BR, Gurley LD (1991) Laser laparoscopic management of large endometriomas. Fertil Steril 55:692–695
Davis A (1936) Intrinsic dysmenorrhoea. Proc Roy Soc Med 29:931
Diamond MP et al. (1987) Adhesion reformation and de novo adhesion formation following reproductive pelvic surgery. Fertil Steril 47:864
DiNovo JA (1983) Radiofrequency leakage current from unipolar laparoscopic electrocoagulators. J Reprod Med 28:565–575
Donnez J (1989) $CO_2$ laser laparoscopy in infertile women with adnexal adhesions and women with tubal occlusion. J Gynecol Surg 5:47–53
Donnez J, Casanas-Roux F (1986) Prognostic factors of fimbrial microsurgery. Fertil Steril 46:200–204
Donnez J, Nisolle M (1989) Carbon dioxide laser laparoscopic surgery: adhesolysis, salpingostromy, laser uterine nerve ablation and tubal pregnancy. In: Sutton CJG (ed) Laparoscopic surgery. Bailliere's Clinical Obstetrics and Gynaecology, Vol 3, no 3, pp 525–544
Einstein A (1917) Zur Quantumtheory der Strahlung. Physio Z 18:121–128
Evers J (1989) The second look laparoscopy for the evaluation of the results of medical treatment of endometriosis should not be performed during ovarian suppression. Fertil Steril 52:502–504
Feste JR (1985) Laser laparoscopy. A new modality. J Reprod Med 30:413–418
Fisher JC (1987) Basic laser physics and interaction of laser light with soft tissue. In: Shapshay SM (ed) Endoscopic laser surgery handbook. Marcel Dekker Inc, New York, p 118
Gomel V (1977) Microsurgery in infertility. Little, Brown and Co., Boston, Toronto, pp 225–236
Gomel V (1983) Salpingo-ovariolysis by laparoscopy in infertility. Fertil Steril 40:607–611
Gomel V, James C (1991) Intraoperative management of ureteral injury during operative laparoscopy. Fertil Steril 55:416–419
Gomel V, Swolin K (1980) Salpingostomy: microsurgical techniques and results. Clin Obstet Gynaecol 23:1243–1258
Guzicks DS, Wilkes C, Jones HW (1986) Cumulative pregnancy rates for in-vitro fertilisation. Fertil Steril 46:663–667
Halme J, Becker S, Haskill S (1987) Altered maturation and function of peritoneal macrophages; possible role in pathogenesis of endometriosis. Am J Obstet Gynecol 156:783–789
Haney AF (1991) The risks/benefits of laparoscopic cautery for endometriosis. Fertil Steril 55:243–245
Jansen RPS, Russell P (1986) Nonpigmented endometriosis: clinical, laparoscopic and pathologic definition. Am J Obstet Gynecol 155:1154–1159
Jenkins S, Olive DL, Haney AF (1986) Endometriosis: pathogenetic implication of an atomic distribution. Obstet Gynecol 67:325–338
Keckstein J (1989) Laparoscopic treatment of polycystic ovarian syndrome. In: Sutton CJG (ed) Laparoscopic surgery. Bailliere's Clinical Obstetrics and Gynaecology. Vol 3, No 3, pp 563–582
Keckstein J (1992) Tissue effects of different lasers and electro-diathermy. In: Sutton CJG, Diamond M (eds) Endoscopic surgery for gynaecologists. WB Saunders, London

Keckstein J, Finger A, Steiner (1988) Laser application in contact and non-contact procedures: sapphire tips in comparison to "bare fibre," argon laser in comparison to Nd-YAG laser (In German). Lasers Med Surg 4:158–162
Kelly RW (1990) Laser surgery of the fallopian tube. In: Keye WR (ed) Laser surgery in gynaecology and obstetrics. Year Book Medical Publishers, Chicago, pp 166–186
Kelly RW, Roberts DK (1983) Experience with a $CO_2$ laser in gynaecological microsurgery. MJ Obstet Gynaecol 146:285–288
Keye WR, Dixon J (1983) Photocoagulation of endometriosis by the argon laser through the laparoscope. Obstet Gynecol 62:383–386
Latarjet A, Roget P (1922) Le plexus hypogastrique chez la femme. Gynecol Obstet 6:225
Lichten EM, Bombard J (1987) Surgical treatment of dysmenorrhoea with laparoscopic uterine nerve ablation. J Reprod Med 32:37–42
Luciano AA, Maier D, Koch E, Nillsen J, Whitman F (1989) A comparative study of postoperative adhesions following laser surgery by laparoscopy versus laparotomy in the rabbit model. Obstet Gynecol 74:220–224
Macdonald R, Sutton CJG (1992) Adhesions and laser laparoscopic adhesiolysis. In: Sutton CJG (ed) Lasers in gynaecology. Chapman and Hall, London, pp 95–113
Mage G, Bruhat MA (1983) Pregnancy following salpingostomy: comparison between $CO_2$ laser and electrosurgery procedures. Fertil Steril 42:
Maiman TH (1960) Stimulated optical radiation in ruby masers. Nature 187:493–494
Marrs RP (1991) The use of the KTP laser for laparoscopic removal of ovarian endometrioma. Am J Obstet Gynecol 164:1622–1626
Martin D (1991) Laparoscopic treatment of ovarian endometriomas. Clin Obstet Gynecol 34:452–459
Martin DC, Olive DL (1986) Cited in Olive DL, Haney AF Endometriosis associated infertility. A critical review of therapeutic approaches. Obstet Gynecol Surg 41:538–555
Martin DC, Hubert GD, Vander Zwaag R, El-Zeky F (1989a) Laparoscopic appearances of peritoneal endometriosis. Fertil Steril 51:63
Martin DC, Hubert GD, Levy BS (1989b) Depth of infiltration of endometriosis. J Gynecol Surg 5:55–60
Menzies D, Ellis H (1989) Intra-abdominal adhesions and their prevention by topical tissue plasminogen activator. J Roy Soc Med 82:534–535
Murphy AA et al. (1991) Laparoscopic cautery in the treatment of endometriosis related infertility. Fertil Steril 55:246–251
Nezhat C (1991) Laparoscopic uretero-neocystostomy following ureteral injuries. Abstracts from The Society for Minimally Invasive Surgery. Third International Meeting. Boston, Mass. Mary Ann Liebert Publishers, New York, p 36
Olive DL, Haney AF (1986). Endometriosis-associated infertility: a clinical review of therapeutic approaches. Obstet Gynecol Surg 41:538–555
Olive DL et al. (1985) Expectant management and hydrotubations in the treatment of endometriosis associated infertility. Fertil Steril 44:35
Patel CKN, McFarlane RA, Faust WL (1964) Selective excitation through vibration energy transfer and optical maser action in nitrogen-carbon dioxide. Physiol Rev 8:470–473
Raftery AT (1981) Effect of peritoneal trauma on peritoneal fibrinolytic activity and intraperitoneal adhesion formation. An experimental study in the rat. Eur Surg Res 13:374–401
Reich H (1987) Laparoscopic treatment of extensive pelvic adhesions including hydrosalpinx. J Reprod Med 32:736–742
Reich H, McGlynn F (1986) Treatment of ovarian endometriomas using laparoscopic surgical techniques. J Reprod Med 31:577
Reich H, McGlynn F (1990) Laparoscopic repair of bladder injury. Obstet Gynecol 76 2:909–910
Reid R (1992) Laser surgery on the vulva. In: Sutton CJG (ed) Lasers in gynaecology. Chapman and Hall, London, pp 211–235
Schavlow AL, Townes CH (1958) Infra-red and optical masers. Physiol Rev 112–119
Seibel MM, Berber MJ, Weinstein FG, Taymor ML (1982) The effectiveness of Danazol on subsequent fertility in minimally invasive endometriosis. Fertil Steril 38:534–537
Singhal V, Li T, Cooke ID (1991) An analysis of factors influencing the outcome of 232 consecutive tubal microsurgery cases. Br J Obstet Gynaecol 98:628–636
Sutton CJG (1986) Initial experience with carbon dioxide laser laparoscopy. Lasers in Medical Science 1:25–31
Sutton CJG (1989) Laser uterine nerve ablation. In: Donnez J (ed) Laser operative laparo-

scopy and hysteroscopy. Nauwelaerts Publishers, Leuven, Belgium, pp 43–52
Sutton CJG (1990) The treatment of endometriosis. In: Studd JWW (ed) Progress in obstetrics and gynaecology. 8:293–313. Churchill Livingstone, Edinburgh
Sutton CJG, Hill D (1990) Laser laparoscopy in the treatment of endometriosis. A 5-year study. Br Obstet Gynaecol 97:901–905
Sutton CJG, Hodgson R (1992) Endoscopic cutting with lasers. Minimal Invas Therapy 1:197–205
Swolin K (1975) Electromicrosurgery in salpingostomy: long-term results. MJ Obstet Gynaecol 121:418–419
Thomas EJ, Prentice A (1992) The aetiology and pathogenesis of endometriosis. Reprod Med Review 1:21–36
Tjaden B, Schlaff WD, Kimball A, Rock JA (1990) The efficacy of presacral neurectomy for the relief of mid-line dysmenorrhoea. Obstet Gynecol 76:89–91
Tulandi T (1987) Adhesion reformation after reproductive surgery with and without the carbon dioxide laser. Fertil Steril 47:704–706
Tulandi T, Vilos GA (1985) A comparison between laser surgery and electrosurgery for bilateral hydrosalpinx: a 2-year follow-up. Fertil Steril 44:846–848
Tulandi T et al. (1984) Reconstructive surgery of hydrosalpinx with and without the carbon dioxide laser. Fertil Steril 42:839–842
West CP (1990) Endometriosis. Large scale studies needed to decide on definitive treatment. Editorial. BMJ 301:189–190
Wilson EA (1988) Surgical therapy for endometriosis. Clin Obstet Gynaecol 31:857–865
Winston RM (1980) Microsurgery of the fallopian tube: from fantasy to reality. Fertil Steril 34:521
Winston RML, Magara RA (1991) Microsurgical salpingostomy is not an obsolete procedure. Br J Obstet Gynaecol 98:637–642

Section IV

# Pelvic Inflammatory Disease

Chapter 13

# Pelvic Inflammatory Disease – An Overview

J.M. Pearce

## Introduction

Pelvic inflammatory disease (PID) is inflammation of the upper female genital tract. The disorder includes endometritis, salpingitis, salpingo-oophoritis together with spread as peritonitis and along the paracolic gutters to cause the Fitzhugh–Curtis syndrome of perihepatitis. About one in a hundred women will suffer from at least one attack of PID. This is often poorly diagnosed and incompletely treated, resulting in substantial physical and psychological sequelae. Marital disharmony may result from suspicions that unfaithfulness caused the infection or from the ensuing dyspareunia, menstrual irregularities or childlessness.

## Pathogenesis

Pelvic inflammatory disease is almost always an infection that ascends through the cavities of the cervix, uterus and fallopian tubes; thus histology of the endometrium usually demonstrates infection (Weström 1980; Heinonen et al. 1985). The cervix and vagina are normally colonised by a wide variety of organisms (Table 13.1) whilst the uterus is sterile. The natural barriers to upward spread of organisms are the cervix and the tubal ostia; in addition the organisms of the lower genital tract are not very mobile.

The downward flow of cervical mucus and the small calibre of the cervical os (especially in the nulliparous state) provide a mechanical barrier. This barrier is complete by 8–9 weeks of pregnancy, after which time ascending

**Table 13.1.** Common organisms found in the vagina

| |
|---|
| *Lactobacillus* species |
| Corynebacterium |
| *Bacteroides* species |
| *Mobiluncus curtisii, M. muliensis* |
| *Clostridia* species |
| Actinomyces |
| Lancefield groups A, B, C, D, H & K *Streptococci* |
| Coagulase-negative *Staphylococci* |
| *Gardnerella vaginalis* |
| *Haemophilus* species |
| Enterobacteria |
| Listeria |
| *Trichomonas vaginalis* |
| Yeasts |
| *Mycoplasma hominis* |
| *Ureaplasma urealyticum* |

infection probably never occurs. In addition to the mechanical barrier, the cervical mucus secretes IgA which, as well as its own action, enhances the action of a lysozyme secreted by the cervix thus causing osmotic lysis of bacteria (Cohen et al. 1984).

The cervical barrier may be compromised after miscarriage, abortion, childbirth, cervical surgery and at the time of insertion of an intrauterine contraceptive device. The risk of PID after termination of pregnancy is about 2% but is up to ten times that figure in women with asymptomatic sexually transmitted diseases (Savage 1989). Up to 30% of women undergoing terminations have potential pathogens in the cervical canal (Cohn and Stewart 1992). At least 10% of women undergoing termination harbour *Chlamydia trachomatis* in the cervix (Cohn and Stewart 1992; Ridgway et al. 1983) and some 20%–25% of such women will develop postabortal sepsis (Qvigstad et al. 1983). It has been estimated that it would cost only £8 per patient to screen for *Chlamydia trachomatis, gonorrhoea, Mycoplasma hominis, Ureaplasma urealyticum* and *Trichomonas vaginalis* (Cohn and Stewart 1992) but few centres do this or give the prophylactic antibiotics which seem to be effective in these circumstances (Savage 1989).

The risk of PID in women fitted with an intrauterine contraceptive device (IUCD) has probably been overstated. There is an increased risk at the time of insertion (Mishell et al. 1966). The widely reported increased risk in IUCD wearers is due to a reporting bias with many of the studies being based upon hospital populations (for review see Kessel 1989).

The most common cause of PID, however, is coitus. The common organisms that cause PID are not sufficiently mobile to ascend the genital tract. Two mechanisms have been proposed by which this problem is overcome. At the time of female orgasm uterine contractions occur which may draw both sperm and micro-organisms into the uterine cavity. Immediately post-orgasm pressures as low as −25 cm water have been recorded in the uterus whilst the pressure in the vagina may be up to +35 cm water (Fox et al. 1970). This steep pressure gradient would result in an influx of vaginal contents into the uterine cavity.

The second mechanism that has been proposed is the attachment of microbes to spermatozoa. Relatively immotile organisms such as *N. gonorrhoea* (Gomez et al. 1979), *Ureaplasma urealyticum* (Gnarpe and Friberg 1973), *Chlamydia trachomatis* (Wolner-Hanssen et al. 1982) and many of the anaerobes (Keith et al. 1984) can become attached to sperm. As sperm penetrate the cervical mucus and reach the fallopian tubes it is likely that they act as vectors for these organisms. Women taking the combined oral contraceptive pill produce cervical mucus that is resistant to sperm and this may account for the protective effect of the pill against PID.

*Trichomonas vaginalis* can penetrate the cervical barrier and has been found in both the uterine cavity and the fallopian tubes. Although *T. vaginalis* is frequently found in association with PID it has never been thought to be a causative organism. It has been suggested that it might be a vector, but although *Escherichia coli* will attach to *T. vaginalis* under laboratory conditions there is no evidence that this occurs with sexually-transmitted organisms. In the case of *N. gonorrhoea*, *T.vaginalis* may reduce viability (for review see Keith et al. 1984). The mechanism whereby micro-organisms cause tubal damage has been reviewed by Weström (1989). The damage occurs in two phases:

## *The Acute Phase*

The micro-organisms gain access to the fallopian tubes via the cavities of the cervix and uterus; thus the response to the infection starts in the mucosa. The swelling of this and the submucosa due to inflammation causes rupture of the serosa at the mesosalpingeal margin of the tube, particularly around the ampullary portion. As the distal portion of the tube usually lacks a mesosalpinx the serosa cannot give way, resulting in a fibrous ring through which the fimbria are drawn as the tube shortens as a result of further swelling. The initial inflammation causes tissue damage in the mucosal, muscular, interstitial and serosal layers of the tube as well as the local peritoneal serosa and subserosa.

Viewed down the laparoscope acute PID begins with a reddening and swelling of the tube accompanied by mesosalpingeal injection and a purulent or seropurulent discharge. The tubes appear swollen but are essentially of normal morphology and motility – this is mild disease. Moderate disease is defined as a shortened mesosalpinx with indrawn fimbria and restricted tubal motility. There may also be filmy adhesions to adjacent structures. If the disease becomes severe there may be tubo-ovarian abscess formation and adhesions such that only the uterine fundus may be visualised.

## *Repair*

Repair occurs simultaneously with the infection. The fimbria are close together so as repair occurs they occlude the end of the tube, thus preventing further spread to the peritoneal cavity. The end result depends upon the stage at which the process is interrupted with antibiotic therapy. Table 13.2

**Table 13.2.** Incidence of infertility following one attack of PID (from Weström 1989)

| Severity of attack | Percentage in age group | | Total |
|---|---|---|---|
| | 15–24 | 25–34 | |
| Mild | 5.8 | 7.8 | 6.1 |
| Moderate | 10.8 | 22.0 | 13.4 |
| Severe | 27.3 | 40.0 | 30.0 |

illustrates the number of women who are infertile following one attack of PID.

The end result may be restoration to normal after a mild attack treated early with appropriate antibiotics. More severe attacks may result in deciliation, intratubal adhesions, hydrosalpinx or pyosalpinx. Such tubes are short and immobile. In addition there may be peritubal adhesions to surrounding structures, particularly the ovary.

Arguments still continue (largely between the Americans and the Scandinavians) as to whether PID is most commonly caused by a single organism (Mardh et al. 1977) or multiple organisms (Sweet et al. 1979). The evidence seems to suggest that a primary infection with *C. trachomatis* or *N. gonorrhoea* or both allows opportunistic infection by the other inhabitants of the vagina (see Table 13.1).

## Prevalence

Pelvic inflammatory disease has undoubtedly become more common. In the past two decades *N. gonorrhoea* has become at least three times more frequent throughout the world (Aral and Holmes 1984; Sweet and Gibbs 1985). PID occurs in about 25% of women who acquire gonorrhoea (Weström et al. 1982). In the past decade *C. trachomatis* has become a more important cause of PID in the developed world accounting for more than half the cases of PID seen in Europe (Catterall 1975) and two fifths of women treated for PID in American hospitals (Urquhart 1979). Chlamydial disease has increased in the United Kingdom (World Health Organization 1981). Sexually transmitted diseases account for most cases of PID. In developed countries the incidence of PID is 10–13 per 1000 women with a peak incidence of 20 per 1000 in the 15–24-year age group (World Health Organization 1981).

## Sequelae of Pelvic Inflammatory Disease

Despite the varying criteria for diagnosing PID and the often inadequate follow-up there is clear evidence that the sequelae of PID are both serious and common. Table 13.3 lists the sequelae of a single attack.

**Table 13.3.** Sequelae of a single attack of pelvic inflammatory disease

| Risk | Condition | Reference |
|---|---|---|
| 6–10 × increase | Further attack of PID | Weström 1975 |
| 1 in 6 | Tubal infertility | Urquhart 1979 |
| 7 × increase | Ectopic pregnancy | Urquhart 1979 |
| 1 in 5 | Chronic pelvic pain | Adler et al. 1982 |
| 2 in 5 | Deep dyspareunia | Adler et al. 1982 |
| 4 in 5 | Menstrual disturbances | Adler et al. 1982 |

**Table 13.4.** Criteria for diagnosis of pelvic inflammatory disease (Hager et al. 1983)

| |
|---|
| At least three of the following: |
| Abdominal tenderness, with or without rebound tenderness |
| Tenderness with motion of the cervix or uterus |
| Adnexal tenderness |
| Plus at least one of the following: |
| Gram-negative, intracellular Diplococci in endocervical secretions |
| Temperature of more than 38 °C |
| Leucocytosis of more than 10 000 per mm² |
| Purulent material obtained from peritoneal cavity by laparoscopy or culdocentesis |
| Pelvic abscess or inflammatory complex on bimanual examination or ultrasound |

## Diagnosis

The Society for Infectious Diseases in Obstetrics and Gynecology of the USA has published the diagnostic criteria which are listed in Table 13.4. The system also grades the disease on clinical features as follows:

Grade 1. Uncomplicated, limited to tubes and/or ovaries

Grade 2. Complicated with an inflammatory mass or abscess involving tubes or ovaries

Grade 3. Spread to structures beyond the pelvis, that is a ruptured tubo-ovarian abscess.

These criteria have not been universally adopted in the United Kingdom, which makes comparisons of series impossible.

## Laparoscopy

If the clinical diagnosis of PID is checked by laparoscopy it is confirmed in only 65% of cases (Jacobson and Weström 1984). The second most common diagnosis was acute appendicitis, followed by endometriosis, bleeding from a corpus luteum, ectopic pregnancy and an ovarian tumour. In 23% of cases no cause could be found. There have now been several series that have confirmed the inaccuracy of the clinical diagnosis. Laparoscopy also provides an opportunity for the correct bacterial specimens to be collected. These are as follows:

1. For immunofluorescent monoclonal antibody testing to *C. trachomatis:*
   urethral swab
   endocervical swab
2. For Gram stain and culture and sensitivity:
   urethral swab
   endocervical swab
   high vaginal swab
   rectal swab
   pharyngeal swab

If laparoscopy is not undertaken then probably the rectal and pharyngeal swabs should be omitted as they cause offence to many patients and only improve the positive culture rate by about 1%.

3. Endometrial biopsy. This should be split into three parts and sent for histology, antibody to *C. trachomatis* examination and culture. The success of culture of organisms from carefully collected endometrial biopsies is high enough to justify performing an out-patient procedure such as a suction curettage if the patient is not to undergo laparoscopy (Heinonen et al. 1985).
4. Pus/aspirate from the fallopian tubes. Pressure on the fallopian tube at the time of laparoscopy may cause pus to be extruded which can be collected by aspiration for culture and antibody testing to *C. trachomatis*.

In addition, several authors have emphasised the value of examining the sexual partner (Gilstrap et al. 1977; Össer and Persson 1982). Organisms can be identified from up to 70% of male partners of women who have PID and in many cases are the only positive source of culture. Close liaison between gynaecologist and genito-urinary physicians is needed to make this effective.

Laparoscopy greatly improves the accuracy of bacteriological diagnosis (Mardh et al. 1977). Most gynaecologists, however, adopt a policy of a 48–72-h trial of antibiotics and only if the patient does not respond is laparoscopy carried out. This is illogical because not only does it destroy the chances of getting a positive culture from the fallopian tubes but also clinical examination is poor in that only 32% of palpated masses are confirmed at laparoscopy and in 10% of cases masses are demonstrated at laparoscopy that were not clinically apparent (Lundberg et al. 1973).

## Treatment

Ideally, all patients with suspected PID should be admitted to hospital to allow laparoscopic diagnosis, frequent observations and parenteral antibiotics. This should include a single dose of ampicillin and probenecid (against *N. gonorrhoea*), a broad-spectrum antibiotic against Gram-negative organisms such as a cephalosporin for 1 week, and metronidazole (against anaerobes) for 1 week. Therapy should be altered if a specific organism is found. All patients, even those with a specific infection should probably have at least a 2-week course of doxycycline or erythromycin to prevent persistence of *C. trachomatis*, even if this organism has not been demonstrated (Sweet et al. 1983). This should be commenced when the patient is free from systemic upset, particularly nausea.

In the United Kingdom, women are usually only admitted to hospital if they are systemically unwell, have a pelvic mass or are pregnant. Patients with mild PID who are treated as out-patients should receive oral tetracyclines, co-trimaxazole and metronidazole. This combination should cover more than 90% of potential organisms (Bell and James 1980). Such patients should be reviewed in 2–3 days and if there is no improvement should be admitted for laparoscopy.

## Continuing Conundrums

*C. trachomatis* is currently the leading cause of PID. It appears that many women carry this organism in their cervix without suffering PID. Precipitating factors are largely unknown. Women with lower abdominal pain and *C. trachomatis* in the cervix or urethra, or both, may still have the organism demonstrated in the upper genital tract even in the absence of laparoscopic evidence of PID (Stacey et al. 1990). This brings into question the accuracy of laparoscopic diagnosis of PID. It also raises the question of whether such women would develop PID if untreated. Undoubtedly, the response to *C. trachomatis* in the upper genital tract varies from woman to woman. It may well be that the tubal damage is due to a local immunological reaction, or the failure of such a reaction.

Recurrence of PID is reduced if women stop having intercourse but as yet there is no evidence that condom usage reduces attacks or sequelae.

## Summary

PID was defined in a recent leading article (Pearce 1990) as a sexually transmitted disease with potentially serious sequelae that is often poorly treated. As the consequences are rarely life-threatening the disease has yet to be taken seriously by the gynaecological community. Hospital admission, accurate diagnosis and aggressive treatment of PID needs to adopted on a wide-scale basis.

## References

Adler MW, Belsey EM, O'Connor BH (1982) Morbidity associated with pelvic inflammatory disease. Br J Ven Dis 58:151–157

Aral SS, Holmes KK (1984) Epidemiology of sexually transmitted disease. In: Holmes KK, Mardh P-A, Sparling PF, Wiesner PJ (eds) Sexually transmitted disease. McGraw-Hill, New York, pp 127–141

Bell TA, James JF (1980) Computer assisted analysis of the therapy of acute salpingitis. Am J Obstet Gynecol 138:1048–1054

Catterall RD (1975) The situation of gonococcal and non-gonococcal infections in the United Kingdom. In: Danielsson D, Juhlin L, Mardh P-A (eds) Genital infections and their complications. Almquist and Wiksel, Stockholm, pp 5–13

Cohen MS, Black JR, Proctor RA, Sparling PF (1984) Host defences in the vaginal mucosa. In: Mardh P-A, Taylor-Robinson D (eds) Bacterial vaginosis. Almquist and Wiksell, Stockholm, pp 13–22

Cohn M, Stewart P (1992) Preavalence of potential pathogens in cervical canal before termination of pregnancy. Br Med J 304:1479

Fox CA, Wolff HS, Baker JA (1970) Measurements of intravaginal and intrauterine pressures during human coitus by radio-telemetry. J Reprod Fertil 22:243–251

Gilstrap LC, Herbert WNP, Cunningham FG, Hauth JC, Van Patten HG (1977) Gonorrhoea screening in male consorts of women with pelvic infection. JAMA 238:965–966

Gnarpe H, Friberg H (1973) *T. mycoplasmas* on spermatozoa and infertility. Nature 245:97–98

Gomez CI, Stenback WA, James AN, Criswell BS, Williams RP (1979) Attachment of *N. gonorrhoea* to human sperm. Br J Ven Dis 55:245–255

Hager WD, Eschenmbach DA, Speme MR, Sweet RL (1983) Criteria for diagnosis and grading of salpingitis. Obstet Gynecol 61:113–114

Heinonen PK et al. (1985) Anatomical sites of upper genital tract infection. Obstet Gynecol 66:384–390

Jacobson L, Weström L (1984) Objectivised diagnosis of acute pelvic inflammatory disease. Am J Obstet Gynecol 150:1088–1098

Keith LG, Berger GS, Edelman DA (1984) On the causation of pelvic inflammatory disease. Am J Obstet Gynecol 149:215–223

Kessel E (1989) Pelvic inflammatory disease with intrauterine device use: a reassessment. Fertil Steril 51:1–11

Lundberg WI, Wall JE, Mathers JE (1973) Laparoscopy in the evaluation of pelvic pain. Obstet Gynecol 42:872–876

Mardh P-A, Ripa T, Svensson L, Weström L (1977) *Chlamydia trachomatis* infection in patients with acute salpingitis. New Engl J Med 296:1377–1379

Mishell DR, Bell JH, Good RG, Moyer DL (1966) The intrauterine contraceptive device:a bacteriological study of the endometrial cavity. Am J Obstet Gynecol 96:119–123

Osser S, Persson K (1982) Epidemiological and serodiagnostic aspects of chlamydial salpingitis. Obstet Gynecol 59:206–209

Pearce JMF (1990) Pelvic inflammatory disease. Br Med J 300:1090–1091

Qvigstad E, Skaug K, Jerve F, Fylling P, Ulstrup JC (1983) Pelvic inflammatory disease associated with *Chlamydia trachomatis* infection after therapeutic abortion. A prospective study. Br J Ven Dis 59:189–192

Ridgway GL, Mumtaz G, Stephens RA, Oriel JD (1983) Therapeutic abortion and chlamydial infection. Br Med J 286:1478–1479

Savage W (1989) Therapeutic abortion. In: Turnbull AC, Chamberlain GVP (eds) Obstetrics. Churchill Livingstone, Edinburgh, pp 430–431

Stacey C et al. (1990) *Chlamydia trachomatis* in the fallopian tubes of women without laparoscopic evidence of salpingitis. Lancet 336:960–963

Sweet RL, Gibbs RS (1985) Sexually transmitted disease. In: Sweet RL, Gibbs RS (eds) Infectious diseases of the female genital tract. Williams and Wilkins, Baltimore, pp 17–52

Sweet RL, Mills J, Hadley KW (1979) Use of the laparoscope to determine microbiological etiology of acute salpingitis. Am J Obstet Gynecol 134:68–74

Sweet RL, Schachter J, Robbie MO (1983) Failure of beta lactam antibiotics to eradicate *Chlamydia trachomatis* in the endometrium despite clinical cure of acute salpingitis. JAMA 250:2641–2645

Urquhart J (1979) Effects of the venereal disease epidemic on the incidence of ectopic pregnancy – implications for the evaluation of contraceptives. Contraception 19:455–480

Weström L (1975) Effects of acute pelvic inflammatory disease on fertility. Am J Obstet Gynecol 121:707–713

Weström L (1980) Incidence, prevalence and trends of acute pelvic inflammatory disease and its consequences in industrialised countries. Am J Obstet Gynecol 138:880–892

Weström L (1989) Long-term consequences of pelvic inflammatory disease. In: Hare MJ (ed) Genital tract infection in women. Churchill Livingstone, Edinburgh, pp 350–367
Weström L, Svensson L, Wolner-Hanssen P, Mardh P-A (1982) Chlamydial and gonococcal infections in a defined population of women. Scand J Infect Dis 32:157–162
Wolner-Hanssen P, Mardh P-A, Moller B, Weström L (1982) Endometrial infection in women with chlamydia salpingitis. J Sex Trans Dis 9:84–88
World Health Organization (1981) Pelvic inflammatory disease. WHO Tech Rep Ser 660:98–100

Section V

# Surgical Techniques for Female Sterilisation

Chapter 14

# Novel Techniques in Tubal Contraception

K. Wamsteker, S. de Blok, M.H. Emanuel and
C.G.W.A. Stappers-de Kuijer

## Introduction

Many different techniques to occlude the fallopian tubes for permanent female contraception have been described and clinically applied. In his "Lectures on the Principles and Practice of Midwifery", presented in 1842 at Guy's Hospital in London, Dr. James Blundell suggested partial salpingectomy during caesarean section and interval sterilisation by minilaparotomy (Blundell 1842; Siegler and Grunebaum 1983). In 1849 Froriep described a transcervical sterilisation method with the application of silver nitrate in the uterine cavity causing chemical cauterisation of the tubal orifices. In 1880 Lungren published the first tubal ligation performed with silk during repeat caesarean section. Female sterilisation procedures became more popular after the publication of a technique of tubal resection through anterior colpotomy by Kehrer from Germany in 1897.

The first use of hysteroscopy for tubal sterilisation was published by Mikulicz-Radecki and Freund in 1927, who used a probe to cauterise the intramural part of the tube. Power and Barnes published the use of laparoscopy for sterilisation in 1941 with electrocauterisation of the tubes. From the early 1970s to the present, laparoscopic techniques to obliterate the fallopian tubes have developed into safe and effective methods for voluntary sterilisation, which has become by far the most prevalent method of permanent female contraception today.

However, since introduction of hysteroscopy with $CO_2$ distension of the uterine cavity by Lindemann in 1971, several methods for non-incisional transcervical hysteroscopic tubal occlusion have been developed. This chapter will focus on the use of these transcervical techniques for contraception.

# Transcervical Hysteroscopic Tubal Contraception

Several techniques for transcervical hysteroscopic tubal occlusion have been investigated: cauterisation of the intramural part of the tubes, application of chemical caustic agents and application of intratubal devices.

## Cauterisation of the Intramural Part of the Tubes

Tubal occlusion by means of hysteroscopic electrocauterisation of the intramural part of the tubes was originally described by Lindemann in 1973. A high-frequency electroprobe, introduced into the uterine cavity through the working channel of the hysteroscope, was placed into the tubal ostium and the intramural part of the tube was cauterised from inside the tubal lumen. Secondary fibrosis resulted in occlusion of the intramural part of the tube. However, a large multicentre study of this technique under the auspices of the World Health Organization failed to establish its effectiveness and safety (Darabi and Richart 1977). The overall occlusion rate was 35.5% and the mean failure rate was 50%. In addition, pregnancies occurred after proven occlusion and serious complications were recorded, such as uterine perforation, intestinal burns, peritonitis and cornual pregnancies. Lindemann confirmed the discouraging results from his own series in 1975. Of his patients, 5.3% became pregnant after proven occlusion. Using thermocauterisation instead of electrocauterisation did not improve the results (Wamsteker 1984).

## Application of Chemical Agents

The non-visual intrauterine or intratubal application of chemical caustic agents, such as silver nitrate, zinc chloride, copper sulphate and formaldehyde, have been tested in animal studies (Richart 1983; Wamsteker 1977). The majority were not successful nor were results improved with other chemical agents such as strong acids and bases (sulphuric acid, salicylic acid, phenol and sodium hydrochloride), sclerosing agents (sodium morrhuate) and granuloma-producing agents (e.g., talc, asbestos, beryllium nitrate). The most promising cytotoxic agent in animal studies was quinacrine. However, in human studies, the results were discouraging. In studies with tissue adhesives, only methyl-2-cyanoacrylate (MCA) and gelatine resorcinol-formaline (GRF) appeared to produce a reasonable rate of tubal occlusion (Richart 1983).

Quinacrine and methyl-2-cyanoacrylate (MCA) have also been investigated in the human with transcervical hysteroscopic intratubal application under direct visual control. However the results failed to justify these techniques as useful clinical methods. Non-visual intrauterine application of quinacrine pellets (Guzman-Serani et al. 1983; Zipper et al. 1987; Mullick et al. 1987) and MCA with the FEMCEPT (FEMCEPT is a registered trademark for BioNexus, Inc, Raleigh, North Carolina, USA) device (Richart et al. 1983; Shuber 1989) are still under clinical investigation.

## Application of Intratubal Devices (ITD)

Intratubal contraceptive devices are all applied by means of hysteroscopy and can be subdivided into three different types: uterotubal junction devices; devices blocking uterotubal junction (UTJ, P-block); and intratubal formed-in-place silicone devices (Ovabloc: Ovabloc is a registered trademark for Advanced Medical Grade Silicones BV, Rotterdam, The Netherlands).

### *Uterotubal Junction Devices*

Uterotubal junction devices are placed into the uterotubal junction and held in place by lateral "wings" at the distal tip and a loop-size extension of the proximal part. The uterotubal junction is not occluded. This type of device has only been applied in experimental studies and its effectiveness is still uncertain.

### *Blocking Uterotubal Junction Devices*

Blocking uterotubal junction devices occlude the intramural part of the tube. However, this part of the tube is a muscular structure and expulsion or pain are problems that occur frequently. The devices are made of polyethylene or silicone and generally have "wings", which are supposed to penetrate the myometrium to anchor the UTJ device (Hosseinian and Morales 1983). The results of these devices are disappointing.

A special type of UTJ device is the P-block, developed by Brundin (1982). The P-block consists of a nylon skeleton with a 4-mm long hydrogel body and two nylon anchoring "wings". After hysteroscopic positioning of the device in the uterotubal junction, the hydrogel expands and occludes the intramural part of the tube. Several different designs have been investigated, the P-block mark 9 being the most recent variant. The gross Pearl index for the total series of 9 different designs is 5, due to rejection of the device. The mark 9 type P-block gives the best results with a Pearl index of 0.3 in 191 patients with a mean follow-up of 21 months, provided the P-block remains properly located (Brudin 1991).

### *Intratubal Formed-in-place Silicone Devices (Ovabloc ITD).*

In extensive studies from 1971 onwards, Erb (1976; Erb and Reed 1979) developed a technique for hysteroscopic intratubal administration of liquid silicone; this is mixed with a catalyst and cures in situ to form rubbery implants. The objective was a non-incisional, non-scarring method for permanent contraception with minimal discomfort to the patient. Clinical testing in humans started in 1978. Reed and colleagues (Erb and Reed 1979; Reed and Erb 1980; Reed et al. 1981) published the first clinical studies and from 1980 until 1985 multicentre phase III clinical trials were performed in the USA and Europe in over 2000 volunteers. The Ovabloc ITD procedure appears to be a very promising and elegant transcervical hysteroscopic method for permanent contraception and will be discussed in more detail.

## The Ovabloc Intratubal Device (ITD) For Permanent Contraception

### Technique

The Ovabloc ITDs are formed in situ after the intratubal administration of liquid medical grade silicone rubber (polydimethyl siloxane) mixed with catalyst (stannous octoate) in a mixer-dispenser (Fig. 14.1). Complete curing of the silicone takes approximately 5 min after mixing with the catalyst.

The silicone is injected through the guide assembly (Fig. 14.1), a double catheter system, which guides the viscous liquid through the working channel of the hysteroscope. At the distal end of the inner catheter, an obturator tip (Fig. 14.2) which is made of cured silicone is placed into the tubal ostium. An opening in the tip allows the silicone material to flow into the oviducts. The liquid silicone mixture is propelled through the catheter system at a pressure of 300 N. After the silicone has reached the obturator tip of the catheter the pressure is allowed to fall to 50 N. The pressure is created by the fluid flow actuator, a mechanical pump (Fig. 14.3). During the curing process a mechanical bond between the obturator tip and the silicone material in the oviduct is formed. The ITD conforms to the shape of the tube with a bulbous ampullary enlargement in its diameter (Fig. 14.4). The

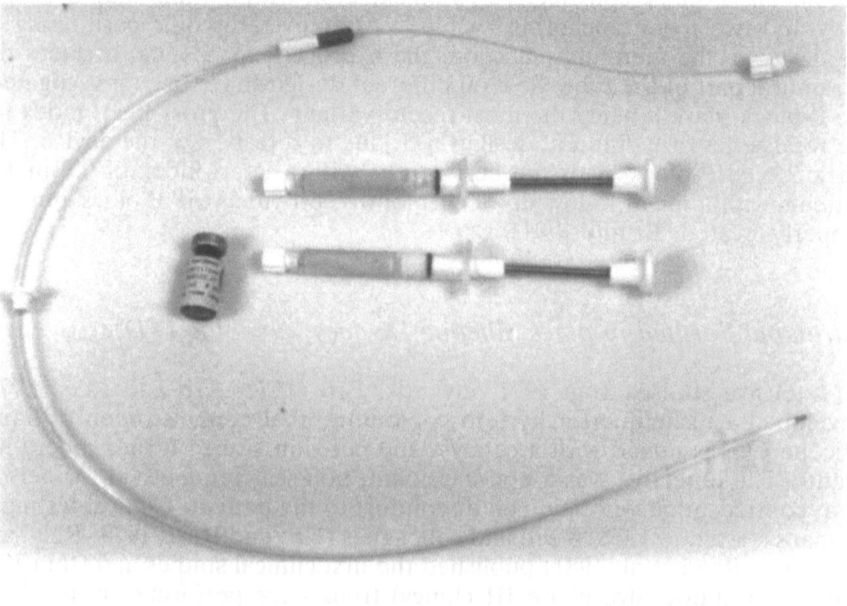

**Fig. 14.1.** Silicone mixer-dispenser, guide assembly and catalyst vial.

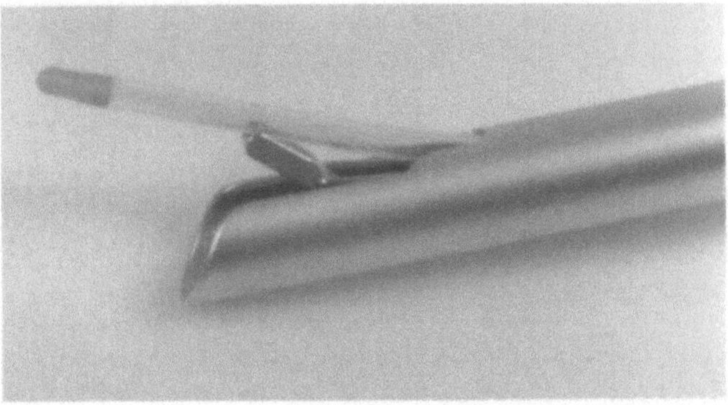

**Fig. 14.2.** Distal end of the operating hysteroscope with Albarran deflecting lever and guide assembly with obturator tip.

total amount of intratubal silicone is approximately 200 mg. After mixing with the catalyst, some silicone is put on a test-plate to follow the curing process outside the body. After completion of the curing as judged on the test-plate, the obturator tip is separated from the catheter, leaving the Ovabloc ITD in situ (Fig. 14.5).

Radio-opaque spherical silver powder is added to the silicone so that the

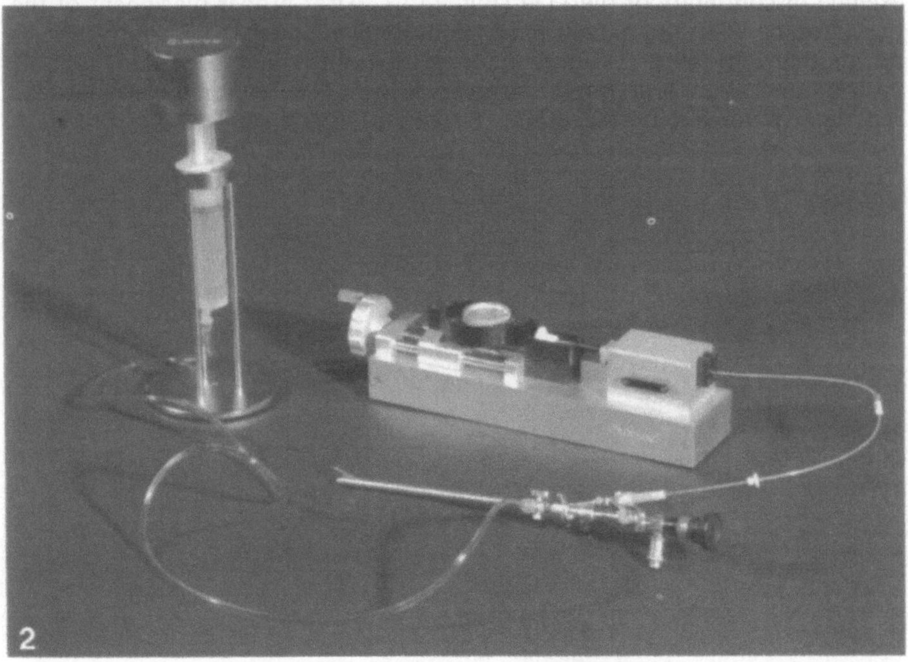


**Fig. 14.3.** Operating hysteroscope with deflecting bridge, mechanical Ovabloc pump for Hyskon® distension and fluid flow actuator with guide assembly.

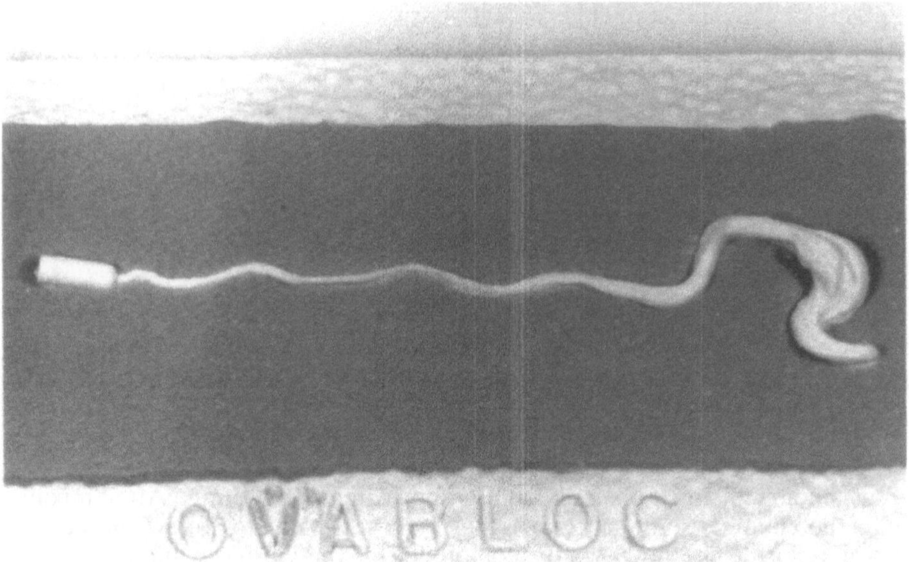


**Fig. 14.4.** Model of a formed-in-situ Ovabloc Intratubal Device.

ITD can be visualised on X-ray, to ensure the ampullary enlargement and to exclude discontinuity of the ITD (Fig. 14.6). After proper placement of the two Ovabloc ITDs the patient has to continue with alternative contraception for another 3 months. A 3-month control X-ray is taken to confirm a stable position and to exclude migration or expulsion. Thereafter the woman can rely on Ovabloc for contraception.

## Method

The Ovabloc procedure is performed on an ambulatory basis with local anaesthesia by means of intra- and paracervical block. The Ovabloc guide

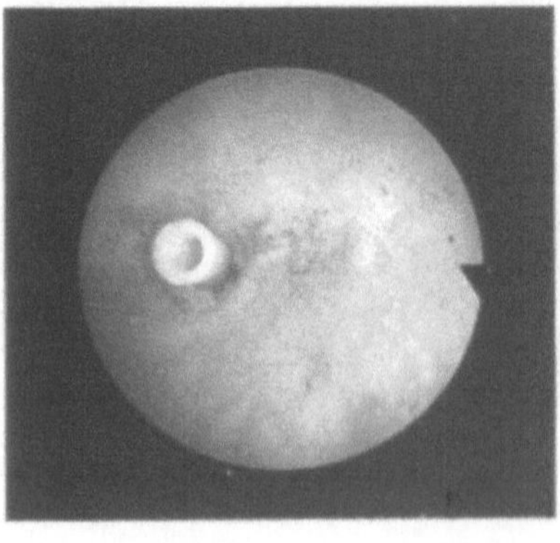

**Fig. 14.5.** Obturator tip with Ovabloc ITD in situ as seen from the uterine cavity.

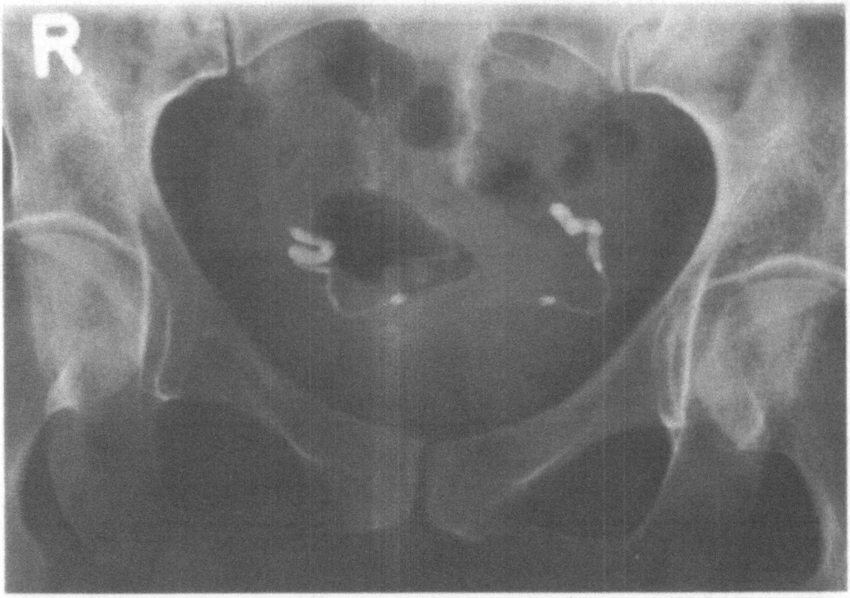

**Fig. 14.6.** X-ray with normal left and right Ovabloc ITD in situ. Note the bulbous ampullary enlargement in diameter.

assembly and the obturator tip are brought into place through the working channel of an operating hysteroscope (Fig. 14.3). During the clinical trials single flow hysteroscopes were used with $CO_2$ or Hyskon® distension of the uterine cavity. For the Ovabloc ITD procedure the operating hysteroscope in equipped with an Albarran deflection bridge (Fig. 14.2) to direct the catheter tip to the tubal ostium. The outer diameter of the operating hysteroscope with the deflection bridge is 7 or 8 mm. The internal cervical os (ICO) must be dilated with half size hegars. The correct positioning of the obturator tip and the patency of the tube are tested with methylene blue injection through the catheter before the silicone mixing and injection are initiated.

In a number of patients, hysteroscopy will reveal very laterally positioned tubal ostia or intrauterine or tubal abnormalities. This prevents proper placement of the obturator tip and in these cases the Ovabloc procedure cannot be performed.

## Phase II and III Clinical Trials: Results

In the original clinical trials some technical and instrumental problems influenced the early results. A "learning curve" can be recognised in these results.

Reed in the USA and de Maeyer in Belgium started their trials in 1978.

**Table 14.1.** Ovabloc ITD clinical trials phase II and III: instillation rates

| Start of study | Reed (USA) 1978 | | de Maeyer (Belgium) 1978 | | Loffer (USA) 1981 | |
|---|---|---|---|---|---|---|
| | n | % | n | % | n | % |
| Patients consented | 443 | | 271 | | 265 | |
| No procedure | 21 | 5 | 9 | 3 | 6 | 2 |
| Instillation attempt | 422 | | 262 | | 259 | |
| Repeat procedures | 123 | 29 | 69 | 26 | 41 | 16 |
| Successful instillation | 366 | 87 | 212 | 81 | 240 | 93 |

Source: CSI/Parexel, Boston, USA, 1989.

**Table 14.2.** Ovabloc ITD clinical trials phase II and III: continuation rate

| Start of study | Reed 1978 | | de Maeyer 1978 | | Loffer 1981 | |
|---|---|---|---|---|---|---|
| | n | % | n | % | n | % |
| Successful instillation | 366 | | 212 | | 240 | |
| Lost to follow-up | 3 | | — | | — | |
| 3-month control X-ray | 363 | | 212 | | 240 | |
| ITD status change at 3 mo. | 19 | 5 | 6 | 3 | 6 | 3 |
| Continuation rate at 3 mo.[a] | 344 | 95 | 206 | 97 | 234 | 97 |
| ITD status change >3 mo.[b] | 24 | 7 | 12 | 6 | 10 | 4 |
| Continuation rate >5 yr | 320 | 88 | 194 | 92 | 224 | 93 |

[a] these patients were classified as "off contraception" and relied on Ovabloc for contraception.
[b] only spontaneous ITD status change; physicians' intervention excluded.
Source: CSI/Parexel, Boston, USA, 1989.

Loffer joined the trial in 1981. In the three trials the Ovabloc procedure could not be performed in 5% (Reed), 3% (de Maeyer) and 2% (Loffer) of cases (Table 14.1). This number of failed attempts in the clinical trials is relatively low, because the patients had to meet stringent inclusion criteria: for example, women with a retroverted uterus were excluded. Successful silicone instillation was accomplished in 366 (87%) of 422 patients by Reed, in 212 (81%) of 262 patients by de Maeyer and in 240 (93%) of 259 patients by Loffer (Table 14.1). The rather high number of repeat procedures (29%, 26% and 16% respectively) reflects the technical and instrumental problems encountered in the early phase of the study and diminished during the course of the study.

From the original number of patients with successful silicone instillation 95% (Reed), 97% (de Maeyer) and 97% (Loffer) were considered able to rely on Ovabloc for contraception after control X-ray at 3 months. They were classified as "off contraception" (Table 14.2) Change of the Ovabloc ITD in the first 3 months was usually uterine or abdominal expulsion or tip separation. The continuation rates for more than 5 years were 88% (Reed), 92% (de Maeyer) and 93% (Loffer). After the 3-months control X-ray, further ITD status changes occurred (Table 14.2), mainly due to tip separation (61% of 46 cases). In phase III of the clinical trials a tip modification

**Table 14.3.** Ovabloc ITD clinical trials phase II and III: pregnancies – Pearl index

| Start of study | Reed 1978 | de Maeyer 1978 | Loffer 1981 |
|---|---|---|---|
| Women months of use[a] | 14.309 | 8.040 | 9.915 |
| Method failure | 10[b] | 2[c] | 1[b] |
| Pearl index | 0.84 | 0.30 | 0.12 |
| Life table index[d] | 0.0093 | 0.0067 | 0.0067 |

[a] calculated from "off contraception", i.e. after 3 months X-ray control.
[b] one pregnancy was ectopic.
[c] one pregnancy was ectopic; one pregnancy was only "biochemical", no intervention.
[d] annualised over 3–5 years.
Source: CSI/Parexel, Boston, USA, 1989.

**Table 14.4.** Ovabloc ITD clinical trials phase II and III: adverse experiences (more than one event) requiring treatment

| | no. of patients | % |
|---|---|---|
| Number of patients with silicone instilled | 943 | |
| Infection | 10 | 1 |
| Abnormal bleeding | 39 | 4 |
| Pain | 29 | 3 |
| Trauma | 3 | 0.3 |

Source: CSI/Parexel, Boston, USA, 1989.

has largely overcome this problem. As a result of these studies, a control X-ray or ultrasonogram is recommended at 12 months.

A total number of 13 pregnancies occurred in patients relying on Ovabloc ITD for contraception, 2 of which were ectopic (Table 14.3). The majority of the pregnancies occurred in the first study group of Reed. In the most recent clinical trial (Loffer) only one pregnancy occurred, resulting in a Pearl index of 0.12. The incidence of adverse effects requiring treatment (Table 14.4) was acceptable. Many of these were probably unrelated to the Ovabloc ITD.

## Clinical Application of Ovabloc ITD for Permanent Contraception: Methods and Results

After approval in The Netherlands the Ovabloc procedure was offered as an alternative method for permanent contraception in the Spaarne Hospital in Haarlem and included in the training programme of our Hysteroscopy Training Centre (HTC-NL). From 1989 up to and including 1991, 171 patients underwent an ambulatory hysteroscopy for Ovabloc ITD contraception. Premedication comprises 500 mg naprosyn (12 h and 1–2 h before the procedure) and 0.5 mg atropine im (10–15 min before procedure). These prevent uterine contractions and vagal reactions. Local anaesthesia was accom-

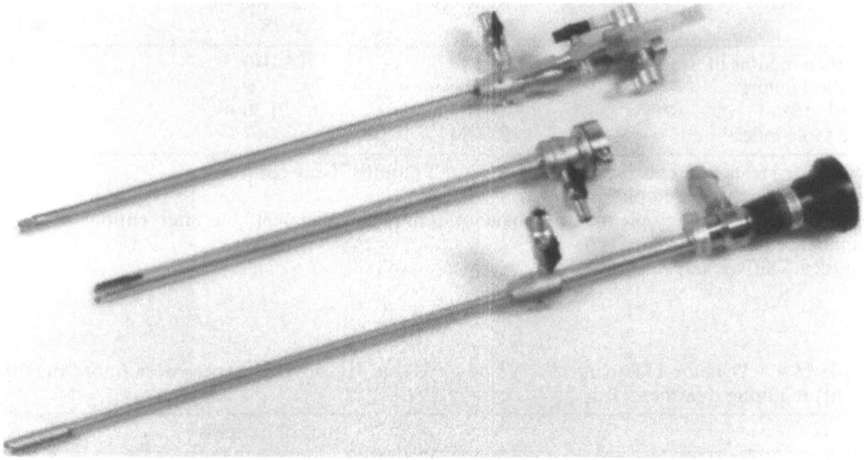

**Fig. 14.7.** The new generation 8-mm continuous-flow Olympus operating hysteroscope with deflecting bridge.

plished by means of an intra- and paracervical block with prilocaine 1% (Citanest®).

The total period of study has been divided into two separate periods: the 1989–1990 period in which the Ovabloc procedures were performed with a 7-mm single flow operating hysteroscope with deflecting bridge and Hyskon® or $CO_2$ for distension of the uterine cavity, and the 1991 period, in which the new 8-mm continuous flow Olympus hysteroscope with deflecting bridge (Fig. 14.7) was used with pressurised low viscosity fluid distension (sorbitol 4%). For $CO_2$ insufflation the Olympus hysteroflator has been used and for the administration of the Hyskon® the mechanical Ovabloc pump (Fig. 14.3). The sorbitol 4% was applied with a continuous infusion pressure of 150 mm Hg, produced by a pressure cuff and an adjustable pump connected to the general pressure line of the hospital (Fig. 14.8). The degree of uterine distension and the flow of the infused sorbitol is controlled by adaptation of the in- and out-flow stopcocks of the CF hysteroscope. No more than 500 ml sorbitol is needed for the complete procedure.

The out-flowing fluid must be collected in a calibrated bottle to permit control of the difference between the infused and the collected return fluid. This difference should never exceed 1500 ml in continuous flow hysteroscopy, as it indicates potential significant intravasation. However, this amount will rarely be used during an Ovabloc procedure. We prefer to insert the outer sheath of the hysteroscope with obturator into the uterine cavity before assembling the working sheath. The proper position and continuity of the Ovabloc ITDs was checked with X-ray immediately after the procedure and after 3 months. An extra X-ray control was scheduled for 12 months.

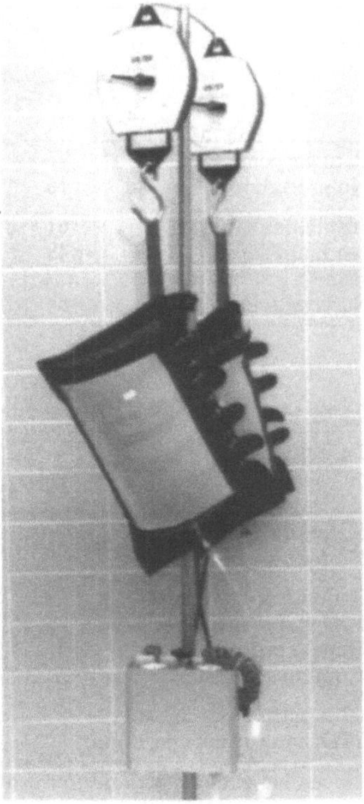

**Fig. 14.8.** Automatic infusion pressure cuffs for low viscosity fluid distension of the uterine cavity during continuous flow hysteroscopy.

In the group of 171 patients who had consented, the Ovabloc procedure could not be performed in 25 patients (15%) (Table 14.5). The introduction of continuous flow hysteroscopy (CFH) in 1991 significantly improved performance and the no-procedure rate diminished from 21% in the 1989–1990 period to 10% in 1991 period (Table 14.5). In addition, the average procedure time was reduced from 40 min with the single flow hysteroscopy to 25 min with continuous flow hysteroscopy. The rate of successful silicone instillation was raised from 89% to 96% with CFH. Also the number of repeat procedures required was reduced significantly by using the CFH system from 13% in the 1989–1990 period to 1% in the 1991 period (Table 14.5).

The overall continuation rate after the 3-months control X-ray in patients with successful instillation was 92% (Table 14.6). The use of CFH raised the continuation rate and number of patients "off contraception" from 89% to 94%. A control X-ray at 12 months was taken in 32 patients. In two women from the 1989–1990 period an ITD status change was noticed: one patient had uterine expulsion and one patient had abdominal expulsion. In both cases the expulsion was unilateral. No tip separations occurred after initial continuity of the ITD. If the ITD shifts alternative contraceptive methods are required. We offer the patients a repeat Ovabloc procedure or laparoscopic tubal occlusion. To date, no pregnancies have occurred in our study group.

In one patient a slow cure of the silicone resulted in an intra-abdominally

**Table 14.5.** Ovabloc ITD instillation rate at Spaarne Hospital, 1989–1991

| Period | 1989–1990 | | Continuous flow hysteroscopy 1991 | | 1989–1991 | |
|---|---|---|---|---|---|---|
| | n | % | n | % | n | % |
| Patients consented | 77 | | 94 | | 171 | |
| No procedure | 16 | 21 | 9 | 10 | 25 | 15 |
| Instillation attempt | 61 | | 85 | | 146 | |
| Normal ITD | 49 | 80 | 81 | 95 | 130 | 89 |
| Repeat procedure | 8 | 13 | 1 | 1 | 9 | 6 |
| Successful instillation | 54 | 89 | 82 | 96 | 136 | 93 |

**Table 14.6.** Ovabloc ITD continuation rates at Spaarne Hospital, 1989–1991

| Period | 1989–1990 | | 1991 (CFH) | | 1989–1991 | |
|---|---|---|---|---|---|---|
| | n | % | n | % | n | % |
| Successful instillation | 54 | | 82 | | 136 | |
| No follow-up | 1 | | 5 | | 6 | |
| 3-month X-ray control | 53 | | 79 | | 132 | |
| ITD status change at 3 mo. | 8 | 15 | 6 | 8 | 14 | 11 |
| Repeat procedure | 4 | 8 | 1 | 1 | 5 | 4 |
| Continuation rate[a] | 47 | 89 | 74 | 94 | 121 | 92 |
| 12-month X-ray control | 24 | | 8 | | 32 | |
| ITD status change at 12 mo. | 2 | | — | | 2 | |

[a] including patients with normal 3-month X-ray control after successful repeat procedure.

located silicone "ball". Subsequently a normal ITD was placed in the same tube. As the patient had persisting abdominal pain, the silicone "ball" was removed by laparoscopy, resulting in complete relief of the complaints. The silicone appeared to be located in the Pouch of Douglas without any adhesions or any obvious reaction of the surrounding peritoneum. No other adverse experiences have been identified in the patients of our study.

## Conclusion

At present the hysteroscopic formed-in-situ silicone Ovabloc ITD procedure appears to be the most reliable and effective method for transcervical hysteroscopic permanent contraception. The initial problems in the phase II and III clinical trials have been largely overcome by technical improvements of the product and the use of the new generation continuous flow Olympus hysteroscope with low viscosity fluid distension.

The Ovabloc ITD procedure is performed on an ambulatory basis without general anaesthesia, does not require any recovery time and is atraumatic. The woman can immediately resume her daily routine. A 3-months X-ray control is mandatory to exclude early expulsion. An extra 12 month X-ray control is strongly recommended. It is likely that vaginal ultrasonography could replace the X-ray follow-up.

As no figures are known on fertility after removal of the ITD the method should be considered to be irreversible. In approximately 10% of the cases the Ovabloc procedure will not be possible due to intrauterine or tubal abnormalities revealed during the hysteroscopic procedure.

# References


Blundell J (1842) Lectures on the principles and practice of midwifery. Edited by C Severn, London

Brundin J (1982) Hysteroscopy for sterilization. In: Hafez ESE, van Os WAA (eds) Contraceptive delivery systems, vol 3. Elsevier, Amsterdam, pp 63–74

Brundin J (1991) Transcervical sterilisation in the human female by hysteroscopic application of hydrogelic occlusive devices into the intramural parts of the fallopian tubes: 10 years experience of the P-block. Eur J Obstet Gynecol Reprod Biol 39:41–49

Darabi KF, Richart RM (1977) Collaborative study on hysteroscopic sterilization procedures; preliminary report. Obstet Gynec 49:48

Erb RA (1976) Silastic: a retrievable custom-molded oviductal plug. In: Sciarra JJ, Droegemueller W, Speidel JJ (eds) Advances in female sterilization techniques. Harper and Row, Philadelphia, p 259

Erb RA, Reed TP (1979) Hysteroscopic oviductal blocking with formed-in-place silicone rubber plugs. I: method and apparatus. J Reprod Med 23:65

Froriep R (1849) Zur Vorbeugung der Notwendigkeit des Kaiserschnitts und der Perforation. Notiz a d Geburtshilfe d Naturund Heilk 11:9

Guzman-Serani R, Bernales A, Cole LP (1983) Clinical report: quinacrine-fused pellets. In: Zatuchni GI, Shelton JD, Goldsmith A, Sciarra JJ (eds) Female transcervical sterilization. Harper and Row, Philadelphia, pp 100–104

Hosseinian AH, Morales WA (1983) Clinical application of hysteroscopic sterilization using uterotubal junction blocking devices. In: Zatuchni GI, Shelton JD, Goldsmith A, Sciarra JJ (eds) Female transcervical sterilization. Harper and Row, Philadelphia, pp 234–239

Kehrer FA (1897) Sterilisation mittels Tubendurchschneidung nach vorderem Scheidenschnitt. Zentralbl Gynaekol 21:961

Lindemann HJ (1971) Eine neue Untersuchungsmethode für die Hysteroskopie. Endoscopy 4:194

Lindemann HJ (1973) Transuterinen Tubensterilisation per Hysteroskop. Geburtsh u Frauenheilk 33:709

Lindemann HJ (1975) Tagung der Niederrhein.-Westfäl. Ges f Gynäk u Geburtsh, Düsseldorf

Lungren SS (1880) Cesarean section. Trans Am Inst Homeopathy, 33rd session, June 15–18, p 432

Mikulicz-Radecki F, Freund A (1927) Ein neues Hysteroskop und seine praktische Anwendung in der Gynäkologie. Z Geburtshilfe Gynaekol 92:13

Mullick B, Mumford SD, Kessel E (1987) Studies of quinacrine and of tetracycline for nonsurgical female sterilization. Adv Contracept 3: 245–254

Power FH, Barnes AC (1941) Sterilization by means of peritoneoscopic tubal fulguration. Am J Obstet Gynecol 41:1038

Reed TP, Erb RA (1980) Hysteroscopic oviductal blocking with formed-in-place silicone rubber plugs. II: clinical studies. J Reprod Med 23:69

Reed TP, Erb RA, de Maeyer J (1981) Tubal occlusion with silicone rubber: an update 1980. J Reprod Med 26:534

Richart RM (1983) The use of chemical agents in female sterilization. In: Zatuchni GI, Shelton JD, Goldsmith A, Sciarra JJ (eds) Female transcervical sterilization. Harper and Row, Philadelphia, pp 24–35

Richart RM et al. (1983) The effectiveness of the FEMCEPT method and preliminary experience with radiopaque MCA to enhance clinical acceptability. In: Zatuchni GI, Shelton JD,

Goldsmith A, Sciarra JJ (eds) Female transcervical sterilization. Harper and Row, Philadelphia, pp 212–218

Siegler AM, Grunebaum A (1983) A short history of tubal sterilization. In: Phillips JM (ed) Endoscopic female sterilization: a comparison of methods. Am Ass Gyn Lap, Downey, pp 3–8

Shuber J (1989) Transcervical sterilization with use of methyl-2-cyanoacrylate and a newer delivery system (the FEMCEPT device). Am J Obstet Gynecol 160:887–889

Wamsteker K (1977) *Hysteroscopie*. Thesis, University of Leiden.

Wamsteker K (1984) Hysteroscopic tubal sterilization with electrocoagulation and thermocoagulation. In: Siegler AM, Lindemann HJ (eds) Hysteroscopy: principles and practice. Lippincott, Philadelphia, pp 243–246

Zipper J, Cole LP, Rivera M, Brown E, Wheeler RG (1987) Efficacy of two insertions of 100-minute releasing quinacrine hydrochloride pellets for non-surgical female sterilization. Adv Contracept 3:255–261

Chapter 15

# The Consequences of Surgical Tubal Occlusion

G.M. Filshie and G. Robinson

## Introduction

Surgical tubal occlusion is the commonest method of female sterilisation. Approximately 70 000 patients undergo female sterilisation each year in England and Wales (Wellings 1986), and an estimate of the prevalence of the procedure suggests that in some parts of the country over 30% of married couples over the age of 35 have contraception provided for by female sterilisation (McCracken 1986). For such a common surgical procedure in the community, it is not unreasonable to account for its consequences.

## Surgical Consequences of Tubal Occlusion

The immediate consequences of the operation, which include surgical difficulties and complications, are well recognised. However, haemorrhage, perforation of visceral structures, and sepsis have also been reported (Chamberlain and Brown 1985). Late complications are rare, but there are a number of reports implicating the existence of a post-sterilisation syndrome, which involves increased menstrual loss accompanied by an increase in dysmenorrhoea. It has been suggested that this syndrome is related to changes in ovarian function resulting from disturbances of the ovarian vasculature that accompany destruction of the tube at occlusion, with the amount of vascular disturbance being proportional to the amount of tubal damage (DeStefano et al. 1985). However, controversy and debate still surround the syndrome, confounded by the fact that menorrhagia, dysmenorrhoea and other problems relating to periods increase with the age of the woman. Other late complications include torsion of the fallopian tube, unexplained pain, and the formation of hydrosalpinges (Frishman and Brest 1992) and pyosalpinges (Bledin et al. 1984). Up to 5% of the patients regret the operation, and approximately 1% of patients subsequently request a reversal. For a patient to undergo a reversal procedure, it is important to understand the pathological consequences of tubal occlusion.

## Pathological Consequences of Tubal Occlusion

The isthmic part of the tube is ideal for tubal occlusion, as the success of reversal procedures appears to depend on the intactness of the ampulla and fimbriae. The greater the amount of tube that is damaged, removed or cauterised at operation, the less tube there is available for examination and for reconstruction should it be required. Thus, methods that cause minimal tubal damage, such as clips and rings, have a higher successful pregnancy rate following reanastomosis than methods that sacrifice a variable to large amount of tube, such as partial salpingectomy and tubal diathermy. Although the latter can be minimal if "one place" endocoagulation is performed, cautery (both mono- and bipolar) is usually performed at 3 points. This is often very destructive to the tube, with the effects of the intense thermal heat generated involving far more of the mesosalpinx than can be inspected visually. The pathological changes in the fallopian tube subsequent to sterilisation with cautery have been reported by Vasquez et al. (1980), who showed that only small or insignificant portions of the proximal isthmic and distal ampullary tube remained intact after cautery. As a result of the extensive damage produced by electrocautery many patients are unsuitable for tubal microsurgical reversal, and the probability of a successful outcome for those who are operated on is poor (Phillips et al. 1977).

In Nottingham, where Filshie Clips have been the dominant method of female sterilisation for the past 10 years (with approximately 2000 pairs of clips being applied annually), considerable data have been obtained regarding the pathological changes in the fallopian tube subsequent to sterilisation with this device. To a lesser degree, data have also been obtained regarding the changes subsequent to sterilisation with the Hulka Clip and Falope–Ring Band. For these studies, specimens of the right and left fallopian tubes, which contained the site of tubal occlusion, and the tubal tissue proximal and distal to this site, were obtained at either total abdominal hysterectomy, bilateral salpingectomy or reversal of sterilisation from 164 patients who had been sterilised with Filshie Clips, 21 patients who had been sterilised with Hulka Clips, and 2 patients who had been sterilised with Falope–Ring Bands.

## Filshie Clip

### *Macroscopy*

At the macroscopic level, there was evidence of peritonealisation and fibrosis around the clip in all the specimens. The degree of peritonealisation and fibrosis was variable in patients who had been sterilised for less than 1 year, but in patients who had been sterilised for longer the clip was usually completely peritonealised and totally encapsulated in a fibrous sheath. The thickness of the fibrous sheath did not appear to be correlated to the length of time that the patient had been sterilised and, in the majority of specimens, the clip was clearly visible beneath the encapsulating tissues. Macroscopically, dilatation of the fallopian tubes was evident in 22% of the proximal segments and 1% of the distal segments. However, it was considered to be of pathological significance in the proximal segment of one only specimen.

In 5 patients, one of the tubes had been transected at the site of sterilisation. In 3 of these patients, the clip was still attached to one of the ends of the tube. In the remaining 2 patients, the clip had become detached and was found in the Pouch of Douglas. However, occlusion of the tubes had been accomplished in all of these patients. Detachment and subsequent migration of clips has also been noted with the clips, if in evidence, being located in the omentum, Pouch of Douglas, or pericolic gutter (Filshie, unpublished observations). In all of these patients, migration of the clip was not associated with any clinical symptoms. Although the mechanisms involved in migration are not known, it is possible that in some patients necrosis of the tube between the jaws of the clip leads to separation of the tubes prior to peritonealisation of the clip, which detaches before it is anchored in position by the peritonealisation process.

### *Microscopy*

By microscopy, changes in tubal morphology were evident at the site of occlusion and in the tubal tissue proximal and distal to this site. The principal pathological features are outlined in Table 15.1.

**Table 15.1.** Principal pathological features subsequent to sterilisation with the Filshie Clip

| |
|---|
| Site of occlusion |
| Fibrosis |
| Muscular atrophy |
| Inflammatation |
| Proximal tube |
| Plical attenuation and fibrosis |
| Luminal dilatation |
| Deciliated cuboidal epithelium |
| Distal tube |
| Plical attenuation and fibrosis |

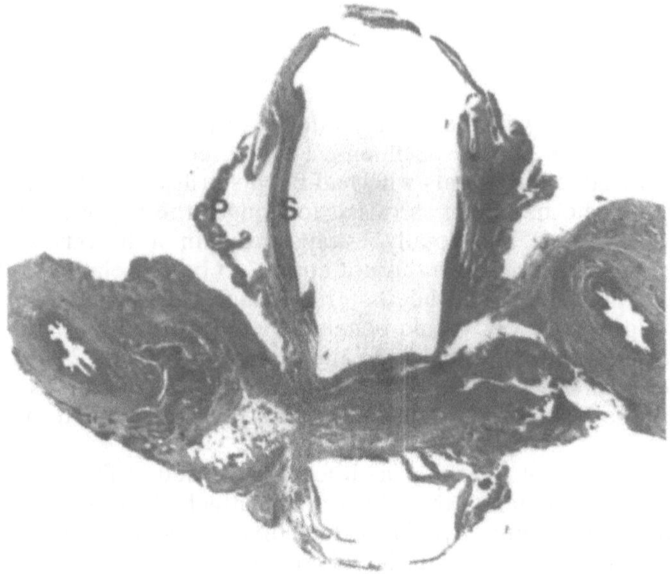


**Fig. 15.1.** A transverse section through a site of sterilisation showing the fibrous sheath (S) and peritoneal covering (P) that encased the Filshie Clip. ×8

*Site of occlusion.* At the site of occlusion, the clip was surrounded by a connective tissue sheath which, in turn, was overlain by the peritoneum (Fig. 15.1). The connective tissue sheath comprised a densely packed admixture of collagen fibres and spindle-shaped fibroblasts, with the former being predominant. Overall, the sheath ranged in width from 0.05 mm to 0.72 mm, but in the majority of specimens it was less than 0.4 mm. The clip was entirely surrounded by this sheath in specimens obtained 14 months or more post-sterilisation, but there appeared to be no correlation between the thickness of the sheath and the length of time that the patient had been sterilised. Immediately adjacent to the occlusion site, the longitudinal and circular smooth muscle had atrophied and been replaced by a vascularised, loose connective tissue. Atrophy of the muscle layers, however, was not total, and in all the specimens small bundles of smooth muscle cells were scattered throughout the loose connective tissue. In general, the bundles became more frequent towards the occluded end of the lumen which, in all the specimens, was delineated by a well-developed band of smooth muscle that was continuous with the normal musculature of the tube. In approximately 10% of the specimens, the loose connective tissue adjacent to the occluded end of the tubal lumen contained one or more isolated glands lined by tubal epithelium (Fig. 15.2). Serial sectioning revealed that there were continuities between these glands and the tubal lumen proper. The majority of the specimens were diffusely and focally infiltrated with small lymphocytes. Lymphocytic foci were most frequent at the outer, i.e. peritoneal, aspect of the connective tissue sheath surrounding the clip (Fig. 15.3) and within the sheath itself and, in an occasional specimen, in the smooth muscle layers at the occluded end of the lumen. Polymorphonuclear leucocytes, eosinophils,

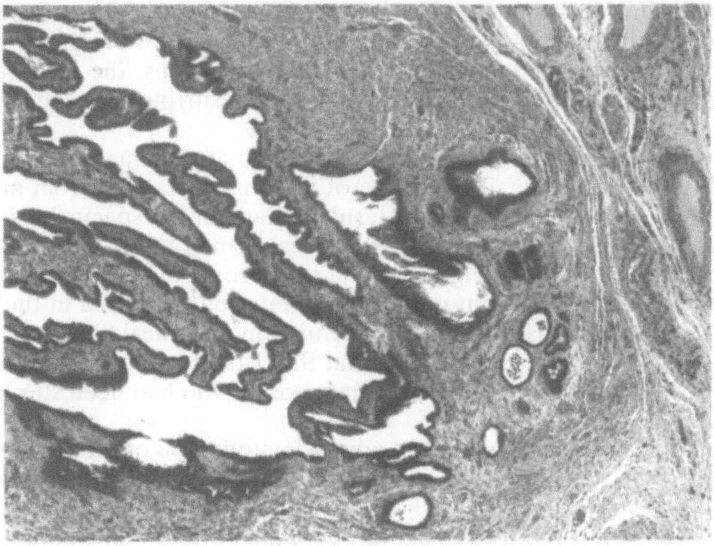

**Fig. 15.2.** A longitudinal section through a proximal tubule segment from a patient sterilised with Filshie Clips showing epithelial-lined glands at the end of the occluded lumen. ×60

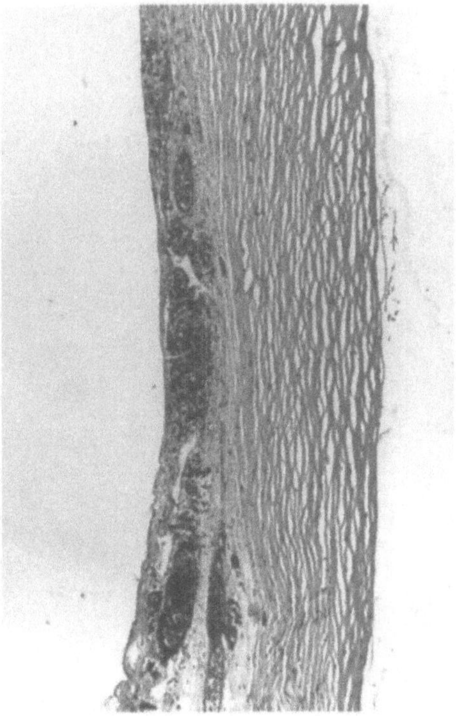

**Fig. 15.3.** Foci of small lymphocytes at the peritoneal aspect of the fibrous sheath that surrounded a Filshie Clip. ×105

plasma cells and macrophages were present in less than 15% of the specimens and usually formed a minor part of the infiltrate. Foreign body giant cells were found in 2 specimens only. In both specimens, the cells occurred on the inner aspect of the connective tissue sheath surrounding the clips.

*Proximal tube.* Plical attenuation was present in approximately 66% of the proximal tubule segments. The degree of attenuation ranged from mild to a complete loss of the normal fold pattern. In many of the specimens in which there was a significant flattening of the plicae, small polyp-like outgrowths protruded into the lumen (Fig. 15.4). Plical fibrosis was evident in 39% of the specimens. It ranged from mild to moderate, but was mild in the majority of affected specimens. Both plical attenuation and plical fibrosis appeared to be correlated to the length of time that the patient had been sterilised and was most pronounced in specimens from patients who had been sterilised for more than 5 years.

Luminal dilatation was evident in approximately 22% of the proximal segments, but was considered to be of pathological significance in only one patient.

At the occluded end of the proximal tube, the normal well-ciliated, columnar, secretory epithelium was replaced by a poorly ciliated, agranular, cuboidal epithelium (Fig. 15.5). In the majority of specimens, there was a return to normal tubal epithelium within 2 mm to 5 mm of the occluded end of the lumen.

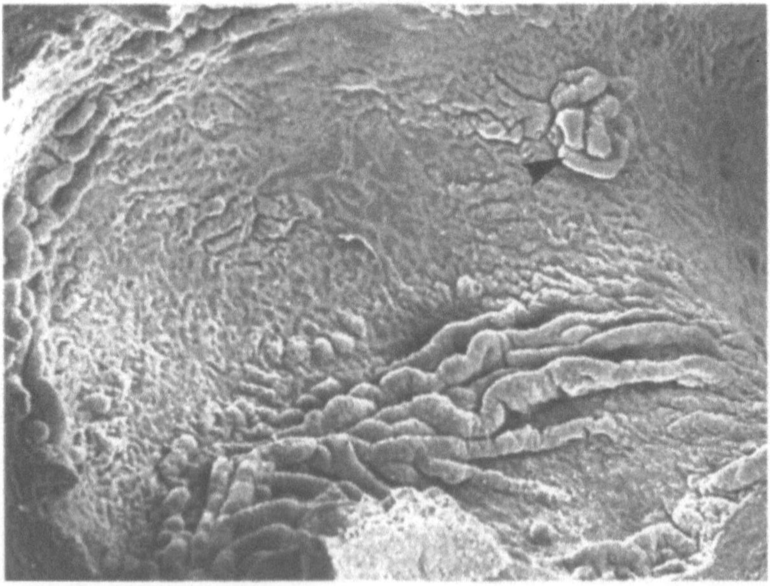

**Fig. 15.4.** A polyp-like protrusion (arrow) in the proximal tubal segment of a Filshie Clip patient 43 months post-sterilisation. Attenuation and flattening of the plicae are also evident. ×22

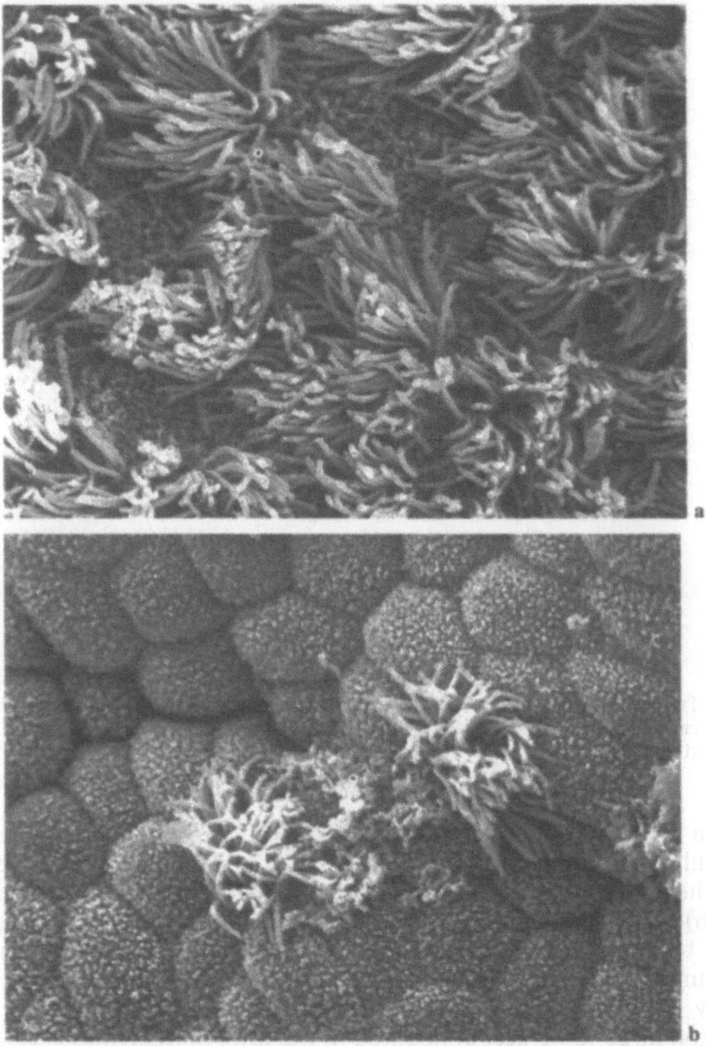

**Fig. 15.5.** **a.** The well-ciliated epithelium in the isthmic region of normal fallopian tube. ×1875. **b.** The deciliated epithelium in the isthmic region of a proximal tubule segment from a Filshie Clip patient 28 months post-sterilisation. ×1875

*Distal tube.* Plical attenuation was present in 54% of the specimens, and plical fibrosis was evident in 23%. In all the specimens, the changes were mild in form and no polyp-like protrusions were found.

## *Failures of Sterilisation*

A total of eight cases of failed sterilisation were studied. In 5 patients one lumen was patent and in the remaining 3 patients both of the lumens were

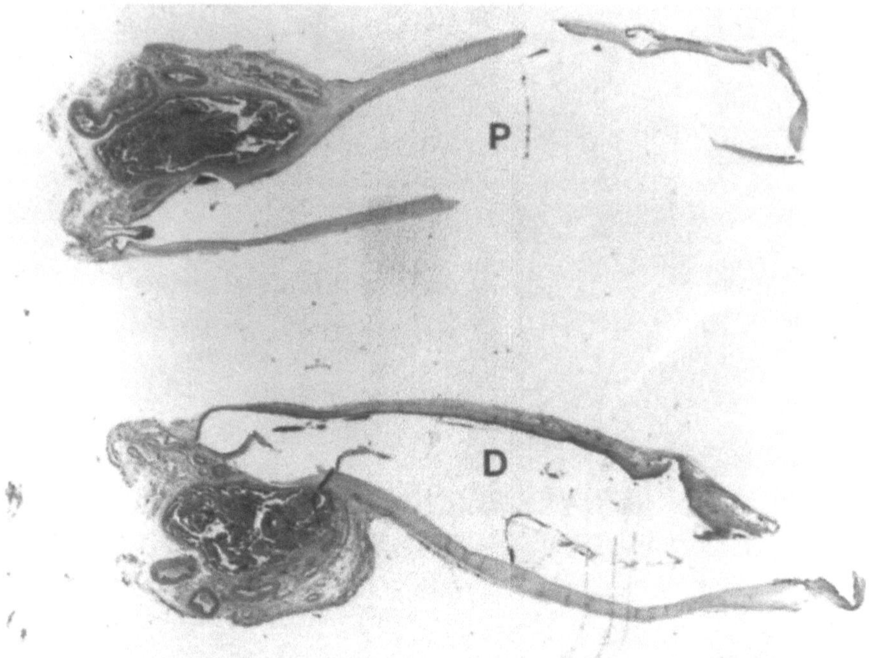


**Fig. 15.6.** Transverse sections through the proximal (P) and distal (D) tubal segments at the site of application in a failed sterilisation. The Filshie Clip has been misapplied and the tube passes behind the clip. ×10

patent. In 7 of the patients, as the devices had been applied to the mesosalpinx only, it is assumed that either the tube had slipped out of the jaw of the clip during closure or the surgeon had not identified the fallopian tube (Fig. 15.6). In the remaining patient, in whom both tubes were patent, the clips had been applied approximately 1 cm from the fimbriae and only part of the lumen had been occluded. The diameter of the tubal lumen immediately adjacent to the sites of sterilisation was approximately 7 mm, which is too large to be accommodated in the jaws of the clips.

## Hulka Clip

Except for differences in magnitude, the principal pathological changes subsequent to sterilisation with the Hulka Clip are similar to those produced by the Filshie Clip.

### *Macroscopy*

At the macroscopic level, all the Hulka Clip specimens were completely peritonealised, but it was evident that the underlying connective tissue sheath surrounding the Hulka Clip was thicker than its counterpart in the

Filshie Clip specimens as the majority of devices were not visible through the overlying tissue layers. Macroscopically, dilatation of the fallopian tubes was evident in 20% of the proximal segments, but it was not considered to be of pathological significance in any of them. The distal tube was not dilated in any of the specimens.

## *Microscopy*

*Site of occlusion.* By microscopy, it was evident that the connective tissue sheath surrounding the Hulka Clip was more extensive than that around the Filshie Clip. Overall, it ranged in width from 0.2 mm to 2 mm, being greater than 0.6 mm in the majority of specimens (Fig. 15.7). With the Hulka Clip, the width of the sheath appeared to be correlated to the length of time since the patient had been sterilised. The pattern of muscular atrophy was similar to that seen with the Filshie Clip, i.e. replacement of the musculature immediately adjacent to the site of sterilisation with a vascularised, loose connective tissue. Isolated glands lined by tubal epithelium were found in this

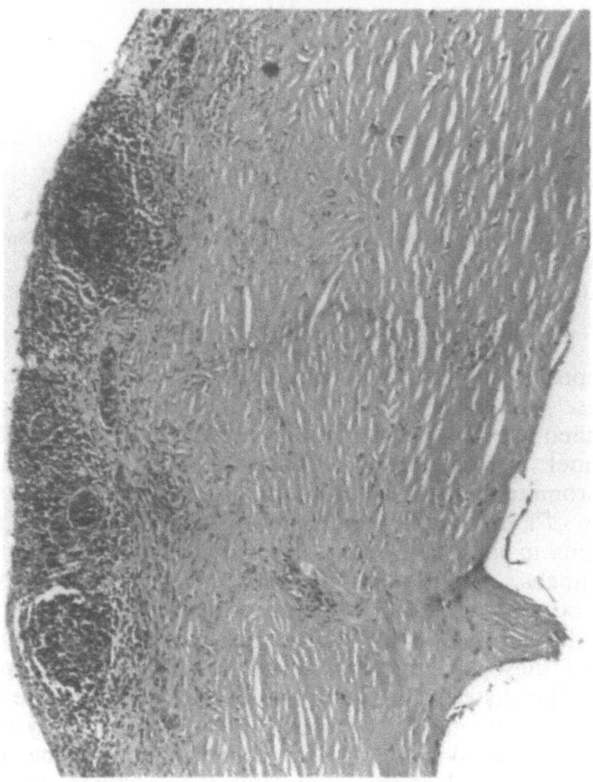

**Fig. 15.7.** Granulomata at the peritoneal aspect of the fibrous sheath that surrounded a Hulka Clip. (cf. Fig. 15.1.) ×105

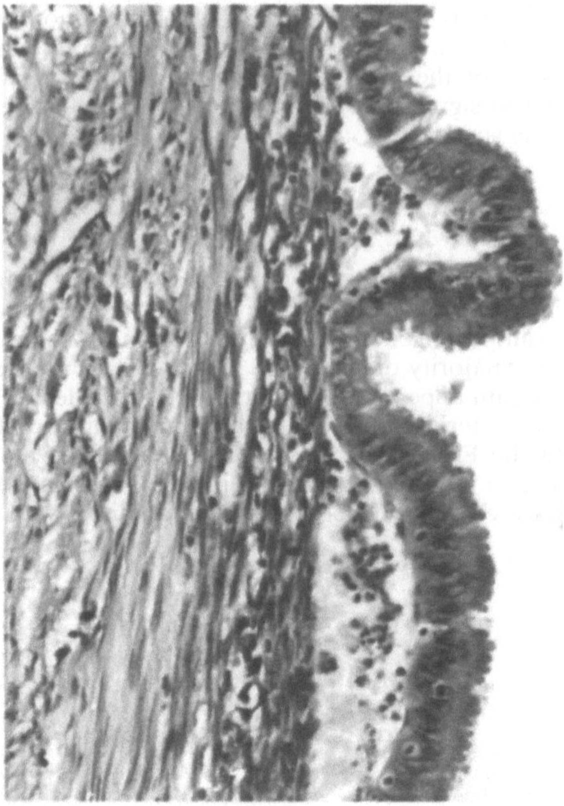

**Fig. 15.8.** Tubal epithelium lining the inner aspect of the connective tissue sheath that surrounded a Hulka Clip. ×345

tissue in approximately 30% of the specimens. As with the Filshie Clip, many of these glands were shown by serial sectioning to be continuous with the tubal lumen. In two specimens, tubal epithelium was also found partially lining the inner, i.e. clip, aspect of the connective tissue sheath (Fig. 15.8). The most prominent histological feature of the Hulka Clip specimens was the presence of a chronic inflammatory response, which was predominantly granulomatous in nature. There was evidence of chronic inflammation in all the specimens, and granulomata were present in 19 of the patients (15 bilaterally and 4 unilaterally). All the granulomata were cuffed by aggregates of small lymphocytes and, although inflammatory foci occurred more frequently in these specimens than in the Filshie Clip specimens, they showed a similar distribution. Multinucleate giant cells were not a common finding in the granulomata, but aggregates of foreign body giant cells were frequently encountered in the loose connective tissue at the site of occlusion and at the inner aspect of the connective tissue sheath. In two specimens, the remnant tissue between the jaws of the clip was associated with abundant foreign body giant cells.

*Proximal tube.* Plical attenuation and plical fibrosis were present in 75% of the specimens. These changes were predominantly mild to moderate in degree, and were most evident in patients who had been sterilised for 3 or more years. The changes in the tubal epithelium were similar to those outlined for the Filshie Clip, i.e. replacement of the normal tubal epithelium by a poorly ciliated, cuboidal epithelium at the occluded end of the lumen and a return to normal epithelium within 2–5 mm of the occluded end.

*Distal tube.* Plical attenuation was found in 75% of the specimens, and plical fibrosis was evident in 62% of the specimens. In all the specimens, the changes were mild in form and no polyp-like protrusions were found.

### *Failures of Sterilisation*

No cases of failed sterilisation involving the Hulka Clip were seen during the study.

## Falope–Ring Band

In the single case obtained from a successful sterilisation with the Falope–Ring Band, the principal pathological changes were minimal fibrosis around the devices themselves and a diffuse and focal inflammatory response of small lymphocytes. In magnitude, these responses were similar to those following sterilisation with the Filshie Clip. There was no evidence of luminal dilatation, plical attenuation, plical fibrosis or epithelial changes.

### *Failure of Sterilisation*

In the Falope–Ring Band sterilisation that failed, a tubo-peritoneal fistula was found on the superior surface of the right proximal tube. As the pregnancy was uterine, it is assumed the ovum gained access via this fistula.

# Discussion

The Filshie Clip, Hulka Clip and Falope–Ring Band have all proved to be safe and efficient methods of tubal sterilisation. Although none of the devices were originally designed with reversibility primarily in mind, they are finding increasing favour over other methods as they are proving to have a high potential for reversibility. The results of this study add support to previous reports which suggest that the success of sterilisation reversal is related to the amount of tubal damage incurred at and arising subsequent to sterilisation (Vasquez et al. 1980, 1983; Walz et al. 1980; Siegler et al. 1985). For the Filshie Clip, the pregnancy rate following microsurgical reanastomosis is 80%–90% (Filshie, unpublished observations).

The principal histological changes subsequent to sterilisation with the Filshie Clip are compatible with the pathological processes occurring following trauma, and there is no evidence to suggest that the constituents of the clip cause a reactive process. However, the presence of a granulomatous reaction in the Hulka Clip specimens is possibly indicative of an adverse tissue reaction to one of the constituents of this clip. Although there appears to be no documented case of an adverse tissue reaction to Lexan (the plastic constituent), allergic reactions to gold, including a case in which the Hulka Clip was implicated, have been reported (Cowan 1960; Elgart 1970; Elgort and Higdon 1971; Trathen and Stanley 1985).

When a sterilisation fails, it is often difficult to establish the exact cause of the failure. Macroscopic visualisation of mechanical devices by laparoscopy may show clear evidence of misapplication. Sometimes, however, it is inconclusive and histological examination of the site of sterilisation is required. In this study, all of the failures of sterilisation involving the Filshie Clip resulted from misapplication of the device. In all but one of the cases, the clip had been applied to the correct region of the tube, i.e. in the mid-isthmic portion approximately 3 cm from the cornua, but the tube had either slipped out of the jaws of the clip when it was being closed or the surgeon had not visualised the tube correctly. In the remaining case, the clips had been applied to the ampullary portion on both tubes, and both tubes had been incompletely occluded as the lumen in this region of the tube is too large to be accommodated by the clip. Although incomplete occlusion of the fallopian tube following correct application has been reported with the Mk. 4 Filshie Clip (Filshie 1985), no pregnancies due to this type of failure have been reported for the current Mk. 6 version.

# References

Bledin KD, Cooper JE, Mackenzie S, Brice B (1984) Psychological sequelae of female sterilisation: short-term outcome in a prospective controlled study. A report from the UK Field Research Centre of a WHO Collaborative Project.

Chamberlain G, Brown JC (1985) The report of the working party of the confidential enquiry into gynaecological laparoscopy. Royal College of Obstetricians and Gynaecologists, London

Cowan MA (1960) Contact dermatitis due to gold. Br J Dermatol 72:348

DeStefano F, Periman JA, Peterson HB, Diamond FL (1985) Long term risk of menstrual disturbances after tubal sterilisation. Am J Obstet Gynecol 152:835

Elgart ML (1970) Allergic contact dermatitis to gold. Arch Dermatol 106:254

Elgart ML, Higdon RS (1971) Allergic contact dermatitis to gold. Arch Dermatol 109:649

Filshie GM (1985) *The development of the TitaniumlSilicone rubber clip for female sterilisation.* DM Thesis, University of Nottingham

Frishman GN, Brest NA (1992) Hulka clip application as a potential cause of chronic pelvic pain. Contraception 45:325

McCracken JS (1986) Contraceptive care and family planning in an urban general practice. J R Coll GP 36:13

Phillips J, Hulka B, Hulka J, Keith D, Keith L (1977) American Association of Gynecological Laparoscopists 1976 membership survey. J Reprod Med 21:3

Siegler AM, Hulka J, Peterz A (1985) Reversibility of female sterilisation. Fertil Steril 43:499

Trathen WT, Stanley RJ (1985) Allergic reaction to Hulka Clips (Case Report). Obstet Gynecol 66:743

Vasquez G, Winston RML, Boeckx W, Brosens IVO (1980) Tubal lesions subsequent to sterilisation and their relation to fertility after attempts at reversal. Am J Obstet Gynecol 138:86
Vasquez G, Winston RML, Boeckx W, Baroness IA (1983) The epithelium of human hydrosalpinges: a light optical and scanning electron microscopic study. Br J Obstet Gynaecol 90:764
Walz KA, Ludwig H, Metzger H, Goudpasture JC, Genz HJ (1980) Morphology of the fallopian tubes removed from a patient after failure of clip sterilisation. Arch Gynecol 230:123
Wellings K (1986) Sterilisation trends (Editorial). BMJ 292:1029

Section VI

# Gamete and Embryo Transfer into the Fallopian Tube

Chapter 16

# Transabdominal Gamete Intrafallopian Transfer

J. Yovich

## Introduction

Gamete intrafallopian transfer (GIFT) appeared at a timely phase in the development of assisted reproduction. Although successful in-vitro fertilisation (IVF) had been achieved 6 years before, those pioneer clinics which were subsequently established were having difficulty establishing credible and consistent live-birth rates.

Indeed, international, multicentre data to the end of 1986, when collected by independent authorities, showed that the live-birth rate per IVF procedure was less than 10% and many clinics were generating occasional pregnancies only (Yovich et al. 1989c). However those clinics which adopted the GIFT procedure rapidly achieved consistent pregnancy rates and many well-established units showed that the live-birth rate achieved in their GIFT programme was significantly higher than in the IVF programme. GIFT was therefore adopted enthusiastically as an infertility treatment procedure and indeed some clinics which could not establish a comprehensive IVF service found they could conduct GIFT procedures quite successfully.

Although GIFT was introduced as a treatment mode for unexplained infertility, it was soon being explored for all types of infertility, including male factor and sub-occlusive tubal disease – categories for which it is now clear that GIFT is unsuitable. Furthermore as IVF and other procedures such as ovarian stimulation and intrauterine insemination (IUI) programmes are becoming more effective, and cost factors are assuming an increasing significance, GIFT is experiencing a lower profile in infertility management. However a number of developments are occurring such as transcervical catheterisation of the fallopian tubes enabling ambulatory, non-general anaesthesia procedures, and improved methods of preparing semen samples. These may lead to a re-emergence of the GIFT procedure.

The past, current and future eras in the evolution of GIFT can be categorised approximately as follows:

1984–1987 Period of enthusiastic initiation

1988–1991 Period of rationalisation

1992–1995 Period of reduced role

1996–1999 Period of rediscovery

This chapter will review the literature and available data with respect to these periods.

## Period of Initiation of GIFT

From discussions it is clear that many of us, including Patrick Steptoe, had transferred retrieved oocytes to the fallopian tubes, sometimes with prepared sperm, during the 1970s and early 1980s when undertaking reconstructive tubal surgery following ovarian stimulation and course timing of the procedure (Perone 1991). However the first successful case, undertaken as a definitive procedure, was that reported by Ricardo Asch and his colleagues (Asch et al. 1984). In a patient having controlled ovarian stimulation with human menopausal gonadotrophin (hMG) and human chorionic gonadotrophin (hCG) 36 h before, they described a laparoscopic approach to both oocyte retrieval and tubal transfer with 2 oocytes transferred to each fallopian tube using a polyurethane catheter. The sperm and oocyte segments within the conveying catheter were separated by an air space. The twin pregnancy which resulted was both a real advance in infertility management; and an opening for Catholic workers keen to explore the advances of assisted reproduction.

Catholic workers had until then been restricted from exploring new reproductive technologies as the Vatican would not tolerate either the process of artificially bringing egg and sperm into contact outside the body, or the action of masturbation to collect the semen sample (or even the collection of semen by sexual intercourse into a condom unless there be no barrier to the possibility of natural conception) (Vatican 1987). Industrious Catholic workers have developed suitable GIFT protocols as modifications of the Asch model which enable Catholic clinics around the world to undertake the procedure without contravening religious tenets (Garcea et al. 1989).

Although the first successful GIFT procedure was performed using laparoscopic techniques, the next report, again by Asch and his co-workers (Asch et al. 1986), described a series of cases using both laparoscopic and minilaparotomy procedures. They generated 4 pregnancies from a series of poorly explained cases of infertility, including moderate male factor cases – 6 of the 10 cases were managed by minilaparotomy for both egg recovery and transfer. Of 4 pregnancies achieved, 2 progressed to term. Of interest Asch and his group still often perform minilaparotomy collections, whereas most other groups now use either laparoscopy for both oocyte retrieval and

**Table 16.1.** Randomised study comparing GIFT and IVF-ET undertaken at PIVET during 1985–86 for a range of infertility disorders. (With kind permission of International Journal of Fertility.)

| | IVF-ET | | GIFT | |
|---|---|---|---|---|
| | number | % | number | % |
| Unexplained | 8/60 | 13 | 20/69 | 29 |
| Tubal | 78/550 | 14 | 21/74 | 28 |
| Endometriosis III and IV | 3/93 | 3 | 18/54 | 33[a] |
| Negative PCT | 2/22 | 9 | 18/58 | 33 |
| ASABs – semen | 5/18 | 28 | 2/12 | 19 |
| – female | 4/20 | 24 | 0/2 | – |
| Ovulatory disorders | 2/31 | 6 | 6/30 | 20 |
| Failed DI | 4/23 | 17 | 13/43 | 30 |
| Oligospermia | 9/75 | 12 | 0/17 | – |
| | | | 11/49 | 22 |
| Total | 132/873 | 15 | 109/408 | 27[b] |

[a] $p<0.01$
[b] $p<0.001$

tubal transfer; or transvaginal ultrasound-directed oocyte recovery followed by laparoscopic transfer.

The potential for GIFT to improve the chance of pregnancy for infertility failing to respond to conventional therapies was explored widely over the ensuing years. One early study over the period of 1985–1986 explored the effectiveness of GIFT in all cases previously enrolled in an IVF programme, but where patency had been demonstrated in at least one fallopian tube (Yovich and Matson 1990). A randomisation process was adopted where patients were given the opportunity to select the established method (IVF) or choose the new technique (GIFT) with its uncertain effectiveness, as only the initial report had appeared at that stage. The data are shown in Table 16.1 and indicate a significantly higher chance of pregnancy with GIFT than with conventional IVF and embryo transfer (ET).

In comparing the subcategories, GIFT was seen to be better for unexplained infertility, severe pelvic endometriosis, cases with poor sperm/mucus interaction (negative post-coital tests (PCTs) performed 8–12 h p.c.), some ovulatory disorders and failed donor insemination (DI). However it was not useful for cases in which the female partner had antispermatozoal antibodies (ASABs) or where there was any degree of male factor disorder, either oligozoospermia, asthenozoospermia or ASABs in the semen. Subsequently it was shown that a modification of the Asch protocol could achieve reasonable rates of pregnancy in moderate oligozoospermic cases if 2–5 times the standard numbers of progressively motile spermatozoa could be harvested for transfer (Matson et al. 1987a). This is in keeping with current knowledge that sperm from male factor cases have functional disorders (e.g. a reduced rate of acrosome reactivity); raising the numbers can improve the chance of fertilisation without necessarily increasing multipronuclear development. It can also be seen that subocclusive tubal infertility is also amenable to GIFT. Pregnancy outcomes were not significantly different in the series (Table 16.2) although there was a trend for fewer blighted ovum pregnancies but more ectopics among the GIFT cases.

**Table 16.2.** Pregnancy outcomes for comparative randomised study of IVF-ET and GIFT at PIVET during 1985–86. (With kind permission of International Journal of Fertility.)

| | IVF–ET | | GIFT | |
|---|---|---|---|---|
| | number | % | number | % |
| Biochemical | 12 | 9.1 | 9 | 8.3 |
| Blighted ovum | 18 | 13.6 | 8 | 7.3 |
| Miscarriage | 3 | 2.35 | 6 | 5.5 |
| Ectopic | 9 | 6.8 | 9 | 8.3 |
| Delivered >20 wks | 90 | 68.2 | 77 | 70.6 |
| Total | 132 | | 109 | |
| Women's ages | | | | |
| range | 22–44 | | 21–42 | |
| mean | 32.5 ± 4.5 | | 32.7 ± 3.7 | |

Data from other clinics (Craft et al. 1988) (Table 16.3) including that of a multinational co-operative study (Asch 1989) (Table 16.4) were consistent showing successful fertilisation and subsequent implantation rates per oocyte transferred ranging from 8%–13%. At that time IVF units were reporting implantation rates per embryo transferred to the uterus as 4%–11% (Yovich et al. 1987a). Craft suggested a flexible approach to oocyte numbers transferred indicating that older women could have 10 or more eggs transferred with minimal risk of high-order multiple pregnancy. However a closer look at the data (Table 16.3) reveals an excessive risk of triplets which is greater when more than 4 oocytes are transferred; this persists even for older women.

An additional indication for GIFT is that of ovum donation which appeared to give very high pregnancy rates, possibly related to the younger age of the donors and their higher responsiveness to stimulation. However others preferred to stagger the treatment days for donor and recipient in order to maintain the confidentiality aspect, e.g. by a blend of GIFT and IVF techniques in the procedures of pronuclear stage tubal transfer (PROST) and tubal embryo stage transfer (TEST) (Yovich et al. 1987a).

**Table 16.3.** Segment of data from a large series of GIFT procedures in a single unit (Humana Wellington, London) with a flexible approach to treatment. The data compare egg numbers transferred with the age of the patient and chance of multiple pregnancy. (With kind permission of Lancet.)

| Number of oocytes | Number of patients | Pregnancies | Pregnancy rate (%) | Pregnancy rate by age | | Multiples 3+ (%) |
|---|---|---|---|---|---|---|
| | | | | 35–39 (%) | 40+ (%) | |
| 1–2 | 115 | 16 | 14 | 11 | 5 | 0 |
| 3–4 | 263 | 65 | 25 | 21 | 18 | 5 |
| 5–6 | 310 | 118 | 38 | 36 | 29 | [a]7 |
| 7–8 | 243 | 104 | 43 | 47 | 24 | [a]12 |
| 9–10 | 108 | 41 | 38 | 50 | 15 | [b]15 |
| >10 | 32 | 16 | 50 | 50 | 25 | 6 |
| Total | 1071 | 360 | 34 | 34 | 19 | 8 |

[a]2 quads and [b]1 quin in 35–39 yr age group

**Table 16.4.** GIFT results from a multinational co-operative study co-ordinated by R. Asch

| Aetiology | Number of cases | Number of pregnancies | Pregnancy rate (%) |
|---|---|---|---|
| Unexplained infertility | 796 | 247 | 31 |
| Male | 397 | 61 | 15 |
| Endometriosis | 413 | 132 | 32 |
| Failed DI | 160 | 66 | 41 |
| Tubal/peritoneal | 210 | 61 | 29 |
| Cervical | 68 | 19 | 28 |
| Immunological | 30 | 5 | 10 |
| Premature ovarian failure | 18 | 10 | 56 |
| Total | 2092 | 601 | 29 |

These latter procedures are preferable to GIFT as increasingly donor oocytes are fertilised and stored for a quarantine period prior to transfer.

## Period of Rationalisation

From the annual reports of the Australian Institute of Health (AIH) National Perinatal Statistics Unit (NPSU) which maintains a comprehensive register of all IVF and GIFT procedures performed in Australia in concert with the Fertility Society of Australia (FSA) (Lancaster 1991), it can be seen that most of the expansion of assisted reproduction in recent years has been with GIFT (Fig. 16.1). However an overall peak for assisted reproductive procedures was reached in 1988. The 1989 data reveals that GIFT procedures resulted in a live-birth pregnancy rate more than double that of IVF-ET.

Scrutiny of the NPSU data for pregnancy outcome of GIFT procedures with respect to the infertility subcategory shows a very high ectopic pregnancy rate in cases with known tubal disease (Table 16.5). Others have previously reported excessive ectopic rates for any tubal transfer procedure in cases of suspected or known tubal disorder even where the tubes appear normal and patent (Yovich 1990). There is some reduction in the rate over the 2 years depicted and it is likely that tubal infertility will disappear completely from the list of disorders treated by GIFT in future.

Male factor cases have generally fared poorly when treated by GIFT. Even those amenable to the modified technique of inseminating higher numbers appear to have higher early pregnancy wastage (Rodriguez-Rigau et al. 1989; Yovich et al. 1989a). Currently, the preferred approach to male factor infertility is to conduct IVF with sperm motility enhancers such as pentoxifylline (Yovich et al. 1990c) and micromanipulation procedures such as subzonal insemination (SUZI) (Ng et al. 1988), partial zona dissection (PZD) (Cohen et al. 1989) or intracytoplasmic sperm injection (ICSI) (Palermo et al. 1992). Thereafter fertilised oocytes can be selected for transfer by PROST or cleaved embryos transferred by ET or TEST for which the results are significantly better (Yovich et al. 1989b).

There are variations in international trends for the adoption of GIFT over IVF. Fig. 16.2 shows comparisons of data for IVF, GIFT and frozen embryo

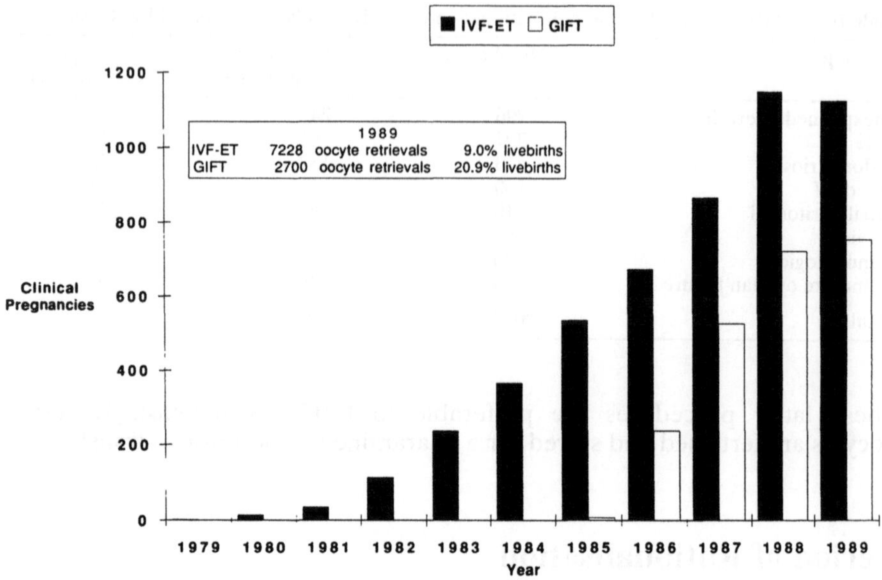


**Fig. 16.1.** Clinical pregnancies reported to the Australian Institute of Health National Perinatal Statistics Unit which maintains the register of cases for all assisted reproduction treatments performed in Australia and New Zealand.

**Table 16.5.** Ectopic pregnancy rates (%) reported from NPSU register and compared according to the main categorisation of infertility aetiology

| | 1988 | 1989 |
|---|---|---|
| Tubal | 19.1 | 17.9 |
| Male | 0.9 | 1.2 |
| Endometriosis | 4.9 | 4.3 |
| Multiple | 2.7 | 3.3 |
| Unexplained | 5.3 | 5.6 |
| Total | 4.8 | 4.6 |

transfer (FET) in Australia (Lancaster 1991), the United Kingdom (Donaldson 1991) and the United States (Medical Research International 1992). Of interest, Australia has a higher rate of procedures per population (1:1600 per annum) than either the UK (1:5000) or the USA (1:12500).

## Procedural Protocol

The procedure of GIFT has been modified little from that described in the original report of 1984. At PIVET the following protocol was current in 1988/89:

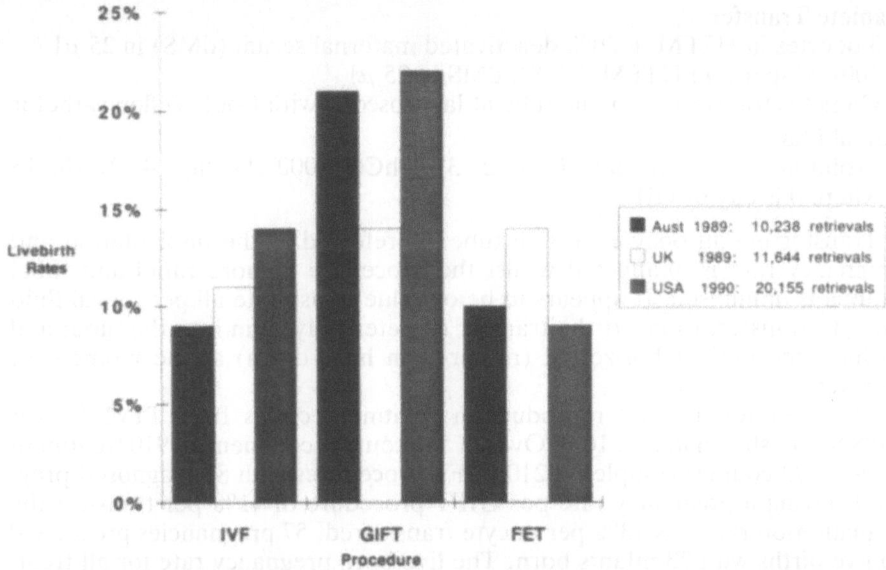


**Fig. 16.2.** Live-birth rates per oocyte retrieval procedure reported from the national registries of three countries. The data include the results from frozen embryo transfer (FET) procedures in addition to IVF and GIFT.

Indications:
- Where up to 4 treatments of IUI has failed for –
  - unexplained infertility
  - poor sperm/mucus interaction
  - endometriosis
  - failed DI

Ovarian stimulation
- CC/hMG
  - hCG 10 000 IU 6th day of E2 rise
- Lucrin/hMG (down regulation preferred)
  - hCG 10 000 IU 7th day of E2 rise

Oocyte recovery
- 36 h after hCG trigger
- Transvaginal ultrasonography directed recovery
- PIVET-Cook aspiration/flushing needle

Laboratory
- Semen collected 2 h before
- Oocytes graded over 4 points
- Supernumerary oocyte options
  - fertilisation and cryopreservation
  - donation to another couple or approved research
  - discard

Gamete Transfer

3 oocytes in HTFM + 20% deactivated maternal serum (dMS) in 25 μl

100 000 sperm in HTFM + 20% dMS in 25 μl

Gametes transferred to one tube at laparoscopy with Cook Teflon catheter

Luteal Phase

Proluton 50 mg imi days 0, 1, 2, 3, 4 hCG 1000 IU days 4, 7, 10, 13 where 0 is day of GIFT

Transferring all oocytes to one tube is preferred as the implantation and pregnancy rate is unaffected whilst the procedure is more rapid and tubal trauma is minimised. It appears to be of value to aspirate all peritoneal fluid prior to transfer; to insert the transfer catheter fully 4 cm into the tube; and to have the patient horizontal (rather than head-down) at the moment of transfer.

The data for assisted reproduction treatment cycles from PIVET over 1988/89 are shown in Fig. 16.3. Overall 581 couples commenced 910 treatment cycles. 172 couples completed 210 GIFT procedures with 87 diagnosed pregnant, giving a pregnancy rate per GIFT procedure of 41% per transfer; the implantation rate was 13% per oocyte transferred. 57 pregnancies proceeded to live births with 73 infants born. The live-born pregnancy rate for all treatments commenced during the period was 24.5% for GIFT (233 cycles commenced), 16.3% for IVF-ET (276 cycles commenced), 17.4% for PROST (172 treatment cycles commenced) and 14.9% for TEST (229 treatment cycles commenced). The latter two procedures contained the majority of severe male factor cases with relatively high rates of failed fertilisation, and pregnancy rates of 36% and 31%, respectively, per embryo transfer.

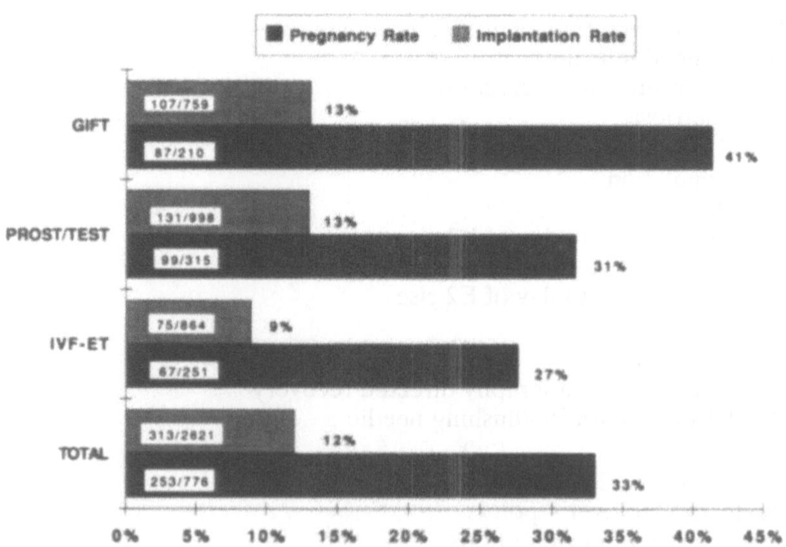


**Fig. 16.3.** The pregnancy rates (βhCG positive) per transfer procedure and the implantation rates (gestational sacs on ultrasound at 8 weeks per oocyte or embryo transferred) of all assisted reproduction procedures conducted at PIVET during 1988/89. The implantation rate from uterine transfer is significantly lower than from tubal transfers ($p < 0.001$).

When up to 4 oocytes were transferred the multiple pregnancy rate for GIFT was 30%, reducing to around 20% when a limit of 3 oocytes was enforced by State Government regulation. These data conform closely to the binomial model for pregnancy and multiple pregnancy rates expected (Yovich et al. 1990a). In the ensuing years there has been a slight reduction in the pregnancy rates to around 30%–33%, probably due to the blanket reduction on oocytes transferable. This effect has been shown in several prominent clinics. However there is also a trend in the data suggesting that GIFT-generated embryos have a higher implantation rate over PROST embryos which in turn have a higher rate over TEST embryos. This indicates that earlier return to the fallopian tube confers an advantage, possibly highlighting deficiencies in laboratory culture methods. All tubal transfer embryos implant at a higher rate than uterine transfers (Yovich et al. 1990a) implying one or all of the following:

1. There is a tubal factor which is beneficial to embryo growth.
2. The early post-ovulation uterine environment is hostile to embryos causing demise of all but the most robust embryos.
3. The tubal environment is physically more secure for transferred embryos.

The question of luteal support in GIFT has been extensively debated. Higher pregnancy rates than IVF can be achieved by GIFT without luteal support so generally it has not been applied. However a carefully conducted, prospective, randomised and controlled study in a GIFT series where cases were selected as least likely to require luteal support showed positive benefit (Yovich et al. 1991). The use of hCG or progesterone significantly improved the chance of pregnancy and highly significantly improved the chance of a live birth. Modelling techniques showed the effect to be greatest for poorer quality oocytes and embryos. There was an apparent benefit in combining the hCG and progesterone, particularly to minimise the need for additional early pregnancy hormonal support.

## Period of Reduced Role

The world-wide activity in the field of assisted reproduction over the past decade has emphasised less invasive and less expensive treatments to generate pregnancies. The same clinics which were established to conduct IVF and GIFT procedures were able to introduce more comprehensive diagnostic facilities to investigate the underlying male and female factors.

Detailed clinical evaluation of both partners can significantly improve the chance of pregnancy in non-tubal infertility (Yovich and Grudzinskas 1990). Furthermore, some previous teachings concerning infertility management no longer hold true e.g., regarding ovarian stimulation.

Not all "normal" menstrual cycles display the hormone levels required for conception. Daily serum oestradiol (E2) indicates that peak E2 should be above 650 pmol/l at the commencement of the luteinising hormone (LH) surge and that pre-surge cervical mucus should score 6 points or more on the Insler rating. Pre-ovulatory PCTs always show a positive score (<10 progressively motile sperm per high power field) when evaluated before the LH surge and when E2 levels are measured to be greater than 500 pmol/l. The PCT should be performed at least 8 h p.c. and evaluated in mucus derived from high in the cervical canal. The midluteal (7–10 days after LH surge) serum progesterone (P4) level should be greater than 30 nmol/l and E2 is usually above 500 pmol/l. The least consistent parameter in conception cycles is the size of the ovarian follicle on transabdominal or transvaginal ultrasound. In over 100 spontaneous conception cycles evaluated the average follicle diameter ranged from 14 to 27 mm when measured within 1 day of the LH surge.

Assessment cycles failing to conform to hormonal criteria are deemed Disordered Ovulatory Cycles if not frankly anovulatory. These are responsive to ovarian stimulation, either with clomiphene citrate (CC) and/or human menopausal gonadotrophins combined with hCG trigger and luteal boosts (Yovich et al. 1987b). CC cycles require careful tracking as up to 22% will display cervical mucus inhibition which will necessitate discontinuation of CC (Matson and Yovich 1987b). Cycles with raised basal LH levels (>10 IU/l) and hyperandrogenism should also avoid CC. Pure FSH is then preferred for ovarian stimulation and down regulation with a gonadotrophin releasing hormone analogue (GnRHa) may also be required. Pregnancy rates average 20% per treatment cycle and the risk of multiple pregnancy can be held below 5% by keeping peak E2 levels below 3500 pmol/l.

Where the PCT is negative, even after ovarian stimulation, intrauterine insemination (IUI) of precapacitated sperm can be effective (Yovich and Matson 1988). The insemination of 0.5 ml of culture medium containing 5–$10 \times 10^6$ high-grade motile sperm 38–42 h after the hCG trigger in stimulated cycles can yield pregnancy rates of 15%–25% per treatment cycle in suitable categories. These are cases of unexplained negative PCTs, mild oligospermia, semen ASABs and female ASABs. Cases with asthenozoospermia are not suitable and those with active underlying endometriosis fare poorly. Cases of unexplained infertility may respond to IUI but the pregnancy rates are only of the order of 10%. High pregnancy rates (around 25%) are seen in donor insemination programmes employing donor IUI exclusively or after a series of failed intracervical inseminations (Patton et al. 1992). Generally 3 or 4 straws are required to generate sufficient sperm numbers.

The samples for IUI using either husband or donor sperm can be derived by sperm swim-up, sedimentation or discontinuous Percoll filtration methods. It is advisable to use whichever method will provide the cleanest possible sample as well as the highest number of highly motile spermatozoa. For asthenozoospermic cases, sperm motility enhancement can be used e.g. with pentoxifylline.

Where couples are considered to have a relatively poor prognosis in IUI, they may still wish to persist with it as a less invasive and cheaper form of treatment. The chance of pregnancy can be improved by 2 inseminations, adding a second the previous day around 18 h post-hCG (Silverberg et al. 1992). Pregnancy rates of the order of 50% can be achieved.

A comparative study between GIFT and ovarian stimulation, with or without IUI, shows a significant benefit and overall cost-effectiveness for GIFT (Table 16.6) (Wessels et al. 1992). However, high pregnancy rates

**Table 16.6.** Comparative pregnancy rates (%) per treatment cycle for GIFT or ovarian stimulation with or without intrauterine insemination. Asterisk marks infertility subgroups where GIFT was shown to be more cost-effective. (With kind permission of Fertility and Sterility.)

| | GIFT (161 cycles) | Ovarian stimulation with or without intrauterine insemination (185 cycles) | |
|---|---|---|---|
| Idiopathic | 23.6 | 36.8 | |
| Endometriosis* | 31.6 | 5.3 | p<0.01 |
| Cervical factor* | 28.6 | – | |
| Anovulation | 50.0 | 26.3 | p<0.01 |
| Immunological* | 25.0 | 15.8 | |
| Multifactorial | 14.3 | 10.5 | |
| Total* | 26.7 | 9.7 | p<0.0001 |

were achieved in the simpler programmes when the subcategory was unexplained infertility or ovulation disorder, indicating the need for rationalisation and individual selection. This view is enhanced by a study showing that the cumulative probability of conception for GIFT or PROST is similar regardless of whether IUI treatment cycles had been conducted beforehand (Robinson et al. 1992).

In clinical practice, patients and clinicians tend to be most comfortable (in an ethical sense) progressing through treatment options in a staged fashion, electing for the least complex, least invasive and least expensive treatment mode which confers a reasonable chance of pregnancy. For some patients age and distance factors may predicate towards GIFT or IVF as an early option but for the majority, GIFT is an early option only in cases of pelvic endometriosis and those with cervical disorders (e.g. post-laser ablation or cone biopsy). Most other non-tubal cases will prefer a trial of ovarian stimulation with or without IUI in the first instance. Cases of male factor infertility and female ASABs will prefer to be treated by IVF then PROST or TEST.

# The Future: Rediscovering GIFT

The advantages of GIFT relate to its high degree of effectiveness; its single event treatment procedure (egg collection and gamete transfer); its close approximation to natural fertilisation; and the double benefit of possible fertilisation with cryopreservation of the supernumerary oocytes.

The disadvantages of GIFT are its ineffectiveness in certain types of infertility; the need to be absolutely certain about normality of the fallopian tubes; the need for complex anaesthesia; the need for high-order operative facilities and skills; and the need for a reasonably sophisticated laboratory to prepare the gametes and deal with the supernumerary oocytes.

These disadvantages are not insurmountable and there are already developments which may swing the pendulum back towards GIFT. These are given below.

### *Ineffectiveness in Certain Types of Infertility*

Improved diagnostic procedures in male factor cases, e.g. the acrosome reaction to ionophore challenge (ARIC) test (Cummins et al. 1991); hyperactivation determined by computer-assisted semen analysis (CASA) (Burkman 1990); and the detection of reactive oxygen species (ROS) in semen (Aitken 1989), permit improved sperm preparations for assisted reproduction. Pentoxifylline and 2-deoxyadenosine appear not only to stimulate sperm motility, but also suppress ROS and improve the acrosome reactivity of defective specimens. At PIVET a number of pregnancies have now been achieved by IUI and GIFT where such sperm preparations have been performed following favourable laboratory results on the ARIC test and CASA.

Where ASABs are present in semen, improved techniques have been reported for their removal; this could also lead to improved results for GIFT (Grundy et al. 1992). However it is difficult to envisage overcoming the barrier for circulating female ASABs except by binding sperm to oocyte or by preliminary sperm microinjection prior to transfer.

### *Normality of Fallopian Tubes*

It is good practice to evaluate all aspects of the female genital tract in the investigation of infertility. Ideally this will include a hysteroscopy and laparoscopy. Any case with a tubal disorder should not have GIFT except in the presence of minimal or unilateral disease. However, given the financial costs of such an exercise patients may prefer to bypass the investigation and rely on out-patient hysterosalpingography or defer to IVF-ET as the less complex option. Out-patient hysteroscopy and falloposcopy (Kerin et al. 1990) procedures are evolving and should make routine investigations more readily acceptable and probably more clinically relevant.

### *Complex Anaesthesia*

Laparotomy and laparoscopy both require general anaesthesia. This usually includes neuromuscular paralysing drugs as well as intubation for effective airway control. The use of propofol as the inducing agent and the newer laryngeal airways which obviate the need for endotracheal intubation, have improved the acceptability of general anaesthesia. Cases are now conducted on a day-care basis but this is still far short of the ambulatory theatre arrangement which is suitable for IVF-ET.

### *Operation Facilities*

The laparoscopy and minilaparotomy techniques also constitute a limitation to the appeal of GIFT from the informed patient's perspective. The development of transcervical cannulation techniques without general anaesthesia will help to expand the potential of GIFT. "Blind" cannulations, with or without ultrasound assistance, have not been satisfactory. Indeed, they may be quite difficult, thereby compromising the outcome of the treatment cycle

(Yovich et al. 1990b). Hysteroscopic or falloposcopic cannulations may prove more satisfactory but few cases have been performed to date.

### *Laboratory Facilities*

The handling of gametes for GIFT requires the same degree of sophistication as that for IVF. In particular oocytes should not be allowed to undergo cooling which can cause irreversible damage, and gamete handling within culture solutions should enable strict control over pH and osmolality. The actual GIFT procedure can be performed with basic laboratory facilities, even mobile facilities. However, the effectiveness is often compromised and there are major limitations to the handling of supernumerary oocytes, when compared to GIFT procedures performed adjacent to a conventional IVF embryology laboratory (Matson and Yovich 1987b).

### *Supernumerary Oocytes*

The fate of the supernumerary oocytes arising from GIFT poses technical and ethical questions. Fertilisation of supernumerary oocytes as a diagnostic guide in the GIFT procedure is only useful if fertilisation occurs. Various reports have confirmed the first observation that the presence or absence of fertilisation in the supernumerary oocytes has no predictive value for either pregnancy or failure of the GIFT procedure in that cycle (Matson et al. 1987b). The fertilisation rate of supernumerary oocytes is less than 50% (Yovich et al. 1989a), as opposed to 75% in normospermic IVF cases, which indicates that the current selection criteria for oocytes to be transferred at GIFT are appropriate.

Many workers in assisted reproduction programmes have expressed disquiet at the process of simply discarding healthy oocytes and believe that facilities should be available to offer fertilisation with subsequent cryopreservation of the pronuclear oocytes or resulting embryos for the couple's subsequent use. Alternatively the woman should be able to donate her oocytes to another couple or an approved research programme. Some GIFT clinics do not have such laboratory support facilities but at least one group has learnt to function successfully as a satellite of a "mother" IVF unit. Gametes are transferred by intravaginal culture tube (Ranoux et al. 1988) or portable incubator.

Other units, e.g. Catholic centres, may restrict oocyte numbers collected to match those which will be transferred. This may cause a dilemma when overstimulation results in the potential for additional oocytes to be released spontaneously. The simple puncture of additional follicles may reduce the risk of high-order multiple pregnancies in that situation.

## Conclusion

GIFT is the most effective treatment for a range of infertility disorders but is not commonly applied as the first treatment. Following its initial enthusiastic introduction the pendulum has tended to swing away from GIFT in many situations.

For the moment GIFT will probably remain as the preferred treatment for non-tubal, non-male factor infertility if there are no detectable ASABs in the female circulation, and if ovarian stimulation with or without IUI treatment has been tried without success. Highly successful IVF units (i.e. with overall pregnancy rates consistently above 20%) may often not consider GIFT except for cases of severe endometriosis or recurrent IVF failures in which embryo quality is consistently poor. There may be special advantages for GIFT in those situations. Sometimes GIFT will also be preferred as a treatment option where the patient's age, time considerations, geographical dislocation and convenience factors may dictate particular needs.

The future should see GIFT results improve for male factor disorders, particularly with better definition of sperm disorders and better semen preparations e.g. using pentoxifylline or 2-deoxyadenosine enhancement. However the main barriers to the utilisation of GIFT relate to the need for high-grade operating facilities and skills, and the concomitant need for complex anaesthesia. Major benefits will apply in favour of GIFT should effective out-patient transcervical procedures become established.

## References

Aitken RJ (1989) The role of free oxygen radicals and sperm function. Int J Androl 12:95–97

Asch RH (1989) GIFT: Indications, results, problems and perspectives. In: Capitanio GL, Asch RH, De Cecco L, Croce S (eds) GIFT: From basics to clinics. Raven Press, New York, pp 209–228

Asch RH et al. (1984) Pregnancy following translaparoscopic gamete intrafallopian transfer (GIFT). Lancet 2:1034

Asch RH et al. (1986) Preliminary experiences with gamete intrafallopian transfer (GIFT). Fertil Steril 45:366–371

Burkman LJ (1990) Hyperactivated motility of human spermatozoa during in vitro capacitation and implications for fertility. In: Gagnon C (ed) Controls of sperm motility: biological and clinical aspects. CRC Press, Boca Raton, pp 303–329

Cohen J et al. (1989) Partial zona dissection of human oocytes when failure of zona pellucida penetration is anticipated. Hum Reprod 4:435–442

Craft I et al. (1988) Analysis of 1071 GIFT procedures – the case for a flexible approach to treatment. Lancet 1:1094–1098

Cummins JM et al. (1991) A test of the human sperm acrosome reaction following ionophore challenge (ARIC): relationship to fertility and other seminal parameters. J Androl 12:98–103

Donaldson M (1991) The sixth report of the Interim Licencing Authority for human in-vitro fertilisation and embryology (6). Interim Licencing Authority.

Garcea N et al. (1989) Is the GIFT a possibility for Catholics in the Assisted Reproduction field? Raven Press, New York, pp 313–319

Grundy CE et al. (1992) Establishment of pregnancy after removal of sperm antibodies in vitro. BMJ 304:292–293

Kerin J et al. (1990) Falloposcopy: a microendoscopic technique for visual exploration of the human fallopian tube from the uterotubal ostium to the fimbria using a transvaginal approach. Fertil Steril 54:390–400

Lancaster P (1991) Assisted Conception Australia and New Zealand 1989 (ISSN 1030–4711). AIH National Perinatal Statistics Unit

Matson PL, Yovich JL (1987a). Changes in cervical mucus following ovarian stimulation for in vitro fertilization. Infertility 10:267–277

Matson PL, Yovich JL (1987b) Gamete intrafallopian transfer in a non-IVF unit. Lancet 1:111–112

Matson PL et al. (1987a) The role of gamete intrafallopian transfer (GIFT) in the treatment of oligospermic infertility. Fertil Steril 48:608–612

Matson PL et al. (1987b) The in vitro fertilization of supernumerary oocytes in a gamete intrafallopian transfer (GIFT) program. Fertil Steril 47:802–806

Medical Research International and The American Fertility Society Special Interest Group, (1992) In vitro fertilization-embryo transfer (IVF-ET) in the United States: 1990 results from the IVF-ET registry. Fertil Steril 57:15–24

Ng SC et al (1988) Pregnancy after transfer of sperm under zona. Lancet 2:790

Palermo G et al. (1992) Pregnancies after intracytoplasmic injection of single spermatozoon into an oocyte. Lancet 340:17–19

Patton PE et al. (1992) Intrauterine insemination outperforms intracervical insemination in a randomised controlled study with frozen, donor semen. Fertil Steril 57:559–564

Perone N (1991) Gamete intrafallopian transfer (GIFT): historic perspective. J In Vitro Fert Embryo Transfer 8:1–4

Ranoux C et al. (1988) A new in vitro fertilization technique. Fertil Steril 49:654–657

Robinson D, Syrop CH, Hammitt DG (1992) After superovulation-intrauterine insemination fails: the prognosis for treatment by gamete intrafallopian transfer/pronuclear stage transfer. Fertil Steril 57:606–612

Rodriguez-Rigau LJ et al. (1989) Relationships between the results of sperm analysis and GIFT. J Androl 10:139–144

Silverberg KM et al. (1992) A prospective randomised trial comparing two different intrauterine insemination regimens in controlled ovarian stimulation cycles. Fertil Steril 57:357–361

Vatican (1987) Instruction on respect for human life in its origin and on the dignity of procreation. Congregation for the Doctrine of the Faith

Wessels PH et al. (1992) Cost-effectiveness of gamete intrafallopian transfer in comparison with induction of ovulation with gonadotrophins in the treatment of infertility: a clinical trial. Fertil Steril 57:163–167

Yovich JL (1990) Tubal transfers: PROST & TEST. In: Asch RH, Balmaceda JP, Johnston I (eds) Gamete physiology. Serono Symposia USA, Norwell, USA, pp 305–317

Yovich JL, Grudzinskas JG (1990) The management of infertility: a practical guide to gamete handling procedures. Heinemann, London

Yovich JL, Matson PL (1988) The treatment of infertility by the high intrauterine insemination of husband's washed spermatozoa. Hum Reprod 3:939–943

Yovich JL, Matson PL (1990) The influence of infertility aetiology on the outcome of in vitro fertilization (IVF) and gamete intrafallopian transfer (GIFT) treatments. Int J Fertil 35:26–33

Yovich JL et al. (1987a) Pregnancies following pronuclear stage tubal transfer. Fertil Steril 48:851–857

Yovich JL et al. (1987b) Ovarian stimulation for disordered ovulatory cycles. Asia-Oceania J Obstet Gynaecol 13:457–463

Yovich JL et al. (1989a) The usefulness of simultaneous IVF and GIFT in predicting fertilization and pregnacy. In: Capitanio GL, Asch RH, De Cecco L, Croce S (eds) GIFT: from basics to clinics. Raven Press, New York, pp 321–332

Yovich JL et al. (1989b) Dyspermiae and GIFT of PROST & TEST. In: Capitanio GL, Asch RH, De Cecco L, Croce S (eds) GIFT: from basics to clinics. Raven Press, New York, pp 411–424

Yovich JL et al. (1989c) In-vitro fertilization today. Lancet 2:688–689

Yovich JL et al. (1990a) The benefits of tubal transfer procedures. In: Mashiach S, Ben-Rafael Z, Laufer N, Schenker JG (eds) Advances in assisted reproductive technologies. Plenum Press, New York, pp 271–285

Yovich JL et al. (1990b) Transcervical tubal embryo-stage transfer (TC-TEST). J In Vitro Fert Embryo Transf 7:137–140

Yovich JM et al. (1990c) Influence of pentoxifylline in severe male factor infertility. Fertil Steril 53:715–722

Yovich JL, Edirisinghe WR, Cummins JM (1991) Evaluation of luteal support therapy in a randomized controlled study within a GIFT program. Fertil Steril 55:131–139

Chapter 17

# Transvaginal Gamete Intrafallopian Transfer

R.P.S. Jansen and J.C. Anderson

## Indications and Anatomical Considerations

If the fallopian tubes are normal, it is appealing to use them when conception is to be assisted clinically (Jansen and Anderson 1992b). The advantages are several. First, an early intratubal location for gametes (Asch et al. 1985) or embryos (Yovich et al. 1987; Balmaceda et al. 1988) provides a better, or at least a more reliable, environment for embryonic development than might be expected with fertilisation and embryo culture in vitro. Second, the timing of embryo entry into the uterus will be determined more by endocrine events affecting the genital tract than by the operator's judgement. And third, the direction of entry of embryos into the uterus will be from the tubes, not from the cervix. Several studies have shown that gamete intrafallopian transfer (GIFT), as well as early embryo transfer to the tubes, as conventionally practised through the fimbrial end of the tube at laparoscopy, produce higher rates of pregnancy than do embryo transfers through the cervix to the uterus (Yovich et al. 1988; Devroey et al. 1989).

Despite the advantages of tubal transfers of gametes (or embryos) at laparoscopy, clinical IVF since 1984 has increasingly rested on transvaginal, ultrasound-guided follicle aspiration for obtaining oocytes, often with local anaesthesia alone (Dellenbach et al. 1985), rendering IVF and uterine embryo transfer (ET) an ambulatory, out-patient procedure in many clinics. The need to keep to laparoscopy and general anaesthesia for gamete or embryo transfer to the tubes therefore has perpetuated a disadvantage. We reported a transvaginal approach to catheterising the tubes for gamete (or embryo) transfer in 1987 (Jansen and Anderson 1987) and, since then, have described pregnancies after using this system to deliver gametes or embryos to the fallopian tubes without operation (Jansen et al. 1988a,b; Jansen and Anderson 1989, 1990, 1992a,b).

The extrauterine part of the tube has an average length of 11 cm, the medial 2–3 cm of which forms the tubal isthmus (Woodruff and Pauerstein 1969). The medial isthmus is the narrowest part of the tube, with an average diameter of 0.4 mm (range 0.1–1.0 mm), mucosa that occupies 3–6 primary folds, and with a firm, thick muscular wall (Lisa et al. 1964). The interstitial or intramural part of the tube joins the isthmus to the funnel-shaped (Lisa et al. 1964) angle of the endometrial cavity. The interstitial tube takes a convoluted course in most specimens dissected after fixation (Sweeney 1961; Rocker 1964), but when intraluminal pressure or the flow of fluid is directed laterally from the uterine angle or funnel there are only minor deviations in its course (Rubin 1928). The tubal isthmus at the time of ovulation produces highly acidic mucus glycoproteins (Jansen 1980, 1984), which may be expected to lubricate and perhaps to protect the mucosa. Lateral to the isthmus, the tubal ampulla is wide and thin-walled.

Between the vagina and the ampullary-isthmic junction lie the cervix, the uterine cavity, the uterotubal junction and the tubal isthmus, where the tube is narrowest. To catheterise the tube from the vagina, a fine enough catheter needs to be delivered to the uterotubal junction after negotiating an anteroposterior curve in the sagittal plane through the endocervix and a lateral curve in the coronal plane between the internal cervical os and the internal tubal ostium.

## Catheter System and Techniques

As a basis for devising a catheter suitable to be passed along the fallopian tube we accepted that plastic splints of about 0.6 mm have been used successfully during operative anastomosis of the isthmus of the fallopian tube (Winston 1977).

Several procedures have now been devised to image and to reach the fallopian tubes from the vagina with catheters, including radiography with contrast medium (Platia and Krudy 1986), hysteroscopy (Confino et al. 1986; Possati et al. 1991), ultrasound (as described by us and by others (Bustillo and Schulman 1989; Scholtes et al. 1990; Yovich et al. 1990)), and indeed with no imaging and, instead, reliance just on tactile sensation (Bauer et al. 1990; Pratt et al. 1991; Risquez et al. 1990; Ferraiolo et al. 1991). Of these, ultrasound is the only objective way to image the catheter in the tube without otherwise disturbing the anatomy and function of the mucosa.

The catheter system we now use is the KJITS-2000 model (William Cook Australia, Brisbane Technology Park, Queensland 4113, Australia – Fig. 17.1), which has a bulb-tip on the outer cannula for ease of passage through the cervix and endometrial cavity to the uterotubal junction (UTJ). The technique of transvaginal catheterisation of the tube is illustrated in Figs. 17.2, 17.3 and 17.4 (Jansen and Anderson 1987). In each of our cases, transvaginal ultrasound images have been obtained (a) of the outer cannula in the

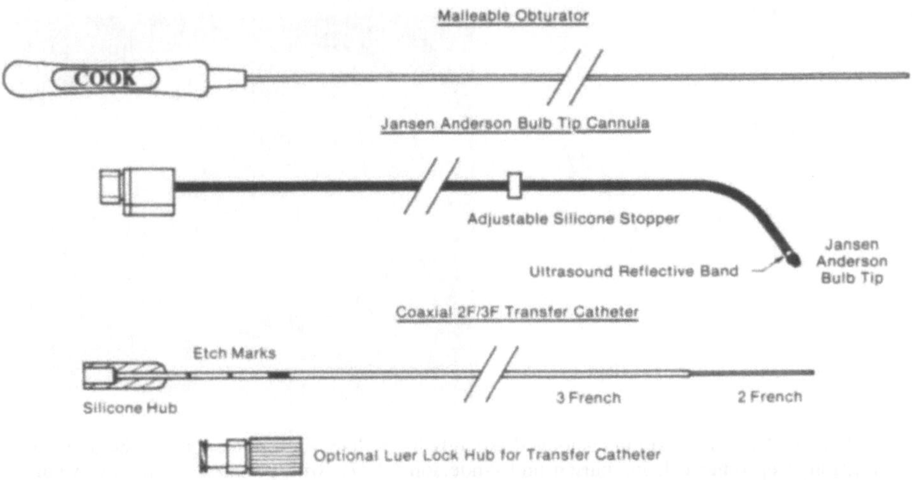


**Fig. 17.1.** Components of the Model KJITS-2000 fallopian catheterisation set, by courtesy of William Cook (Aust.) Pty Ltd, Brisbane Technology Park, Queensland 4113, Australia.

lateral angle of the uterine cavity (Fig. 17.3) and (b) of the 2-F inner catheter in the fallopian tube among the adnexal echoes (Fig. 17.4).

We have recently compared our experience with the KJITS-2000 catheter system used this way during 1991 with a contemporary series of laparoscopic GIFT (LAP–GIFT) procedures. For each case of transvaginal GIFT (TV–GIFT) there were three cases of LAP–GIFT controlled for age, number of

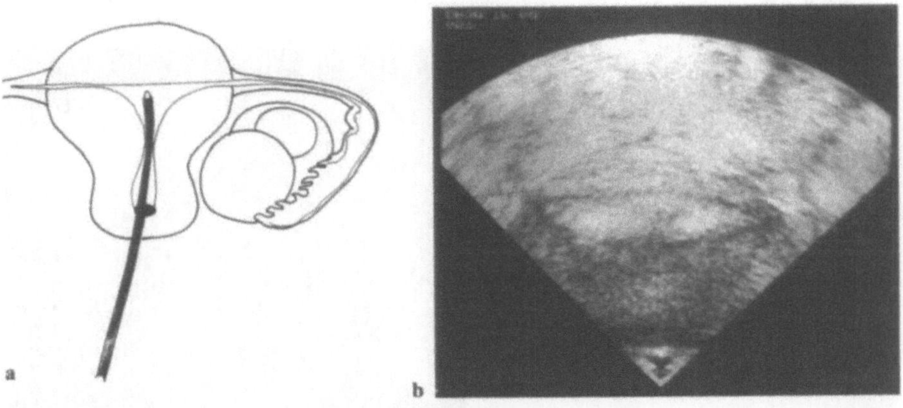

**Fig. 17.2. a.** Passage of the outer cannula, with or without a malleable obturator, through the cervix from the vagina. Reproduced from Jansen and Anderson (1987), with permission. **b.** Coronal ultrasound scan of the endometrium (echogenic) obtained from an anteflexed uterus with the probe situated anterior to the cervix; for a retroflexed uterus a similar image is obtained with the probe posterior to the cervix. The usual image has been inverted for comparison with **a.** Reproduced from Jansen and Anderson (1992b), with permission.

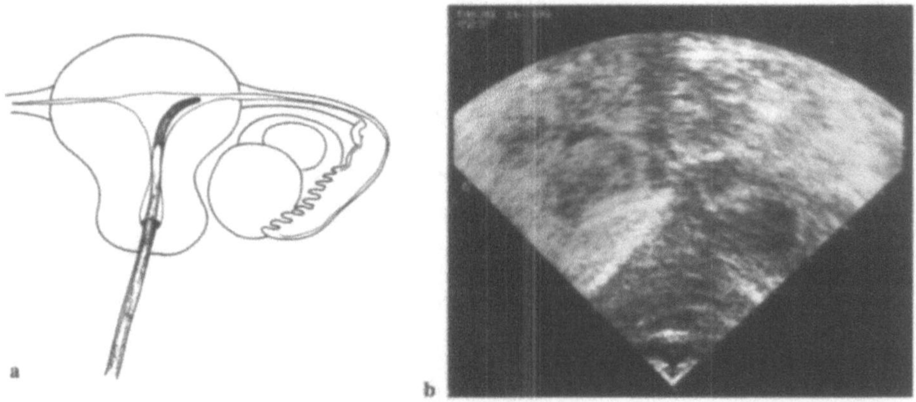
a b

Fig. 17.3. **a.** The outer cannula is lodged securely in the lateral uterine angle, at the uterotubal junction. Reproduced from Jansen and Anderson (1987), with permission. **b**. Transvaginal ultrasound image of the outer cannula positioned in the lateral angle of the endometrial cavity. The transducer has been rotated from the coronal plane clockwise (for an anteflexed uterus; anticlockwise for a retroflexed uterus) towards the sagittal plane. Inverted image. Reproduced from Jansen and Anderson (1992b), with permission.

previous GIFT cycles, number of eggs obtained from follicle aspiration and number of eggs transferred (Jansen and Anderson 1992b). Semen parameters were the same in the two groups, but because the volume of fluid transferred was, by design, less with TV–GIFT there were fewer spermatozoa transferred this way (Table 17.1). Oocytes were dissected partly of their cumulus in order further to reduce the volume of medium needed for transfer. The catheter was passed to a depth of 2–3 cm from the UTJ to effect transfer.

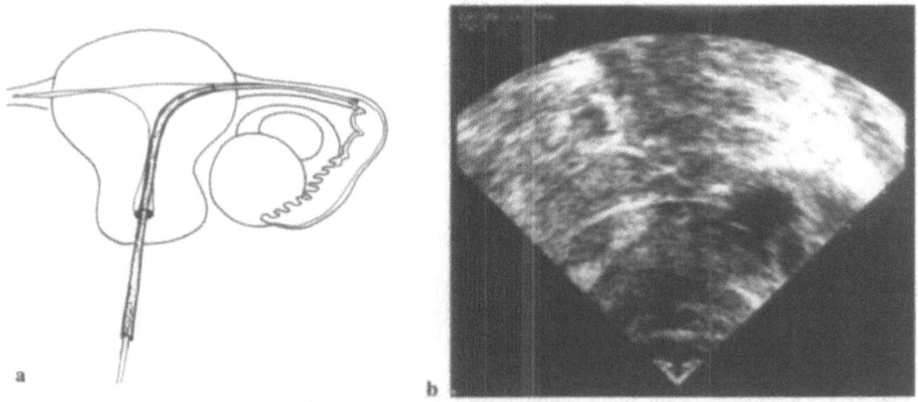
a b

**Fig. 17.4.** The inner catheter is passed down the fallopian tube isthmus. Reproduced from Jansen and Anderson (1987), with permission. **b.** With further rotation of the probe, the inner catheter is seen in the fallopian tube among the adnexal echoes. Inverted image. The more anteverted the uterus, the more posteriorly directed the tubes are, and the more sagittal the plane of the transducer needs to be to image the catheter. Reproduced from Jansen and Anderson (1992b), with permission.

**Table 17.1.** Comparison of patient and cycle characteristics among 20 TV–GIFT procedures and 60 matched LAP–GIFT controls. From Jansen and Anderson (1992b)

| | TV–GIFT | LAP–GIFT |
|---|---|---|
| Number of procedures | 20 | 60 |
| Mean age[a] (years) (range) | 36.7 (31.9–43.1) | 34.9 (24.1–44.7) |
| Mean duration of infertility (years) | 2.8 | 3.8 |
| Mean cycle order[a] | 1.41 | 1.36 |
| Sperm density after prep. (× 1000/30 μl) | 181.9 | 118.2 |
| Sperm motility after prep. (%) | 98 | 96 |
| Mean eggs obtained[a] | 8.8 | 8.7 |
| Mean eggs transferred[a] | 2.8 | 2.7 |
| Mean total transfer volume (range) | 38 μl (16–75 μl) | 71 μl[b] (35–135 μl) |
| Mean total sperm transferred | 118 000 | 247 000[b] |
| Total eggs transferred | 54 | 162 |
| Total sacs | 5 | 25 |
| Implantation rate (%) | 9.3 | 15.4 |
| Clinical pregnancies | 4 | 21 |
| Clinical pregnancy rate (%) | 20.0 | 35.0 |

[a] Variables controlled by the experimental design.
[b] $p < 0.01$.

We do not know yet if this preparative method and depth and volume of gamete transfer is optimal.

# Outcome

Table 17.1 gives details of this case-controlled retrospective study of TV–GIFT versus LAP–GIFT. Table 17.2 compares this study with other reported TV–GIFT series.

The clinical pregnancy rate among LAP–GIFT procedures in this study (35.0 %) was consistent with that in an earlier, larger series of ours (Jansen et al. 1990) and shows why it has not been simple to recruit candidates for

**Table 17.2.** TV–GIFT: summary of published results

| Author | Number of pregnancies | Number of cycles | Pregnancy rate (%) |
|---|---|---|---|
| *KJITS-1000 or KJITS-2000* | | | |
| Bustillo and Schulman (1989) | 1 | 14 | 7.1 |
| Lucena et al. (1989) | 3[a] | 7 | 42.9 |
| Ferraiolo et al. (1991) | 7[a] | 26 | 26.9 |
| Jansen and Anderson (1992a) | 7[a] | 28 | 25.0 |
| Jansen and Anderson (1992b) | 4 | 20 | 20.0 |
| Total | 22 | 95 | 23.2 |
| *$CO_2$-Hysteroscopic TV–GIFT* | | | |
| Possati et al. (1991) | 7 | 26 | 26.9 |

[a] each including one ectopic pregnancy.

TV–GIFT, with results less certain than with LAP–GIFT. Although the total number of TV–GIFT procedures reported is still limited, our data and those of others (Table 17.2) indicate that, despite the supposed advantages to patients of avoiding exposure to general anaesthesia and laparoscopy, pregnancy rates with TV–GIFT seem to be two-thirds those of LAP–GIFT (Jansen and Anderson 1992b).

# Complications

## Infection

In the first 100 fallopian catheterisations there were 2 patients who developed fever and unilateral pain several days after the procedure (Jansen and Anderson 1992b). In both cases endocervical cultures were negative, but antibiotics were administered and clinical resolution took place. In one of these cases conception and uterine pregnancy has since occurred after LAP–GIFT. In the other case hysterosalpingography has shown both tubes to be patent. Among 168 cases of transcervical intratubal insemination, Bieber, Pratt and co-workers (Bieber 1991; Pratt et al. 1991) reported one case of severe salpingitis requiring salpingectomy. Routine culture of the endocervix is probably unnecessary in the absence of clinical cervicitis (which we define as yellow mucus on a cervical swab), but it is important to remember that persistent unilateral discomfort on the side of catheterisation is abnormal and should indicate antibiotic therapy.

## Ectopic Pregnancy

In a previous review of our procedures there were 57 conceptions during the cycle of fallopian catheterisation (donor semen, n = 11; husband's semen, n = 5; TV–GIFT, n = 9; embryos, n = 32); there were three tubal pregnancies, in two of which there was a past history of contralateral ectopic pregnancy but no hysterosalpingographic indication of disorder on the catheterised side. The four further pregnancies among our most recent series of TV–GIFT procedures (Jansen and Anderson 1992a) were all uterine. Among TV–GIFT pregnancies reported (Table 17.2) (Lucena et al. 1989), there have been three ectopic pregnancies (3.3 %), a rate similar to that with LAP–GIFT.

## Pain and Vaso-vagal Reactions

Pain during passage of the catheter is usually mild, but can sometimes be substantial and accompanied by vaso-vagal hypotension. Premedication with a narcotic analgesic and atropine is sometimes advisable. One patient on two occasions experienced bilateral cramps that lasted for several days after bilateral catheterisations: a later laparoscopy showed no sign of trauma, both tubes were patent, and the patient has since delivered a baby after LAP–GIFT.

# Conclusions

Further experience with TV–GIFT may simply narrow the gap between its results and those now expected with LAP–GIFT. However, it seems reasonable to look at the factors that might reduce the success rates. Although there may be mechanical disadvantages in passing a gamete delivery catheter through the fallopian tube isthmus, which is normally closed at the time of ovulation (Jansen 1980), the low rate of ectopic pregnancy reported after TV–GIFT and transvaginal tubal embryo transfer procedures, and the protective mucus usually present in the isthmus at ovulation, would make it unlikely that mucosal trauma is a factor; moreover, because of their bulk, oocytes in cumulus would seem less likely than embryos to follow the withdrawn catheter down the uterus and be lost.

Volumes of fluid transferred into the tubes for GIFT were significantly smaller for TV–GIFT (trans-isthmic) procedures than for LAP–GIFT (trans-fimbrial) procedures (Table 17.1), mainly to reduce the chance that transferred oocytes might be expelled from the end of the fallopian tube. It may be that limiting transfer volumes by sacrificing some of the cumulus and by decreasing the total number of sperm transferred is wrong. The occurrence of pregnancies after transfer of oocytes-in-cumulus directly into the cul-de-sac (Coulam et al. 1991) implies that the fimbrial end is likely to recover most oocytes-in-cumulus that pass beyond it: the risk of losing such oocytes through the fimbrial end of the tube if TV–GIFT volumes are higher may have been overstated.

It remains to be shown (a) whether increasing the number of spermatozoa transferred will improve pregnancy rates, and (b) whether there is a real advantage in using ultrasound to place the fallopian catheter in comparison with simply positioning it in the tube by tactile sensation (Bauer et al. 1990; Pratt et al. 1991; Risquez et al. 1990; Ferraiolo et al. 1991). The results reported here indicate, however, that TV–GIFT is a reasonable alternative to other ambulatory, non-anaesthesia-requiring forms of assisted conception, such as ovarian stimulation and washed-semen intrauterine insemination (Silverberg et al. 1992) and follicle aspiration with direct intraperitoneal sperm and oocyte transfer (Coulam et al. 1991). For the limited number of eggs transferred at TV–GIFT, the pregnancy rate is at least comparable and the hazard of occasional high-multiple pregnancy can be avoided.

*Acknowledgements.* We thank Dr. Tom Boogert, Dr. Paul Sutherland and Dr. Warwick Birrell for carrying out some of the TV–GIFT procedures, and Mr. Geoff Reeves, William Cook (Aust.) Pty Ltd, for developing the KJITS series of catheter sets.

# References

Asch RH, Balmaceda JP, Ellsworth LR, Wong PC (1985) Gamete intra-fallopian transfer (GIFT): a new treatment for infertility. Int J Fertil 30:41–45

Balmaceda JP, Borrero C, Castaldi C, Ord T, Remohi J, Asch RH (1988) Tubal embryo transfer as a treatment for infertility due to male factor. Fertil Steril 50:476–479

Bauer O, Van der Ven H, Diedrich K, Al-Hasani S, Krebs D, Gembruch U (1990) Preliminary results on transvaginal tubal embryo stage transfer (TV-TEST) without ultrasound guidance. Hum Reprod 5:553–556
Bieber R (1991) Transvaginal intratubal insemination by tactile sensation. Presented at the 7th World Congress on In Vitro Fertilization and Assisted Procreations (sic). Paris, France, June 30 to July 3
Bustillo M, Schulman JD (1989) Transcervical ultrasound-guided intrafallopian placement of gametes, zygotes and embryos. J In Vitro Fert Embryo Transf 6:321–324
Confino E, Friberg J, Gleicher N (1986) Transcervical balloon tuboplasty. Fertil Steril 46:963–966
Coulam CB, Peters AJ, Gentry M, Gentry W, Critser ES, Critser JK (1991) Pregnancy rates after peritoneal ovum-sperm transfer. Am J Obstet Gynecol 164:1447–1452
Dellenbach P, Nissand I, Moreau L, Feger B, Plumere C, Gerlinger P (1985) Transvaginal sonographically controlled follicle puncture for oocyte retrieval. Fertil Steril 44:656–662
Devroey P et al. (1989) ZIFT: indications and limitations. In: Capitanio GL, Asch RH, De Cecco L, Croce S (eds) GIFT: from basics to clinics. Raven Press, New York, pp 333–337
Ferraiolo A et al. (1991) "Blind" transcervical transfer of gametes in the fallopian tube: a preliminary study. Hum Reprod 6:537–540
Jansen RPS (1980) Cyclic changes in the human fallopian tube isthmus and their functional importance. Am J Obstet Gynecol 136:292–308
Jansen RPS (1984) Endocrine response in the fallopian tube. Endocr Rev 5:525–551
Jansen RPS, Anderson JC (1987) Catheterisation of the fallopian tubes from the vagina. Lancet 2:309–310
Jansen RPS, Anderson JA (1989) Transvaginal gamete and embryo transfer to the fallopian tubes. In: Capitanio GL, Asch RH, De Cecco L, Croce S (eds) GIFT: from basics to clinics. Raven Press, New York, pp 383–389
Jansen R, Anderson J (1990) New routes of gamete and embryo transfer. In: Asch RH, Balmaceda JP, Johnston I (eds) Gamete physiology. Serono Symposia USA, Norwell, Massachusetts, pp 331–342
Jansen RPS, Anderson JC (1992a) Transvaginal gamete and embryo transfer to the fallopian tubes. In: Confino E, Risquez F (eds) Transcervical procedures on the fallopian tubes. Blackwell Scientific Publications, Cambridge MA
Jansen RPS, Anderson JC (1992b) Transvaginal versus laparoscopic GIFT: a case-controlled retrospective comparison. Fertil Steril 59:836–840
Jansen RPS, Anderson JC, Radonic I, Smit J, Sutherland PD (1988a) Pregnancies after ultrasound-guided fallopian insemination with cryostored donor semen. Fertil Steril 49:920–922
Jansen RPS, Anderson JC, Sutherland PD (1988b) Nonoperative embryo transfer to the fallopian tube. N Engl J Med 319:288–291
Jansen RPS et al. (1990) Outpatient gamete intrafallopian transfer: 710 cases. Med J Aust 153:182–188
Lisa JR, Gioia JD, Rubin IC (1964) Observations on the interstitial portion of the fallopian tube. Surg Gynecol Obstet 99:159–169
Lucena E et al. (1989) Vaginal intratubal insemination (VITI) and vaginal GIFT endosonographic technique: early experience. Presented at the 6th World Congress of In Vitro Fertilization, Jerusalem, Israel, April 2–7
Platia MP, Krudy AG (1986) Transvaginal fluoroscopic recanalization of a proximally occluded oviduct. Fertil Steril 44:704–706
Possati G, Pareschi A, Seracchioli R, Maccolini A, Melega C, Flamigni C (1991) Gamete intrafallopian transfer by hysteroscopy as an alternative treatment for infertility. Fertil Steril 56:496–499
Pratt DE, Shangold G, Bieber E, Vignovic E, Barnes R, Schreiber J (1991) Transvaginal intratubal insemination by tactile sensation: a preliminary report. Fertil Steril 56:984–986
Risquez F et al. (1990) Retrograde tubal transfer of human embryos. Hum Reprod 5:185–188
Rocker I (1964) The anatomy of the utero-tubal junction area. Proc Roy Soc Med 57:707–709
Rubin IC (1928) Observations on the intramural and isthmic portions of the fallopian tubes with special reference to so-called "isthmospasm". Surg Gynecol Obstet 4:87–94
Scholtes MCW, Roozenburg BJ, Alberda AT, Zeilmaker GH (1990) Transcervical intrafallopian transfer of zygotes. Fertil Steril 54:283–286
Silverberg KM, Burns WN, Johnson JV, Schenken RS, Olive DL (1992) A prospective, randomized trial comparing two different intrauterine insemination regimens in controlled ovarian hyperstimulation cycles. Fertil Steril 57:357–361

Sweeney WJ (1961) The interstitial portion of the uterine tube – its gross anatomy, course, and length. Obstet Gynecol 19:3–8

Winston RML (1977) Microsurgical tubocornual anastomosis for reversal of sterilization. Lancet 1:284–285

Woodruff JD, Pauerstein CJ (1969) The fallopian tube. Structure, function, management. Williams & Wilkins, Baltimore, pp 44–66

Yovich JL, Blackledge DG, Richardson PA, Matson PL, Turner SR, Draper R (1987) Pregnancies following pronuclear stage tubal transfer. Fertil Steril 48:851–857

Yovich JL, Yovich JM, Edirisinghe WR (1988) The relative chance of pregnancy following tubal or uterine transfer procedures. Fertil Steril 49:858–864

Yovich JL, Draper RR, Turner SR, Cummins JM (1990) Transcervical tubal embryo-stage transfer (TC-TEST). J In Vitro Fert Embryo Transf 7:137–140

Section VII

# Diagnosis and Treatment of Ectopic Pregnancy

Chapter 18

# Early Diagnosis of Ectopic Pregnancy

B. Cacciatore, P. Ylöstalo and M. Seppälä

## Introduction

The incidence of ectopic pregnancy (EP) has increased rapidly during the past 20 years, but during the same period mortality has decreased. This is largely due to improved diagnostic measures (Mäkinen 1988). In spite of advances, EP still represents a major threat to the reproductive health of a woman at child-bearing age. Depending on whether or not EP was related to the use of an intrauterine contraceptive device (IUD), 50%–80% of the patients will conceive again, while only 30%–50% will have a live birth (Sandvei et al. 1987). Early diagnosis before tubal damage would reduce subsequent morbidity and allow conservative fertility-preserving treatment.

Identification of patients at risk of an EP is important for early diagnosis. In patients with clinically suspected EP the diagnosis is subsequently confirmed in about 50% of the cases (Weckstein 1985; Tuomivaara 1990).

Highly sensitive pregnancy tests can demonstrate the presence or absence of a pregnancy-related disorder in virtually 100% of cases (Seppälä and Purhonen 1987) and, in combination with endovaginal ultrasound, the non-invasive early diagnosis of EP has become widely available (Nyberg et al. 1987; Cacciatore et al. 1989; Timor-Tritsch et al. 1989).

## Clinical Features: Who Is At Risk?

In order to decide who is at risk of ectopic pregnancy, examination of the history is important (Weckstein 1985; Tuomivaara 1990). A previous ectopic pregnancy carries a 8%–27% risk of a recurrence in any subsequent pregnancy (Stabile and Grudzinskas 1990; Tuomivaara 1990). About one-third of women with EP have had previous pelvic surgery, notably tubal surgery. About one-fifth of the patients with EP have a history of pelvic inflammatory disease. An IUD in situ in a symptomatic woman with a positive pregnancy test should always raise a suspicion of EP. Finally, infertile women or women treated with assisted reproductive technology have an increased risk of EP. Early monitoring by ultrasound of these patients is recommended, once pregnancy has been established (Stiller et al. 1989; Shepherd et al. 1990).

The clinical picture of patients with EP varies considerably depending on whether the EP is unruptured or ruptured. In the latter case the diagnosis usually presents no major difficulty, because the symptoms and signs are clear. Much more common and more difficult is the diagnosis when the symptoms are mild and vague (Weckstein 1985; Tuomivaara 1990; Stabile and Grudzinskas 1990). More than one-third of the patients may not have amenorrhoea, particularly if they are IUD users. Abdominal pain is the most common complaint (97%), but it may be diffuse, bilateral or even contralateral to the ectopic site. Irregular bleeding has been reported in 75%–95% of the patients. Many are unaware of being pregnant at all, or are unable to recall the date of the last menstrual period (LMP). Symptoms of early pregnancy, such as nausea and breast tenderness, are present in only 20%–35% of patients.

On clinical examination, abdominal tenderness is found in up to 90% of the patients, whereas an adnexal mass is detected in 63% only and pain on cervical excitation in 50% (Tuomivaara 1990).

## Pregnancy Testing

In order to detect the low levels of hCG present in EP an ideal pregnancy test is highly sensitive, specific, rapid and simple enough to be applicable in an emergency situation. The development of radioimmunoassays (RIA) specific for the beta subunit of hCG can detect EP, but they are too time-consuming for emergency situations. Rapid modifications (Seppälä et al. 1980a) have proved the usefulness of sensitive pregnancy tests in gynaecological emergencies, substantiated by monoclonal antibody technology ushering in a new generation of pregnancy tests (Stenman et al. 1983). These tests have the potential to detect the very low amounts of hCG present in early pregnancy and even in non-pregnant women and men, both in serum and urine (Norman et al. 1985; Stenman et al. 1987).

Simple analyses of hCG can be carried out as qualitative tests on either urine or serum just to demonstrate a pregnancy-related condition, or as quantitative tests to demonstrate changes in hCG concentrations. Immunochromatography-based or enzyme immunoassays are very rapid (5–10 min), sensitive (25 IU/l) and easy to interpret in out-patient and bed-side management, with predictive indices for a pregnancy-related disorder of almost

100%. Thus, they can be reliably used as the first-line pregnancy test in patients suspected of having EP (Nordenskjold et al. 1985; Buck et al. 1986; LeMaistre et al. 1987). Whereas most laboratories now use hCG assays calibrated against the Third International Standard equivalent to the First International Reference Preparation (IRP), some laboratories still use the Second International Standard which gives values about half of the IRP. This difference should be made clear to clinicians who may use absolute hCG values as guidelines for management.

In more difficult cases where the diagnosis is not obvious, highly sensitive RIAs or immunometric assays have been applied to quantify serum hCG concentrations. These methods require a well-equipped laboratory and are therefore more expensive. Many tertiary referral centres admitting emergency patients have this facility. We too have adopted a routine use of time-resolved fluorometry for a two-site sandwich-type immunofluorometric assay by which hCG concentrations as low as 0.02 IU/l can be quantitated within 30 min (Stenman et al. 1983, 1987).

## Serum hCG Levels in Normal and Ectopic Pregnancy

Production of hCG has been demonstrated in the blastocyst stage embryo in vitro (Fishel et al. 1984). In a normal early pregnancy, the first significant rise of hCG in maternal serum is usually detected 8–10 days after ovulation, when the invading trophoblast consolidates with the lumen of maternal blood vessels. In ectopic pregnancy, the hCG level may rise sooner, perhaps resulting from early implantation (Fig. 18.1) (Seppälä et al. 1980b). Thereafter, the serum hCG concentrations rise exponentially. Between conception and 42 days of gestation the hCG concentration increases by at least 66% every 2 days (Braunstein et al. 1973; Pittaway et al. 1985).

In patients with EP, serum hCG levels are usually lower than those in normal pregnancy, probably because ectopic trophoblast produces less hCG than intrauterine trophoblast (Braunstein et al. 1973; Cartwright and DiPietro 1984). Thus, quantitative determination of serum hCG may help to distinguish between normal and ectopic pregnancy. Studies on early pregnancies conceived after in vitro fertilisation (IVF) have shown that a single hCG value on day 9 after embryo transfer, or on day 14 after oocyte collection, may distinguish EP or threatened abortion from a normal gestation (Confino et al. 1986; Okamoto et al. 1987).

If the day of ovulation is unknown, serial hCG determinations allow better distinction between normal and abnormal gestation than a single hCG value (Cartwright and DiPietro 1984; Pittaway et al. 1985). In symptomatic patients, the rise of hCG levels is often attenuated or not taking place at all, due to inadequate growth and shedding of trophoblastic tissue. A rise in serum hCG concentration of less than 66% in 2 days indicates abnormal pregnancy in 70%–90% of cases, but with a 12.5% false-positive rate (Romero et al. 1986). The rate of hCG increase per day has been related to the initial hCG level to give an hCG score (Lindblom et al. 1989). Among women with

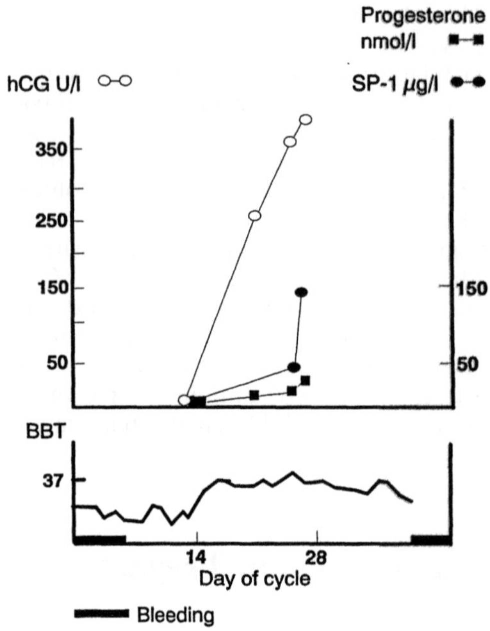


**Fig. 18.1.** Early detection of hCG, SP-1 and progesterone in ectopic pregnancy. BBT, basal body temperature chart.

suspected EP, an hCG score below a given discriminatory curve has yielded a predictive value of 94.7%.

In asymptomatic women, serial hCG determinations are helpful. However, among patients in whom EP was subsequently diagnosed, the hCG level showed a normal rising curve in 64% of cases (Shepherd et al. 1990) suggesting that trophoblast function was normal before the symptoms appeared. In some cases hCG production began to attenuate a few days later (Shepherd et al. 1990). Serial hCG determinations are useful for monitoring the efficacy of treatment, documenting disappearance or persistence of trophoblastic activity.

## Other Biochemical Markers of Early Pregnancy

Besides hCG, other placental proteins have been studied for their value in the diagnosis of EP. However, none of them has proved to be as effective as hCG, and they rarely give additional information to that given by hCG alone (Seppälä and Purhonen 1987; Stabile and Grudzinskas 1990). Like hCG, pregnancy-specific $\beta$-1 glycoprotein (SP-1) is a product of the placental syncytiotrophoblast, and it is detectable in serum within a few days of implantation (Seppälä et al. 1980b) (Fig. 18.1). However, a rapid 2-hour RIA for SP-1 is less effective than a rapid serum hCG RIA (Siiteri et al. 1981).

Pregnancy-associated plasma protein-A (PAPP-A) is also produced by the placental syncytiotrophoblast (Wahlström et al. 1981). In ectopic pregnancy PAPP-A levels are lower than in normal pregnancy (Sinosich et al. 1985). In spite of this, the PAPP-A test has limited value relative to hCG for the diagnosis of EP (Sjöberg 1987; Sauer et al. 1989a; Coddington et al. 1989).

Determination of serum progesterone levels may be useful in the management of early pregnancy complications (Buck et al. 1988). A level below 15 ng/ml (47 nmol/l) in women with a positive pregnancy test may indicate EP or threatened abortion (Hubinont et al. 1987; Sauer et al. 1989a), and EP is unlikely when the progesterone concentration is above that level (Yeko et al. 1987). Hahlin and his co-workers (1990) found viable pregnancy in all patients in whom the serum progesterone level was above 30 nmol/l, whereas progesterone levels below this threshold were found in 88% of EPs and 83% of spontaneous miscarriages.

Early pregnancy factor (EPF) is a substance which may be produced by the blastocyst, even before implantation. Serum concentrations of EPF have been reported as undetectable in 94% of cases of EP or miscarriage (Mesrogli et al. 1988). Serum relaxin levels have also been found to be lower in EP than in normal pregnancy (Garcia et al. 1990), whereas the serum Ca-125 levels are elevated in some ruptured tubal gestations (Sauer et al. 1989b). None of the above markers has been adopted for clinical routine.

## Vaginal Sonography

Detection of hCG in serum or urine indicates a pregnancy-related disorder, but it does not indicate the site of trophoblastic activity. The introduction of endovaginal transducers has brought about significant progress in sonographic evaluation of early pregnancy complications. By operating in close proximity to the pelvic organs the image can be magnified and the examination can be performed with an empty bladder, thus avoiding displacement of pelvic organs. In addition, high-frequency transducers (5–7.5 MHz) can be used, offering higher image resolution as compared with the lower frequency transducers (3.5–5.0 MHz) used in abdominal ultrasound (Wikland et al. 1985; Timor-Tritsch et al. 1988). Endovaginal ultrasound has made a dramatic impact on the diagnosis of suspected EP by allowing early detection of intrauterine pregnancy and by improving imaging of the adnexae (Nyberg et al. 1987; Shapiro et al. 1988; Cacciatore et al. 1989; Timor-Tritsch et al. 1989).

In a prospective study of 200 consecutive women admitted for suspected EP at Departments I and II of Obstetrics and Gynaecology, Helsinki University Central Hospital, we found vaginal sonography to have a 93% sensitivity for EP on admission and 100% after repeat scans; this was associated with high specificity (99%) (Table 18.1). Even very small EPs, less than 1 cm in diameter, were visualised by vaginal scanning. Due to the high efficiency the rate of ruptured EP found in this prospective study was only 7% (Cacciatore et al. 1990a).

**Table 18.1.** Sonographic findings on admission and final outcome in 200 pregnant women with suspected EP (adapted from Cacciatore et al. 1990a)

| Sonography | IUP | EP | Total |
|---|---|---|---|
| IUP (viable embryo/yolk sac, eccentric ring) | 117 | 0 | 117 |
| EP (adnexal ring or mass) | 1 | 63 | 64 |
| Non-diagnostic (no mass, no IUP sac) | 14 | 5 | 19 |
| Total | 132 | 68 | 200 |

IUP = intrauterine pregnancy.

## Diagnosis by Exclusion of Intrauterine Pregnancy

The usual way to diagnose EP by ultrasound is based on adnexal findings. Alternatively, presence or absence of intrauterine pregnancy may be identified. Reliable diagnosis of intrauterine pregnancy is important, because concurrent existence of intrauterine and ectopic pregnancy is rare, although not impossible. This is particularly important after assisted reproduction, where the incidence of combined intrauterine and ectopic pregnancy is 1 in 6800 pregnancies as compared with 1 in 30 000 pregnancies after spontaneous conception (Gambardella and Marrs 1989).

Vaginal sonography allows excellent visualisation of the uterine cavity with two endometrial layers and the detection of the yolk sac and a viable embryo (deCrespigny et al. 1988; Fossum et al. 1988; Cacciatore et al. 1990b). Early intrauterine pregnancy becomes detectable by sonography when the blastocyst cavity can be visualised as a small intrauterine fluid collection surrounded by an echogenic margin, i.e., the gestational sac (Fig. 18.2). In a longitudinal study of 20 women followed up by vaginal sonography and hCG measurements at 2–4-day intervals, between 28 and 45 days of gestation, we could demonstrate a gestational sac at 33 days post-LMP (Cacciatore et al. 1990b). The early sac was identified as a fluid collection of 1–3-mm diameter located within either side of the endometrium, eccentrically with respect to the uterine cavity. The sac was outlined by an echoic contour caused by trophoblast invasion into the decidualised endometrium.

It is not always easy to distinguish a true intrauterine sac from the so-called pseudogestational sac seen in EP (Nyberg et al. 1983; Yeh 1988). The pseudogestational sac can be observed in 10%–20% of EPs, causing a potential false-positive diagnosis of intrauterine pregnancy. Some features of a true intrauterine sac are important for differential diagnosis. Due to intracavitary fluid collection, the pseudosac is usually located centrally in the uterine cavity, i.e., between the two endometrial layers (Fig. 18.3), as opposed to the intrauterine implanted blastocyst cavity which is located within one of the two endometrial layers, and is eccentric with respect to the cavity. Furthermore, the pseudogestational sac is composed of a single decidual layer surrounded by a fluid collection. Thus, a single thin echogenic ring is observed in EP, whereas in intrauterine pregnancy the early gestational sac is surrounded by the chorionic membrane and, around this, by the

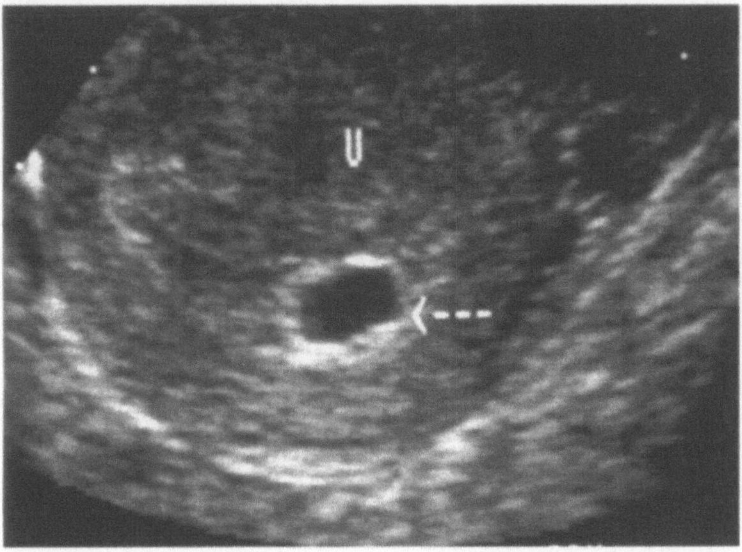


**Fig. 18.2.** Intrauterine pregnancy: the gestational sac is located eccentrically with respect to the uterine cavity.

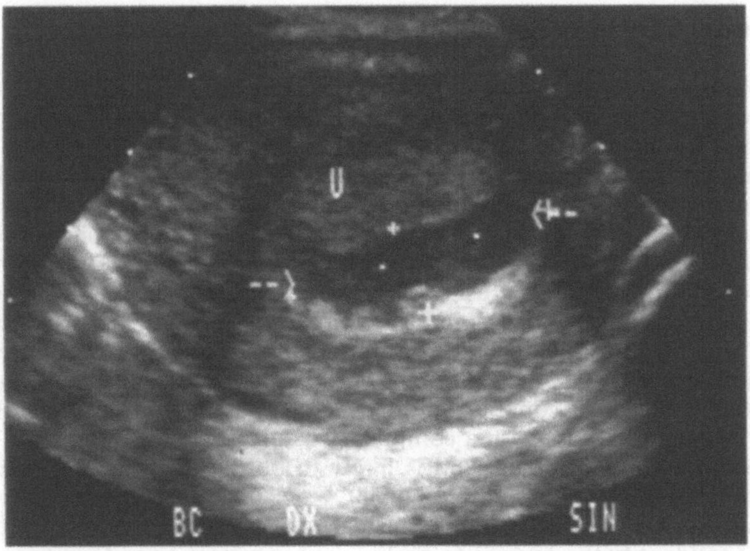


**Fig. 18.3.** Ectopic pregnancy: the pseudogestational sac is located centrally in the uterine cavity, between the two endometrial layers.

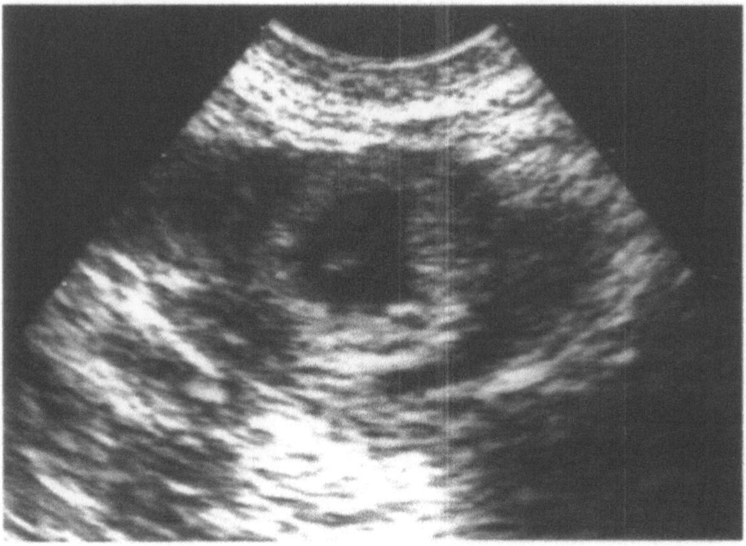

**Fig. 18.4.** Ectopic pregnancy: tubal ring, visualised by vaginal sonography.

decidua parietalis, giving a typical acoustic mismatch in the sonogram (Nyberg et al. 1983; Cadkin and McAlpin 1984; Cacciatore et al. 1990b).

## Diagnosis of Tubal Pregnancy

If no intrauterine sac is seen, or the detected sac is considered pseudogestational, the second phase of the examination consists of scanning of the adnexae. The appearance of an EP depends on its size, on whether it is developing or aborted, whether it is ruptured or unruptured, and whether or not there is intraperitoneal bleeding. Traditionally, evidence obtained by ultrasound has been considered diagnostically reliable only when an ectopic sac is visualised with a viable embryo. This condition can be detected in only about one-fifth of EPs, even using vaginal transducers. If it exists, the adnexal mass is either complex or cystic in most cases. Detection of an adnexal or "tubal ring" with a thick echoic contour is strongly suggestive of an ectopic gestation sac (Fig. 18.4). Among women with EP diagnosed at an early stage this is the most common finding, being present in more than 60% of cases. An adnexal mass with a complex structure (Fig. 18.5) has been found in about one-third of cases, and is likely to be due to a tubal haematoma (Nyberg et al. 1987; Fleischer et al. 1990; Cacciatore 1990).

Before such a mass or a ring is considered to be suggestive of EP, it is important to identify the ovaries to exclude ovarian cysts or endometriomas. A corpus-luteum cyst, supported by hCG in early pregnancy, may look like a gestational sac. A blood clot inside such a cyst may even be mistaken for an embryo, increasing the risk of a false-positive diagnosis. Usually a rim of

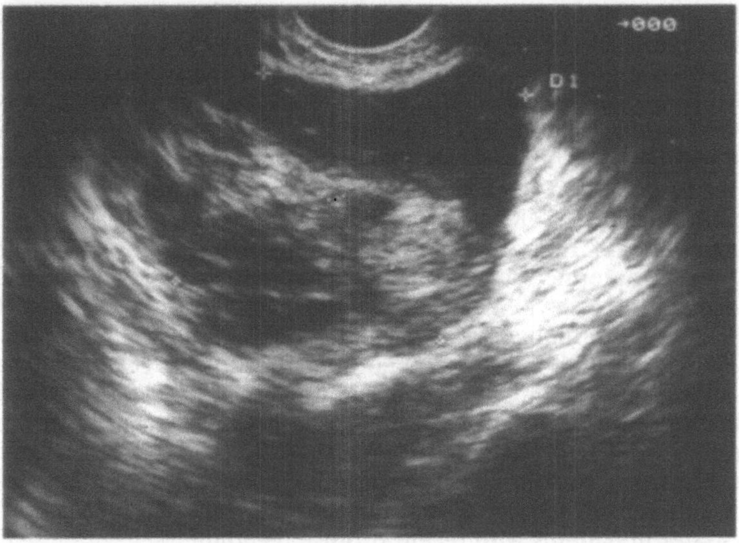


**Fig. 18.5.** Ectopic pregnancy: an adnexal mass with complex structure, visualised by vaginal sonography.

ovarian tissue can be found around the corpus luteum (Fleischer et al. 1990). Another possibility is a bowel loop. This can be ruled out by demonstrating peristalsis. Having excluded these diagnostic problems we found that the detection of an adnexal mass is 99% specific for EP in patients with a positive hCG test (Cacciatore et al. 1990a).

Pulsed doppler and colour flow imaging may help to evaluate a non-specific adnexal mass by detecting high-velocity flow consistent with trophoblastic activity (Kurjak et al. 1989; Dillon et al. 1990).

Free intraperitoneal fluid can be detected in 40%–83% of women with EP. Although up to 20% of patients with intrauterine pregnancy also have peritoneal fluid at sonography, detection of particulate peritoneal fluid seems to have a high predictive value for EP (Nyberg et al. 1991).

## Combined Use of Ultrasound and hCG: the Discriminatory hCG Level

Symptomatic patients with a positive pregnancy test in whom no intrauterine pregnancy, adnexal mass or cul-de-sac fluid is detected by ultrasound represent a diagnostic problem. In such cases a recent complete or incomplete abortion is possible, or an early viable intrauterine or ectopic pregnancy. Surgical intervention on a patient with a normal intrauterine pregnancy is unfortunate, but so is delayed surgery of EP. In such cases serum hCG concentrations have proved to be useful.

In cell cultures hCG production correlates positively with the number and log growth phase of the trophoblast (Braunstein et al. 1973). A linear correlation between hCG levels and the diameter of the intrauterine sac measured by ultrasound has been demonstrated (Nyberg et al. 1986). Attempts have been made to find an hCG level that can distinguish between patients with and without a gestational sac, the aim being to identify a discriminatory hCG level to define those cases in which EP exists in the absence of a detectable intrauterine sac (Kadar et al. 1981; Nyberg et al. 1986).

An hCG value of 1000 IU/l represents a cut-off level above which the absence of an intrauterine sac in vaginal sonography should raise suspicion of an abnormal pregnancy. When tested prospectively in women with suspected EP, this discriminatory level has performed well (Cacciatore et al. 1990a). When the hCG level exceeded that threshold, a gestational sac was seen in all intrauterine pregnancies but in none of the EPs. These results indicate that absence of an intrauterine sac on a vaginal scan when the hCG level exceeds 1000 IU/l (IRP) is strongly suggestive of EP. However, serum levels of hCG may remain elevated for a few hours after spontaneous abortion; it is, therefore, recommended that another hCG be measured one or two days later in patients with recent profuse bleeding.

## Sonographic Criteria of EP: Implications for Management

As an alternative to laparotomy, laparoscopic salpingotomy has become a routine in many centres. In selected cases, local injections of methotrexate or other substances through the laparoscope or under sonographic guidance have been attempted (Fernandez et al. 1988; Stoval et al. 1991; Feichtinger and Kemeter 1989). Careful clinical assessment is crucial. Observation alone may be sufficient in selected cases, when the EP has miscarried and is regressing spontaneously (Ylöstalo et al. 1991); laparoscopic evaluation or injection of drugs may be necessary for treatment of a growing unruptured EP. Serial hCG measurements and/or a diagnostic laparoscopy may be needed to determine the treatment. A study of 120 consecutive proven cases of EP indicates that vaginal sonography provides reliable information of the clinical state of tubal pregnancy (Cacciatore 1990). Compared with operative findings, vaginal sonography accurately predicted the size of the tubal mass; the discrepancy between sonographic and surgical measurements never exceeded 1 cm. A sac-like adnexal ring was found to be highly predictive of a growing ectopic sac within an intact fallopian tube (Fig. 18.4). In fact, none of the women with such a sonographic finding had a ruptured fallopian tube at surgery. Among those women the serum hCG levels were usually high, in excess of 1000 IU/l, and in most cases the hCG level was rising. The complex adnexal mass was usually associated with tubal haematoma or incomplete tubal abortion (Fig. 18.5). Such a hyperechoic mass may be due to a trophoblastic pole from a recently collapsed sac, as suggested by high serum hCG levels in some of these patients.

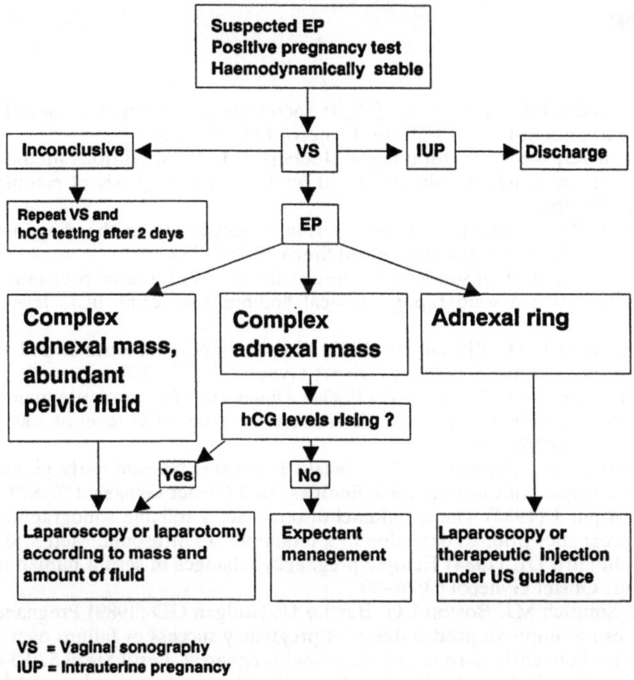


**Fig. 18.6.** Options for management of ectopic pregnancy (EP), based on vaginal sonography (VS) and serum hCG.

# Conclusion

Vaginal sonography in combination with a sensitive pregnancy test is the method of choice for early diagnosis of EP. In the hands of an experienced operator, vaginal ultrasound allows detection of intrauterine pregnancy as early as 4 weeks after the last menstrual period. In the vast majority of patients with EP, the diagnosis can be made on admission, and in virtually all remaining cases after repeated scanning a few days later. Very small EPs can be visualised, allowing diagnosis before tubal rupture has occurred. Studies conducted at Helsinki University Central Hospital support the view that quantitative measurement of serum hCG levels is helpful, both for the diagnosis and for the management of EP. Absence of an intrauterine sac on vaginal sonography, when the hCG level is above 1000 IU/l, is highly suggestive of EP. Finally, vaginal sonography in combination with hCG levels and clinical findings helps the clinician to decide the best course of management (Fig. 18.6). With the advent of this non-invasive approach, measures such as endometrial histology, puncture of the Pouch of Douglas, and even diagnostic laparoscopy are now less frequently needed.

*Acknowledgements*. This work was supported by grants from the Sigrid Jusélius Foundation and the Academy of Finland.

# References

Braunstein GD, Grodin JM, Vaitukaitis J (1973) Secretory rate of human chorionic gonadotropin by normal trophoblasts. Am J Obstet Gynecol 115:447–450

Buck RH, Norman RJ, Reddi K, Moodley J, Joubert SM (1986) Various methods for determining urinary choriogonadotropin evaluated for the early diagnosis of ectopic pregnancy. Clin Chem 32:879–882

Buck RH, Joubert SM, Norman RJ (1988) Serum progesterone in the diagnosis of ectopic pregnancy: a valuable diagnostic test? Fertil Steril 50:752–755

Cacciatore B (1990) Can vaginal sonography predict the status of a tubal pregnancy: a prospective comparison between sonography, surgical findings and serum hCG levels. Radiology 177:481–484

Cacciatore B, Stenman U-H, Ylöstalo P (1989) Comparison of abdominal and vaginal sonography in suspected ectopic pregnancy. Obstet Gynecol 75:770–774

Cacciatore B, Stenman U-H, Ylöstalo P (1990a) Diagnosis of ectopic pregnancy by vaginal ultrasonography in combination with a discriminatory serum hCG level of 1000 IU/L (IRP). Br J Obstet Gynaecol 97:904–908

Cacciatore B, Tiitinen A, Stenman U-H, Ylöstalo P (1990b) Normal early pregnancy: serum hCG levels and vaginal ultrasonographic findings. Br J Obstet Gynaecol 97:899–903

Cadkin AV, McAlpin J (1984) The decidua-chorionic sac: a reliable sonographic indicator of intrauterine pregnancy prior to detection of a fetal pole. J Ultrasound Med 3:539–548

Cartwright PS, DiPietro DL (1984) Ectopic pregnancy: changes in serum human gonadotropin concentrations. Obstet Gynecol 63:76–80

Coddington CC, Sinosich MJ, Boston EG, Bartko JJ, Hodgen GD (1989) Pregnancy associated protein-A does not improve predictability of pregnancy success or failure over human chorionic gonadotropin in early normal and abnormal pregnancy. Fertil Steril 52:854–857

Confino E, Demir RH, Friberg J, Gleicher N (1986) The predictive value of hCG b-subunit levels in pregnancies achieved by in vitro fertilization and embryo transfer: an international collaborative study. Fertil Steril 45:526–531

deCrespigny LCH, Cooper D, McKenna M (1988) Early detection of intrauterine pregnancy with ultrasound. J Ultrasound Med 7:7–10

Dillon EH, Feyock AL, Taylor KJ (1990) Pseudogestational sacs: doppler US differentiation from normal or abnormal intrauterine pregnancy. Radiology 176:359–364

Feichtinger W, Kemeter P (1989) Treatment of unruptured ectopic pregnancy by needling of sac and injection of methotrexate or $PGE_2$ under transvaginal sonography control. Arch Gynecol Obstet 246:85–89

Fernandez H, Rainhorn JD, Papiernik E (1988) Spontaneous resolution of ectopic pregnancy. Obstet Gynecol 71:171–174

Fishel JB, Edwards RG, Evans CJ (1984) Human chorionic gonadotropin secreted by preimplantation embryos cultured in-vitro. Science 223:816–818

Fleischer AC et al. (1990) Ectopic pregnancy: features at transvaginal sonography. Radiology 174:375–378

Fossum GT, Davajan V, Kletzky OA (1988) Early detection of pregnancy with transvaginal ultrasound. Fertil Steril 49:788–791

Gambardella FR, Marrs RP (1989) Heterotopic pregnancy associated with assisted reproduction technology. Am J Obstet Gynecol 160:1520–1524

Garcia AJ, Skurmark JH, Goldsmith LT, Emmi A, Weiss G (1990) Human chorionic gonadotropin and relaxin concentrations in early ectopic and normal pregnancies. Obstet Gynecol 75:779–783

Hahlin M, Wallin A, Sjöblom P, Lindblom B (1990) Single progesterone assay for early recognition of abnormal pregnancy. Hum Reprod 5:662–666

Hubinont CJ, Thomas C, Schwers JF (1987) Luteal function in ectopic pregnancy. Am J Obstet Gynecol 156:669–674

Kadar N, DeVore G, Romero R (1981) Discriminatory hCG zone: its use in the sonographic evaluation for ectopic pregnancy. Obstet Gynecol 58:156–161

Kurjak A, Zalud I, Jurkovic D, Alfirevic Ž, Mijan M (1989) Transvaginal color doppler for the assessment of pelvic circulation. Acta Obstet Gynecol Scand 68:131–135

LeMaistre A, Bracey A, Katz A, Wu AHB (1987) Role of qualitative assays in diagnosis of ectopic pregnancy. Clin Chem 33:1908–1910

Lindblom B, Hahlin M, Sjöblom P (1989) Serial human chorionic gonadotropin determination by fluoroimmunoassay for differentiation between intrauterine and ectopic gestation. Am J Obstet Gynecol 161:397–400

Mäkinen J (1988) *Ectopic pregnancy in Finland in 1966–1986*. MD thesis, University of Turku

Mesrogli M et al. (1988) Tubargraviditäten: early pregnancy factor, progesteron, b-hCG and vaginalsonographie als differentialdiagnostische parameter. Z Geburtsh u Perinat 192:130–133

Nordenskjold F, Ahlgren M, Erreth L, Hultberg B (1985) A sensitive urine pregnancy test as an aid in the diagnosis of ectopic pregnancy. Fertil Steril 43:48–52

Norman RJ, Poulton T, Gard T, Chard T (1985) Monoclonal antibodies to human chorionic gonadotropin: implications for antigenic mapping, immunoradiometric assay, and clinical applications. J Clin Endocrinol Metab 61:1031–1038

Nyberg DA, Laing FC, Filly RA, Uri-Simmonds M, Brooke JR Jr (1983) Ultrasonographic differentiation of the gestational sac of early intrauterine pregnancy from the pseudogestational sac of ectopic pregnancy. Radiology 146:755–759

Nyberg DA, Filly RA, Duarte Filho DL, Laing FC, Mahony BS (1986) Abnormal pregnancy: early diagnosis by US and serum chorionic gonadotropin levels. Radiology 158:393–397

Nyberg DA, Mack LA, Brooke JR Jr, Laing FC (1987) Endovaginal sonography evaluation of ectopic pregnancy: a prospective study. AJR 149:1181–1186

Nyberg DA, Hughes MP, Mack LA, Wang KY (1991) Extrauterine findings of ectopic pregnancy at transvaginal US: importance of echogenic fluid. Radiology 178:823–826

Okamoto SH et al. (1987) Predictive value of plasma human chorionic gonadotropin b-subunit in diagnosing ectopic pregnancy after in vitro fertilization and embryo transfer. Br Med J 294:66–70

Pittaway DE et al. (1985) The efficacy of early pregnancy monitoring with serial gonadotropin determinations and real-time sonography in an infertile population. Fertil Steril 44:190–195

Romero R et al. (1986) The value of serial human chorionic gonadotropin testing as a diagnostic tool in ectopic pregnancy. Am J Obstet Gynecol 155:392–394

Sandvei R, Ulstein M, Wollen A-L (1987) Fertility following ectopic pregnancy with special reference to previous use of an intra-uterine contraceptive device (IUCD). Acta Obstet Gynecol Scand 66:131–135

Sauer MV et al. (1989a) Predictive value of a single serum pregnancy associated plasma protein A or progesterone in the diagnosis of abnormal pregnancy. Hum Reprod 3:331–334

Sauer MV, Vasilev SA, Campeau J, Vermesh M (1989b) Serum cancer antigen 125 in ectopic pregnancy. Gynecol Obstet Invest 27:164–165

Seppälä M, Purhonen M (1987) The use of hCG and other pregnancy proteins in the diagnosis of ectopic pregnancy. Clin Obstet Gynecol 30:148–154

Seppälä M, Tontti K, Ranta T (1980a) Use of a rapid hCG-b subunit radioimmunoassay in acute gynaecological emergencies. Lancet 1:165–166

Seppälä M, Venesmaa P, Rutanen E-M (1980b) Pregnancy-specific beta-1-glycoprotein in ectopic pregnancy. Am J Obstet Gynecol 136:189–193

Shapiro BS, Cullen M, Taylor KJW, DeCherney AH (1988) Transvaginal ultrasonography for the diagnosis of ectopic pregnancy. Fertil Steril 50:425–429

Shepherd RW, Patton PE, Novy MJ, Burry KA (1990). Serial b-hCG measurements in the early detection of ectopic pregnancy. Obstet Gynecol 75:417–420

Siiteri JE, Koistinen R, Ranta T, Stenman U-H, Seppälä M (1981) Use of a rapid radioimmunoassay for pregnancy-specific $\beta$-1 glycoprotein in gynecological emergencies; comparison with routine urinary pregnancy test and a rapid radioimmunoassay for human chorionic gonadotropin. Am J Obstet Gynecol 139:968–972

Sinosich MJ, Grudzinskas JG, Saunders DM (1985) Placental proteins in the diagnosis of the "elusive" early pregnancy. Obstet Gynecol Surv 40:273–282

Sjöberg J (1987) Pregnancy-associated plasma protein-A in pregnancy-related disorders. Hum Reprod 2:615–616

Stabile I, Grudzinskas JG (1990) Ectopic pregnancy: a review of incidence, etiology and diagnostic aspects. Obstet Gynecol Surv 45:335–347

Stenman U-H, Alfthan H, Myllynen L, Seppälä M (1983) Ultrarapid and highly sensitive time-resolved fluoroimmunometric assay for chorionic gonadotropin. Lancet 2:647–649

Stenman U-H et al. (1987) Serum levels of human chorionic gonadotropin in nonpregnant women and men are modulated by gonadotropin releasing hormone and sex steroids. J Clin Endocrinol Metab 64:730–736

Stiller RJ, Haynes de Regt R, Blair E (1989) Transvaginal ultrasonography in patient at risk for ectopic pregnancy. Am J Obstet Gynecol 161:930–933

Stoval YG, Ling FW, Gray LA (1991) Methotrexate treatment of unruptured ectopic pregnancy: a report of 100 cases. Obstet Gynecol 77:749–753

Timor-Tritsch IE, Bar-Jan Y, Elgali S, Rottem S (1988) The technique of transvaginal ultrasonography by the use of a 6.5 MHz transducer probe. Am J Obstet Gynecol 158:1019–1024

Timor-Tritsch IE, Yeh MN, Peisner DB, Lesser KB, Slavik TA (1989) The use of transvaginal ultrasonography in the diagnosis of ectopic pregnancy. Am J Obstet Gynecol 161:157–161

Tuomivaara L (1990) *Ectopic pregnancy. An analysis of aetiological risk factors and subsequent fertility*. MD thesis, University of Oulu

Wahlström T, Teisner B, Folkersen J (1981) Tissue localization of pregnancy-associated plasma protein-A (PAPP-A) in normal placenta. Placenta 2:253–258

Weckstein LN (1985) Current perspective on ectopic pregnancy. Obstet Gynecol Surv 40:259–275

Wikland M, Enk L, Hamberger L (1985) Transvesical and transvaginal approaches for the aspiration of follicles by use of ultrasound. Ann NY Acad Sci 442:182–194

Yeh HC (1988) Sonographic sign of early pregnancy. CRC Critic Rev Diagn Imag 28:181–211

Yeko TR et al. (1987) Timely diagnosis of early pregnancy using a single blood progesterone measurement. Fertil Steril 62:1048–1050

Ylöstalo P et al. (1991) Conservative treatment of ectopic pregnancy. Ann NY Acad Sci 626:516–523

Chapter 19

# Management of Tubal Pregnancy: Transabdominal

V. Gomel

## Introduction

There has been a significant increase in the rate of ectopic pregnancy in the last two decades. In 1985, 78 400 ectopic pregnancies were reported in the United States of America as compared to 17 800 in 1970. This represents a more than fourfold increase in both the number and the rate (from 4.8 to 20.9 per 1000 live births) of ectopic pregnancy since 1970 (Center for Disease Control 1988).

Whereas the risk of death associated with ectopic pregnancy fell significantly from 1970 to 1983 (from 35.2 to 5.3 deaths per 10 000 cases), ectopic pregnancy has become the second leading cause of maternal mortality in the United States. Although death from ectopic pregnancy accounted for 7.8% of all maternal deaths in 1970, this rate doubled (14.7%) in 1982 (National Center for Health Statistics 1984). The latter change is largely associated with the fourfold increase in the number of ectopic pregnancies during the same period.

The single most important cause for the increase in the rate of ectopic pregnancy has been the concomitant rise in the prevalence of pelvic inflammatory disease (PID). Specific and non-specific infections of the oviduct damage its mucosa and muscularis, compromising tubal peristalsis and especially mucosal ciliary function. These changes predispose to the occurrence of a tubal pregnancy unless the tube becomes totally occluded by the inflammatory process. Women with PID, proven laparoscopically, were shown to have a sixfold increase (1/24) in ectopic pregnancy compared to a control group of women (1/146) submitted to laparoscopy for pelvic pain, without evidence of PID (Westrom et al. 1981).

Other factors contributing to this increase include: the wide utilisation of reconstructive tubal surgery and assisted reproductive techniques; frequent use of conservative treatment of tubal pregnancy; the vast number of tubal sterilisations performed each year; and last, but not least, accuracy and ease of diagnosis of ectopic pregnancy especially due to new sensitive diagnostic techniques. In-vitro fertilisation and embryo transfer, a technique designed to by-pass the fallopian tube, has been associated with an unexpectedly high incidence of ectopic pregnancy. Indeed the first human pregnancy obtained from IVF had a tubal implantation (Steptoe and Edwards 1976). With IVF the rate of tubal pregnancy is significantly higher among patients with tubal infertility compared to the non-tubal group (Zouves et al. 1991). Embryonic and endocrine factors may also play a role in the occurrence of tubal pregncy, which would explain such occurrences in fallopian tubes of normal appearance (Poland et al. 1976).

Concurrent with the dramatic increase in the prevalence of tubal pregnancy there have been very significant advances in diagnosis and management.This chapter will primarily review the surgical management of the condition via the transabdominal route.

## Diagnosis

Modern ancillary measures have greatly facilitated and increased the accuracy of the diagnosis of tubal pregnancy. However a high index of suspicion and a thorough history and physical examination remain the key to early diagnosis. The ancillary measures include serial quantitative determination of serum $\beta$-subunit human chorionic gonadotrophin ($\beta$-hCG), serum progesterone assay, ultrasonography (especially using a vaginal sectoscanner) and laparoscopy. Thus, it has become possible to diagnose tubal pregnancies early and in the unruptured state much more frequently. This fact not only helps to avoid complications associated with delayed diagnosis but also facilitates the use of conservative management of the condition.

Diagnostic accuracy is increased when the symptoms (if any) are considered together with the results of the investigation. Serum $\beta$-hCG levels are usually lower in ectopic pregnancy than in intrauterine pregnancy of corresponding gestational age (Sauer et al. 1988). Whereas in normal pregnancy $\beta$-hCG levels double in 1.4 to 2.2 days (Batzer et al. 1981) the rate of increase is usually much slower in ectopic pregnancy. Serial serum $\beta$-hCG determinations also indicate when an intrauterine pregnancy should be detectable by ultrasound. An intrauterine sac becomes visible by abdominal scanning when the serum $\beta$-hCG level is greater than 6500 mIU/ml. However endovaginal scanning allows detection of a sac at levels greater than 1500 mIU/ml (Fossum et al. 1988).

A single serum progesterone determination is a useful diagnostic adjunct; a level greater than 15 ng/ml is usually associated with a normal intrauterine pregnancy whereas lower values suggest an ectopic or failing intrauterine pregnancy (Yeko et al. 1987). Hahlin et al. (1991) demonstrated that a progesterone value under 30 nmol/l combined with an abnormal hCG increase had a positive predictive value for pathological pregnancy of 1.0.

# Treatment

Treatment of tubal pregnancy may be: expectant, medical or surgical.
Asymptomatic tubal pregnancies with low and falling β-hCG levels may be treated expectantly. Such tubal gestations frequently resolve spontaneously.

## Expectant Treatment

In 1955 Lund reported 215 cases of ectopic pregnancy treated between 1930 and 1946 inclusive. Ninety-six of these patients displayed signs of extensive intraperitoneal haemorrhage and were treated by immediate operation. The remaining 119 patients were not acutely distressed on admission; these were termed "subacute cases" and were observed. They all had positive pregnancy tests (Aschheim–Zondek and, later, Friedman's test). Their treatment consisted of confinement to bed with close observation during the first few days when constipation was encouraged by means of opium. The pregnancy test was repeated every 7–10 days and the patients examined regularly. They were kept in bed until the pregnancy test became negative and the pain ceased. With this regime, the condition resolved in 68 out of the 119 patients. The others (51 cases), required surgery, either because of evidence of intra-abdominal haemorrhage or a persistent tender adnexal mass. This was a brave approach considering the lack of sensitive diagnostic means at the time.

In a more recent publication Garcia et al. (1987) reported on 13 patients with unruptured tubal pregnancy managed expectantly. The prerequisites for inclusion were as follows: the patients were clinically stable; they had falling β-hCG levels 48 h apart; and an empty uterus on ultrasonographic examination. They were then submitted to a dilatation and curettage and if there was no gross evidence of conception products a diagnostic laparoscopy was undertaken. Patients with a tubal mass under 4 cm in diameter and without active bleeding were managed expectantly. The patients were followed in hospital with daily serum β-hCG, ultrasonography and haematocrit. If asymptomatic with declining β-hCG levels for 5 consecutive days they were discharged from the hospital. Thereafter β-hCG was monitored three times per week until it was undetectable on two occasions. Only one of the 13 thus treated required a surgical intervention. Her β-hCG level had remained constant for 11 days but she experienced increasing abdominal pain commencing on the ninth post-laparoscopy day. Of the 13 patients, 10 had hysterosalpingography 3 months later: 7 of these had normal appearing patent fallopian tubes, and 3 had a tubal occlusion at the site of the previous gestation. Fernandez et al. (1988) reported on 14 patients with ampullary tubal pregnancy confirmed by laparoscopy, and managed expectantly. In 9 of these (64%), the pregnancy resolved sapontaneously. In 4 (29%) surgical intervention was ultimately necessary, in 2 patients because of rising $\beta$-hCG titres and in 2 because of pain. One patient, included in the series after laparoscopic observation of a tubal pregnancy, was subsequently found to have an ongoing intrauterine pregnancy. Spontaneous resolution occurred more frequently when the initial $\beta$-hCG concentration was less than 1000 mIU per ml. Of the 9 patients who had a spontaneous resolution, 6 had subsequent hysterosalpingography. The tubes were patent in all but one had an ampullary defect, 2 cm in diameter, at the previous gestational site. We have reported on 5 patients with tubal occlusion at the site of an untreated tubal pregnancy (Gomel and Filmar 1987).

Expectant management may have a place in the treatment of tubal pregnancy in a patient who is asymptomatic, with low and falling $\beta$-hCG levels. Otherwise, such management is protracted and expensive, especially if patients require admission to hospital for observation. In addition, it has limitations and a relatively high failure rate.

## Medical Treatment

Medical therapy may be systemic or local. Methotrexate has been used systemically, frequently in conjunction with citrovorum factor. Most protocols include intramuscular administration of methotrexate and citrovorum factor on alternate days, the former at a dosage of 1 mg/kg per day and the latter at a dosage of 0.1 mg/kg per day, for a total period of 8 days. This therapy is contra-indicated in patients who have ultrasonographic evidence of cardiac activity or formed fetal elements. Failure is more likely to occur when $\beta$-hCG levels are above 6500 mIU/ml (Sauer et al. 1987; Stovall et al. 1989).

Methotrexate is a potent drug with many side effects, some of which may be serious. It has several proven indications. However, considering other available proven, effective and safe therapeutic modalities for tubal pregnancy, considering the failure rate, side effects, and rate of tubal occlusion, we view with scepticism the systemic use of methotrexate for this condition. On the other hand, methotrexate has a distinct place in the treatment of retained trophoblast (after conservative surgical management); this requires the use of a much lower dosage, usually 50 mg given in a single injection. Systemic administration of methotrexate may be useful in the treatment of pregnancies of rare ectopic location such as the cervix and the cornu.

Local medical therapy, with injection (under laparoscopic visualisation) of methotrexate (Pansky et al. 1989), prostaglandin $F_{2\alpha}$ (Lindblom et al. 1990), or hypertonic glucose solution (Lang et al. 1990) into the tubal gestation site (and the ovary containing the corpus luteum in the case of prostaglandin $F_{2\alpha}$), appears to be effective in selected patients and is associated with few side effects. However the post-operative period is usually protracted. As long as it is necessary to resort to a laparoscopy to administer the medication, we believe that it is preferable to remove the gestational products instead. Local medical treatment is promising, especially if the drug can be administered transvaginally under ultrasonographic control and local anaesthesia.

## Surgical Treatment

Ectopic pregnancy was regarded as inevitably fatal when, over 100 years ago, Lawson Tait (1884) introduced timely surgical intervention and excision of the involved structures. By accomplishing haemostasis in this manner, Tait was able to save the lives of 33 out of 40 women with ectopic pregnancy. This approach became widely accepted and salpingectomy remained the traditional treatment for tubal pregnancy for nearly a century. Stromme (1953) was the first to describe conservative surgical treatment of tubal gestation. By performing a salpingotomy he was able to remove the ectopic gestation without sacrificing the fallopian tube.

The decision as to whether to employ a radical or a conservative surgical approach depends upon the patient's desire for future fertility and the status of the oviduct at the time of the intervention.

### *Merits of Conservative Surgery*

The subsequent fertility of patients with tubal pregnancy is decidedly impaired. Their reproductive performance appears to be influenced by parity, history of infertility, previous abdominal surgery, the number of prior tubal pregnancies, the operative procedure employed for treatment, and the status of the fallopian tubes at the time of the intervention. These factors individually or collectively contribute to the fertility outcome. The incidence of an ectopic pregnancy increases eightfold or more after an initial episode.

In a study performed in our department the number of prior tubal pregnancies and the status of the contralateral tube at the time of surgical intervention for tubal pregnancy proved to be the only two significant predictors of subsequent fertility outcome. The intrauterine and ectopic pregnancy rates subsequent to one tubal pregnancy were 61% and 7% respectively; after two tubal pregnancies both intrauterine and tubal pregnancy rates became 28%; after three or more tubal pregnancies the intrauterine pregnancy rate was only 14% whereas the rate of ectopic pregnancy rose to 72% (Urman et al. 1991).

Irrespective of whether radical or conservative surgery is employed for the treatment of the index tubal pregnancy, subsequent fertility is influenced by the status of the contralateral tube (Tuomivaara and Kauppila 1988). Earlier studies demonstrated no difference both in intrauterine and ectopic pregnancy rates subsequent to a tubal pregnancy whether treated radically or conservatively (Timonen and Nieminen 1967; DeCherney and Kase 1979). The value of conservative over radical surgery becomes evident in patients with a single fallopian tube treated for tubal pregnancy. Hallatt (1986) reported on the subsequent fertility of 26 patients who had an ectopic pregnancy on their only tube and who were treated conservatively. Of these patients, 10 achieved a subsequent intrauterine pregnancy and 5 another tubal pregnancy. Had these 26 patients been treated in a radical fashion, none would have achieved a subsequent spontaneous pregnancy, intrauterine or otherwise. Valle and Lifchez (1983) reported on the reproductive outcome of 13 women with a single fallopian tube following conservative surgery for tubal pregnancy. One of these women was lost to follow-up, another had intentionally avoided a pregnancy; all of the remaining 11 patients achieved full-term viable deliveries. Other studies fail to report such optimistic outcomes. In 15 patients with tubal pregnancy with only one "functional" fallopian tube treated by salpingotomy DeCherney et al. (1982) reported a subsequent viable pregnancy rate of 53% with a recurrent ectopic pregnancy rate of 20%. In a similar study Oelsner et al. (1986) reported subsequent intrauterine and ectopic pregnancy rates of 48% and 43% respectively. Gomel (1983a) reported on the reproductive outcome of 9 patients submitted to microsurgical tubo-tubal anastomosis subsequent to an ectopic pregnancy on their single tube treated by segmental excision. Of these, 5 achieved a viable pregnancy and 1 patient achieved a recurrent tubal pregnancy. In a more recent survey of 17 such patients, the same author noted that 10 of them had achieved viable pregnancies and 2 had tubal pregnancies. It is noteworthy that none of these patients had prior reconstructive tubal surgery. The reproductive performance, in terms of intrauterine pregnancy, subsequent to conservative treatment of tubal pregnancy in the single remaining tube, in patients with prior tubal surgery, is disappointingly low and the tubal pregnancy rate very high (Urman et al. 1991).

## *Surgical Technique*

*General Principles.* The traditional approach to the surgical treatment of tubal pregnancy is via laparotomy. Unless there is overt haemoperitoneum, a laparoscopy is usually performed before the laparotomy to confirm the diagnosis. A patient with obvious haemoperitoneum and an acute surgical abdomen requires implementation of appropriate resuscitation measures and immediate laparotomy.

Laparoscopy, in addition to confirming the diagnosis, permits assessment of the site and size of gestation; status of the affected tube; status of the ipsilateral ovary; status of the contralateral tube and ovary and of other pelvic structures. If the definitive surgical treatment is to be carried out via laparotomy, the information yielded by the preceding laparoscopy will enable the surgeon to carry out the procedure through a minilaparotomy incision. Manipulation of the uterus via a rigid uterine cannula facilitates the exposure of the affected tube under the incision and the intervention in general. This requires maintenance of the modified Trendelenburg position used during laparoscopy.

Tubal pregnancy may also be treated via laparoscopy, provided the gestational site is accessible and the surgeon has the necessary experience and instrumentation.

Selection of the specific surgical procedure is based upon many factors which include: expectations of the patient regarding future fertility; the haemodynamic status of the patient; the site and size of the tubal gestation; the status of the affected tube and whether or not it had been the site of a prior tubal pregnancy; and the status of the contralateral tube and ovary.

The tenets of microsurgical technique must be observed, especially when the procedure aims to conserve the oviduct. When the approach is via laparotomy, the use of magnification is not mandatory; however, utilisation of low power loops is helpful (Gomel 1983b).

After entry into the peritoneal cavity, the tube containing the conceptus is elevated on a Kerlex pad soaked in lactate–Ringers solution. The same solution is used during the procedure to irrigate exposed serosal surfaces and the implantation site. At the close of the procedure it is essential to remove any conception products that may be present in the pelvis since trophoblastic tissue may implant onto peritoneal surfaces. Therefore all the blood should be suctioned and a thorough pelvic lavage performed with plain or heparinised lactate–Ringers solution.

To prevent serious complications associated with retained products of gestation, the patient must be followed post-operatively with serial serum $\beta$-hCG determinations until the level becomes undetectable.

*Principles of Conservative Surgery.* The prerequisites for conservative surgery of tubal pregnancy include:

1. The patient must desire to retain her fertility
2. She must be surgically stable
3. The tubal gestation must preferably be unruptured, although in most instances rupture does not preclude a conservative approach provided the tube is viable.

The principles of conservative surgery are to excise all gestational tissue; to obtain haemostasis; to conserve as much healthy oviduct as possible; to employ an atraumatic technique and to conclude the procedure by suctioning all the blood and performing a pelvic lavage (Gomel 1983b). The site of tubal gestation is the major determinant in the type of conservative surgery to be employed.

## *Treatment via Laparotomy*

*Salpingectomy.* Salpingectomy has been the traditional surgical approach to tubal pregnancy. Using 3-0 or 4-0 Vicryl or PDS (Ethicon Inc., Sommerville N.J.), the tube is suture ligatured at the tubo-uterine junction and transected. The mesosalpinx is then suture ligatured in sections and divided until complete excision of the tube is achieved. While performing a salpingectomy, the blood supply of the tube, from both uterine and ovarian vessels, must be taken into account. This is important to prevent post-operative bleeding.

*Segmental Excision.* Segmental excision is performed by ligating the tube proximal and distal to the affected portion with 3-0 or 4-0 Vicryl or PDS sutures. The tubal segment containing the gestation is excised by further ligation and transection of the adjacent portion of mesosalpinx.

Segmental excision is the conservative surgical approach of choice in ectopic pregnancies of isthmic location. Segmental excision is also possible with an ampullary pregnancy, either when the affected tubal segment appears irreversibly damaged or when a linear salpingotomy fails to provide appropriate haemostasis.

*Linear Salpingotomy*. Salpingotomy was the first conservative surgical procedure described for the removal of tubal pregnancy, without sacrificing the involved tube (Stromme 1953). Salpingotomy is the conservative surgical procedure of choice in gestations of ampullary location. After immobilisation of the tube, a longitudinal incision is made on the antimesosalpingeal aspect of the involved tubal segment, using a needle electrode and blended current, or a scalpel blade. When placing the incision it is essential to consider that the implantation site is usually on the proximal end of the segment of tube enlarged as a result of the ectopic gestation. Therefore, the incision should be extended proximally to ensure visualisation and removal of all gestational products. After placement of the incision the products of conception commence to extrude. Gentle external pressure, holding the tube between finger and thumb, helps in the extrusion process. The conception products are grasped with a forceps and slowly and gently shelled out of the tube. Care should be taken to avoid grasping endothelial fronds of the tube during this process, since trauma to the endothelium may result in significant bleeding which may be difficult to control without serious damage. The implantation site is irrigated to ensure complete removal of the products of conception and haemostasis. Mild venous oozing from the margins of the tubal incision usually stops spontaneously; more significant bleeders may require individual pin-point electrocoagulation. Persistent bleeding from the implantation site after a period of compression may be treated either by injection of 1.5 to 2 ml of dilute vasopressin solution (10 IU diluted in 60 to 100 ml) into the adjacent mesosalpinx or by serial ligation of the small blood vessels leading to the affected segment of the tube using 5-0 or 6-0 Vicryl or PDS suture. If all of these measures fail to control the bleeding, and if tubal conservation is desired, the affected segment of tube can be excised (segmental excision).

The salpingotomy incision may be closed with 5-0 or 6-0 Vicryl or PDS sutures. If the incision is left open it invariably closes by secondary intention without leaving a significant scar. Occasionally a fistulous opening may remain at this site.

*Tubal Abortion.* When a tubal pregnancy is extruded from the tube through the fimbria the result is a tubal abortion. With pregnancies located in the infundibulum or distal ampulla, spontaneous tubal abortion is a frequent phenomenon. A pregnancy at these locations may be converted to a tubal abortion by expressing and extruding (milking out) the products of conception through the fimbriated end of the tube. A gestation of infundibular location can be shelled out with relative ease and the certainty of having removed all the gestational products. With ampullary pregnancies, even of distal location, one cannot be certain of complete removal of gestational products since trophoblast frequently penetrates the lamina propria and muscularis of the tube and thus the gestation becomes extraluminal (Budowick et al. 1980). Indeed the incidence of post-operative bleeding after this approach is higher than with other conservative procedures. For this reason, with gestations of distal ampullary location we recommend an incision on the antimesosalpingeal aspect of the tube, extending from the fimbriated end to the affected portion of the ampulla. Such an incision permits exposure of the implantation site, and enables complete removal of gestational products, and achievement of haemostasis. This approach is preferable to that of milking out the gestational products.

## Treatment via Laparoscopy

Tubal pregnancy can also be managed via laparoscopy even in the presence of tubal rupture. The general prerequisites for operative laparoscopy must be met. In addition, the patient must be surgically stable, and the gestational site accessible (Gomel et al. 1986). Once the laparoscope has been introduced and the diagnosis made, the contralateral adnexa and the remainder of the pelvis must be assessed carefully. It may be necessary to suction blood accumulated in the pelvis to achieve proper visualisation.

### *General Principles*

The anaesthetised patient is placed in modified lithotomy position. The bladder is emptied and unless contraindicated a rigid uterine cannula is attached to the cervix. Manipulation of the uterus via this cannula enhances visualisation and facilitates surgical manipulation in the pelvis. In addition the uterus can be made to elevate and/or immobilise adnexal structures.

The laparoscope is usually introduced intraumbilically. The ancillary (operative) instruments are inserted through second and third puncture sites placed suprapubically in the midline and at McBurney's point. If the need for an additional instrument arises this is introduced through a fourth puncture site placed at an appropriate site in the left lower quadrant. While the target organ may be immobilised with the use of a probe or an appropriate grasping forceps, the uterus may be manipulated (via the cannula) to elevate and immobilise the tube and/or ovary.

The procedure is performed by viewing a high resolution television monitor which permits appropriate interaction among the surgeon, the assistant and other operating room personnel. We normally locate the television monitor at the caudal end of the operating table. Such placement permits a clear view of the screen for all those involved with the case. At the close of the procedure, blood accumulated in the pelvis is suctioned and the peritoneal cavity is thoroughly lavaged with heparinised (5000 u/l) lactate–Ringers solution, utilising a suction irrigation cannula passed through one of the ancillary puncture sites. A thorough lavage permits the removal of clots, fibrin, debris and any trophoblastic tissue from the peritoneal cavity. Trophoblastic tissue retained in the peritoneal cavity may implant upon serosal surfaces and cause a post-operative rise in β-hCG levels.

Whereas some authors (Mettler and Semm 1988; Donnez and Nisolle 1989) routinely leave an intraperitoneal drain, placed in the Pouch of Douglas for 24 h or longer, this has not been our practice.

Depending on the site, size and status of the tubal pregnancy, and further depending on whether or not the patient is desirous of maintaining fertility, the following laparoscopic approaches are available for surgical management of tubal pregnancy: ablation of gestational site, linear salpingotomy, segmental excision, or salpingectomy.

### Ablation of Gestational Site

Small (up to 1.5 cm) ectopic pregnancies located in the isthmus or proximal ampulla can be dealt with by electrocoagulation, preferably using the bipolar mode. The result is similar to that obtained with tubal sterilisation by electrocauterisation. The tube is grasped with an electrosurgical forceps across the site of the ectopic pregnancy as far as the mesosalpinx, and this segment of the oviduct is electrocoagulated.

A bipolar grasping forceps should be used to perform the procedure with the bipolar mode. Coagulating current is used first until adequate blanching is noted. To ensure desiccation of the full thickness of the tube (including the inner part), the burn is completed with the use of blended or cutting current. Two or three contiguous burns will effectively destroy the ectopic pregnancy together with the segment of oviduct containing it. The principal disadvantage of this technique is the absence of a specimen for histological examination.

### Linear Salpingotomy

Linear salpingotomy is the conservative surgical procedure of choice in gestations of ampullary location. This technique avoids the need for subsequent surgery to restore tubal patency. The tube is immobilised either with a probe or by gently holding it with a grasping forceps proximal to the implantation site.

The use of vasopressin solution (or other vasoconstrictor) is optional, but is advisable in advanced cases. We infiltrate the mesosalpinx, beneath the affected region of the tube, with 1.5–2 ml of a dilute solution of vasopressin. A 20-gauge spinal needle with the stilet in place is introduced through the abdominal wall. The stilet is removed and a 3-ml syringe containing the dilute vasopressin solution is attached to the needle. The tip of the needle is introduced just under the serosa of the mesosalpinx and the solution injected. This approach avoids the introduction of the vasopressin solution into a vessel and thus into the general circulation of the patient.

A pointed (needle) electrode is introduced through a third puncture and a linear incision is placed electrosurgically along the antimesosalpingeal border of the affected segment of tube. The current used for this purpose should be a blend of cutting and coagulation. Alternatively the incision may be effected with scissors or laser energy. Irrespective of the modality employed, the incision should extend more towards the uterus, for reasons noted earlier.

The incision is continued until gestational products are encountered, at which time they start to protrude. Gentle compression of the tube facilitates extrusion of the products of conception. These are grasped with forceps and slowly and gently teased out of the tube. As with laparotomy, it is important to grasp gestational tissue only and not the endothelial fronds. Laceration of these fronds may cause bleeding that is difficult to control without causing damage. Furthermore, undue trauma to the endothelium may result in subsequent tubal occlusion. Another approach for removal of the gestational products is hydrodissection and suction with a laparoscopic suction cannula.

Once the gestational tissues have been removed, they can either be taken out of the peritoneal cavity immediately or placed in the vesico-uterine pouch for subsequent removal. The tubal lumen and implantation site are thoroughly irrigated to ensure complete removal. The edges of the incision are examined for the presence of any bleeding points which may be electrocoagulated with a monopolar or bipolar electrode. Instrumentation with combined capability for suction irrigation and electrocoagulation is available. The salpingotomy incision may be left open. There appears to be no advantage to closing this incision, which usually heals well by secondary intention.

## *Segmental Excision*

Segmental excision is the procedure of choice for gestations located in the isthmus and may also be employed for pregnancies less than 3 cm in diameter situated in the proximal ampulla. Segmental excision may also be used after salpingotomy if there is persistent bleeding despite the administration of vasopressin solution, and if tubal conservation is desired.

While segmental excision via laparoscopy may be effected using suturing techniques similar to that described via laparotomy, this technique is more tedious than electrosurgical procedures. Electrosurgically, either the unipolar or bipolar modality may be used. The bipolar mode offers the assurance of more controlled tissue desiccation and electrical dissipation. When using the monopolar mode, electrocoagulation is achieved with insulated grasping forceps although a similar effect can be obtained by the use of 5-mm insulated laparoscopic scissors. A grasping forceps, introduced through a suprapubic second puncture site placed in the midline, is used to elevate and immobilise the affected tube.

Electrocoagulation and division may be effected by the alternate use of a second pair of insulated grasping forceps and scissors introduced through the third puncture site or simply by accomplishing both functions with a pair of insulated scissors. The affected tube is elevated with the first pair of grasping forceps. It is electrocoagulated and divided both proximal and distal to the implantation site with instruments introduced through the third puncture site. Using the first grasping forceps, the affected portion of tube is grasped near the distal transection site and gently elevated to expose the adjacent mesosalpinx. A series of burns and cuts are placed progressively along the mesosalpinx immediately beneath the margin of the tube from the distal to the proximal transection site until the excision is completed. Thereafter, the mesosalpinx is inspected and any bleeding areas are recoagulated (Gomel 1978; Stangel and Gomel 1980).

The same procedure can be carried out by using the bipolar mode. The tube is elevated as described previously with the forceps introduced through the second puncture site. With the bipolar grasping forceps introduced through the third puncture site, the oviduct is grasped immediately proximal to the gestation site and electrocoagulated. The tube is similarly electrocoagulated immediately distal to the gestation site. The bipolar forceps is replaced with a pair of scissors and the tube is transected over the two coagulated areas. The scissors are replaced with the bipolar grasping forceps. The segment containing the gestation is regrasped with the suprapubic forceps near the distal transection line and is elevated. The mesosalpinx is electrocoagulated along the margin of the ectopic pregnancy. This grasping forceps is once again replaced with the 5-mm scissors, and the electrocoagulated mesenteric margin is transected until excision of the affected portion of tube is completed. The excised segment of tube is removed through one of the cannulae already in place.

The techniques of simple coagulation (ablation) and segmental excision result in an occluded tube. The remaining segments are usually amenable to later microsurgical anastomosis if this proves necessary.

## *Salpingectomy*

The indications for salpingectomy are similar irrespective of whether the procedure is performed via laparotomy or laparoscopy.

Salpingectomy may be effected via laparoscopy by a technique similar to that used via laparotomy. We prefer to use an electrosurgical technique (using the monopolar or bipolar mode) similar to that employed for segmental resection of the tube.

The tube together with the adjacent mesosalpinx is grasped, electrocoagulated and divided at the level of the utero-tubal junction. This obliterates one of the two major sources of blood supply to the tube, via the ascending branch of the uterine artery. The tubo-ovarian ligament is then grasped, electrocoagulated and divided. This obliterates the second major source of blood supply through the ovarian artery. The mesosalpinx is then electrocoagulated and divided until complete excision of the tube. The mesosalpinx may be electrocoagulated in a selective manner taking into account the vessel that reaches the tube at the level of the ampullary isthmic junction.

## *Removal of Gestational Products*

One of the limitations of operative laparoscopy relates to removal of excised tissue from the peritoneal cavity. Removal of gestational products, resected tube or tubal segment may be effected using one of the following approaches.

1. Via the laparoscopic cannula. If a 10-mm laparoscope has been employed, the conception products may be removed through the 11-mm laparoscopic cannula in one of the following ways: a) if an operating laparoscope (with an operative channel permitting the introduction of a grasping forceps) was used for the procedure, the specimen is grasped with a strong grasping forceps introduced through the operative channel of the laparoscope and withdrawn together with the laparoscope through the 11-mm cannula; b) if an operating laparoscope is not available, the 11-mm cannula can be used for the removal of the specimen: the 10-mm laparoscope is removed and a strong grasping forceps (either 10 mm or 5

mm, using an appropriate adapter) is introduced through this cannula. The pelvis is viewed by a 5-mm laparoscope introduced through one of the auxiliary puncture sites.
2. Via an 11-mm cannula introduced suprapubically. When a smaller calibre laparoscope is employed for the procedure, the conception products may be removed by the introduction of an 11-mm trocar and cannula suprapubically. This can be achieved by the use of an adaptor through the existing 5-mm puncture site after the skin incision is enlarged. While the conception products can be removed by simply enlarging the suprapubic incision and pulling them through with an appropriate forceps, this approach carries the risk of trophoblastic implantation in the abdominal wall. Releasing incisions or morcellation will usually permit the removal of the specimen through the 11-mm cannula.

## *Post-operative Care*

After operative laparoscopy patients are usually kept in hospital for a few hours and then discharged home. Since such procedures are usually performed as an emergency in the evening, after the elective operating list, our practice is to keep patients in hospital overnight and discharge them home the next morning. We have not usually found it necessary to keep the patients in hospital for longer periods of time. The mean post-operative hospital stay of patients treated via laparoscopy was 0.87 days compared to 4.03 days in a control group (matched for gestational age, prior tubal pregnancy, tubal surgery or in-vitro fertilisation, clinical presentation, site of implantation, tubal rupture and specific surgical procedure performed to treat the tubal pregnancy) treated via laparotomy (Zouves and Gomel 1989). Some authors (Mettler and Semm 1988) report post-operative hospital stays between 3 and 5 days. Such long hospital stay defeats one of the advantages of the laparoscopic approach, which is the reduction of health-care costs.

The patients must be followed post-operatively by serial quantitative $\beta$-hCG determinations until the level becomes undetectable. This approach permits early detection of patients who have retained trophoblast. Such patients usually respond to a single dose of 40 to 50 mg methotrexate, administered intramuscularly (Gomel and Urman 1990).

## *Advantages of the Laparoscopic Approach*

Surgical treatment of tubal pregnancy via laparoscopy offers numerous advantages. The post-operative hospital stay is significantly shorter as indicated previously. The reduction in hospital stay was estimated to result in average savings of $1500 per patient (Vermesh et al. 1989). In addition, the patients usually return to full activity within one week of the surgery.

In a study of 216 consecutive tubal pregnancies we found that the operating time and the amount of post-operative analgesia was significantly less with patients treated via laparoscopy compared to those treated via laparotomy. There was no difference in the rates of post-operative morbidity and retained trophoblast in the two groups. Furthermore, the subsequent fertility outcome was similar for both groups (Zouves et al. 1992). The additional benefit of the laparoscopic approach is the avoidance of a laparotomy scar; this is cosmetically important to most women.

# References

Batzer FR et al. (1981) Serial B-subunit human chorionic gonadotropin doubling time as a prognosticator of pregnancy outcome in an infertile population. Fertil Steril 35:307

Budowick M, Johnson TRB, Genadry R, Parmley TH, Woodruff JD (1980) The histopathology of the developing tubal ectopic pregnancy. Fertil Steril 34:169–171

Center for Disease Control (1988) Ectopic pregnancy – United States, 1984 and 1985. MMWR 37:637–639

DeCherney A, Kase N (1979) The conservative surgical management of unruptured ectopic pregnancy. Obstet Gynecol 54:451–455

DeCherney A, Maheaux R, Naftolin F (1982) Salpingostomy for ectopic pregnancy in the sole patent oviduct: reproductive outcome. Fertil Steril 37:619–622

Donnez J, Nisolle M (1989) Laparoscopic treatment of ampullary tubal pregnancy. J Gynecol Surg 5:157–162

Fernandez H et al. (1988) Spontaneous resolution of ectopic pregnancy. Obstet Gynecol 71:171–174

Fossum GT, Davajan V, Kletzky OA (1988) Early detection of pregnancy with transvaginal ultrasound. Fertil Steril 49:788–791

Garcia AJ, Aubert JM, Sama J, Josimovich JB (1987) Expectant management of presumed ectopic pregnancies. Fertil Steril 48:395–400

Gomel V (1975) Laparoscopic tubal surgery in infertility. Obstet Gynecol 46:47–48

Gomel V (1978) La laparoscopia en el diagnostico y tratamiento de la gestacion ectopica. Gine Dips 2:85–87

Gomel V (1983a) Microsurgery in female infertility. Little Brown & Co., Boston, pp 242–243

Gomel V (1983b) Microsurgery in female infertility. Little Brown & Co., Boston, pp 253–265

Gomel V, Urman CB (1990) Laparoscopic surgery. Curr Op Obst Gynec 2:303–311

Gomel V, Taylor PJ, Yuzpe AA, Rioux J (1986) Laparoscopy and hysteroscopy in gynecologic practice. Year Book Medical Publishers Inc., Chicago, pp 140–142

Gomel V, Filmar S (1987) Arrested tubal pregnancy. Fertil Steril 48:1043–1047

Hahlin M, Sjöblom P, Lindblom B (1991) Combined use of progesterone and human chorionic gonadotropin determinations for differential diagnosis of very early pregnancy. Fertil Steril 56:492–496

Hallatt JG (1986) Tubal conservation in ectopic pregnancy: a study of 200 cases. Am J Obstet Gynecol 154:1216–1221

Lang PF, Weiss PAM, Mayer HO, Haas JG, Honign W (1990) Conservative treatment of ectopic pregnancy with local injection of hyperosmolar glucose solution or prostaglandin-$F_{2a}$: a prospective randomised study. Lancet 336:78–81

Lindblom B, Hahlin M, Lundorff P, Thorburn J (1990) Treatment of tubal pregnancy by laparoscope-guided injection of prostaglandin $F_{2a}$. Fertil Steril 54:404–408

Lund JJ (1955) Early ectopic pregnancy. J Obstet Gynecol Br Emp 62:70

Mettler L, Semm K (1988) Management of ectopic pregnancy: a shift from laparotomy to pelviscopy. Int J Fertil 33:389–392

National Center for Health Statistics (1984) Final mortality statistics, 1982. Monthly Vital Statistics Report. 33 (Suppl):35

Oelsner G, Rabinovitch O, Morad J, Mashiach S, Serr DM (1986) Reproductive outcome after microsurgical treatment of tubal pregnancy in women with a single fallopian tube. J Reprod Med 31:483–486

Pansky M et al. (1989) Local methotrexate injection: a nonsurgical treatment of ectopic pregnancy. Am J Obstet Gynecol 161:393–396

Poland BJ, Dill FJ, Stylblo C (1976) Embryonic development in ectopic human pregnancy. Teratol 14:315

Sauer MV et al. (1987) Nonsurgical management of unruptured ectopic pregnancy: an extended clinical trial. Fertil Steril 48:752–755

Sauer MV et al. (1988) Rapid measurement of urinary pregnanediol glucuronide to diagnose ectopic pregnancy. Am J Obstet Gynecol 159:1531–1535

Stangel JJ, Gomel V (1980) Techniques in conservative surgery for tubal gestation. Clin Obstet Gynecol 23:1221–1228

Steptoe PC, Edwards RG (1976) Reimplantation of human embryo with subsequent tubal pregnancy. Lancet 1:880

Stovall TG, Ling FW, Buster JE (1989) Outpatient chemotherapy of unruptured ectopic pregnancy. Fertil Steril 51:435–438

Stromme WB (1953) Salpingotomy for tubal pregnancy. Obstet Gynecol 1:472

Tait RL (1884) Pathology and treatment of extrauterine pregnancy. Br Med J 2:317

Timonen S, Nieminen U (1967) Tubal pregnancy, choice of operative method of treatment. Acta Obst et Gynec Scandinav 46:327–339

Tuomivaara L, Kauppila A (1988) Radical or conservative surgery for ectopic pregnancy? A follow-up study of fertility of 323 patients. Fertil Steril 50:580–583

Urman B, Zouves C, Gomel V (1991) Fertility outcome following tubal pregnancy. Acta Europaea Fertil 22:205–208

Valle JA, Lifchez AS (1983) Reproductive outcome following conservative surgery for tubal pregnancy in women with a single fallopian tube. Fertil Steril 39:316–320

Vermesh M et al. (1989) Management of unruptured ectopic gestation by linear salpingostomy: a prospective randomized clinical trial of laparoscopy versus laparotomy. Obstet Gynecol 73:400–403

Westrom L, Bengtsson LPH, Mardh PA (1981) Incidence trends, and risks of ectopic pregnancy in a population of women. Br Med J 282:15

Yeko TR et al. (1987) Timely diagnosis of early ectopic pregnancy using a single blood progesterone measurement. Fertil Steril 48:1048–1050

Zouves C, Gomel V (1989) Tubal pregnancy: management by operative laparoscopy versus laparotomy. Infertil 12:23–29

Zouves C, Erenus M, Gomel V (1991) Tubal ectopic pregnancy after in vitro fertilization and embryo transfer: a role for proximal occlusion or salpingectomy after failed distal tubal surgery? Fertil Steril 56:691–695

Zouves C, Urman B, Gomel V (1992) Laparoscopic surgical treatment of tubal pregnancy. A safe, effective alternative to laparotomy. J Reprod Med 37:205–209

Chapter 20

# Non-surgical Approaches in Ectopic Pregnancy: Systemic Medical Treatment or Local Injection Therapy?

B. Lindblom

## Introduction

It is now some 10 years since the first reports on medical treatment of ectopic pregnancy were published. Tanaka and collaborators (1982) treated a case of interstitial pregnancy by intramuscular injection of methotrexate (MTX). Since then, several reports have confirmed the efficiency of systemic medical treatment, not only for interstitial and tubal implantations but also in cases of cervical and ovarian pregnancy. With proper dosage and combinations with citrovorum factor, this treatment is usually well tolerated although, in individual cases, adverse effects such as severe stomatitis and hair loss may occur. Some 400 cases have been reported, the largest group of cases being that of Stovall et al. (1991). Stovall claims 96% success rate in 100 cases treated by MTX 1 mg/kg/day x 4 days i.m. About 10% of the cases exhibited toxic side effects, although citrovorum factor was given. Available data suggest an approximately 95% success rate of systemic medical treatment. However, no controlled trials, i.e. MTX treatment versus surgery, have been performed to date.

Laparoscopy is the only method with sensitivity and specificity sufficient to establish the diagnosis firmly and direct such a trial, even though it has been claimed that good results can be obtained by diagnostic algorithms (Stovall et al. 1991). Thus, the patient must undergo two types of treatment: anaesthesia and surgery followed by cytotoxic therapy. For this reason, most prefer local injection in conjunction with the diagnostic laparoscopy or laparoscopic surgery alone.

Thus, primary systemic MTX therapy is still unusual in ectopic pregnancy except in those cases in which surgery or general anaesthesia is contraindicated.

**Table 20.1.** Results of systemic primary MTX treatment in unruptured tubal pregnancy

| Author | Success rate |
|---|---|
| Ichinoe et al. 1986 | 21/22 |
| Ory et al. 1986 | 5/6 |
| Sauer et al. 1987 | 20/21 |
| Stovall et al. 1989 | 34/36 |
| Zakut et al. 1989 | 8/10 |
| Total | 88/95 (92.6 %) |

Recently, second-line therapy, i.e. treatment of women with persistent trophoblast after conservative treatment, has become increasingly popular. In these cases, low-dose oral MTX treatment has been used with promising results (Bengtsson et al. 1990, 1993). It should be noted, however, that delayed haemorrhage can occur several days after discontinuation of such therapy (Dumesic and Hafez 1991).

In cervical pregnancy, the cytotoxic drug etoposide has been used successfully as an alternative to hysterectomy (Segna et al. 1990). A new approach to this condition is pre-operative angiographic embolisation of the uterine artery, followed by conservative surgery without hysterectomy (Lobel et al. 1990). There are also reports on other agents for systemic medical treatment. The use of the progesterone antagonist RU486 (mifepristone Roussel UK) has not been encouraging (Keningsberg et al. 1987). Prostaglandin $E_2$ has been used in conjunction with local $PGF_{2\alpha}$ injection (Egarter and Husslein 1988). None of these agents has been tested against a placebo.

Since expectant management is successful in more than 50% of the cases in which levels of hCG are declining (Ylöstalo et al. 1990), a new therapy must show at least this level of effectiveness to be considered as a serious alternative to surgery.

The results presented in Table 20.1 provide a picture of the effectiveness of systemic MTX treatment in tubal pregnancy. The inclusion criteria for these studies varied, as did the dosage of MTX. Most, but not all, included citrovorum rescue. Nevertheless, it can be concluded that the failure rate of this treatment is about 5%, which is similar to the risk of persistent trophoblast after conservative surgery (Di Marchi et al. 1987; Lundorff et al. 1991). Conversely, the risk of failure when a radical measure (salpingectomy or tubal resection) is performed should be considerably lower, probably less than 1%.

## Local Injection Therapy (see Fig 20.1a, b)

### Transabdominal Approach

The success of systemic medical therapy with MTX has prompted our group to consider local injection of drug, under laparoscopic control, for selected cases of tubal pregnancy. Because of the problems with systemic MTX treat-

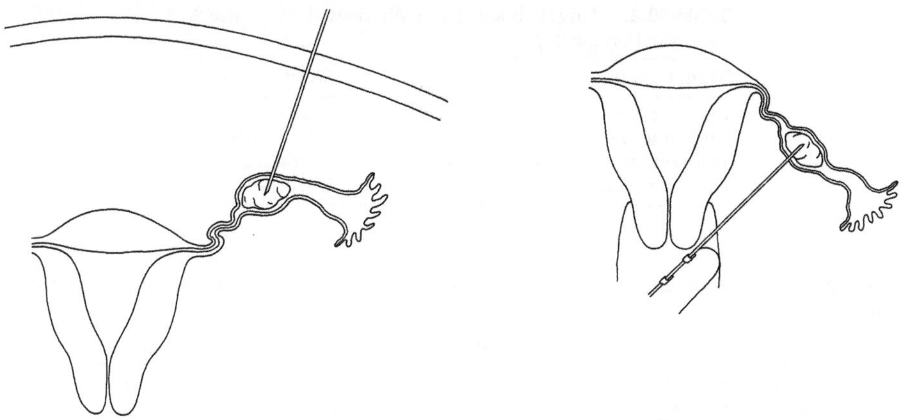


**Fig. 20.1.** **a.** Laparoscope-guided transabdominal injection therapy in ectopic pregnancy. The procedure requires general anaesthesia but is very simple from a technical viewpoint. A needle 10–15-cm long with an outer diameter of 0.5–1.0 mm is used. Proper visualisation is of utmost importance to avoid leakage at the injection site. **b.** Transvaginal injection into a tubal pregnancy using an endovaginal ultrasound transducer equipped with a needle guide.

ment, we intentionally searched for another principle of medication. Based on in-vitro experiments on the human fallopian tube and ovary, we considered prostaglandins (PG) to be a candidate for this application (Hahlin et al. 1987). The low incidence of ectopic pregnancies in women treated by systemic PG for legal first trimester abortion gave further support to this theory (Borten and Friedman 1985). Our first trials with a laparoscopically-guided injection of $PGF_{2\alpha}$ were conducted in 1986 (Hahlin and Lindblom 1986; Lindblom et al. 1987). Two Austrian groups also proposed local injection of drug as a treatment for ectopic pregnancy. Feichtinger and Kemeter (1987) published one case of ectopic pregnancy treated by "aspiration under ultrasonographic control and injection of MTX". Egarter and Husslein (1988) used $PGF_{2\alpha}$ for injection under laparoscopic control and added a $PGE_2$-analogue systemically. Serious side effects, i.e. pulmonary oedema and cardiac arrythmia, occurred in several cases. These adverse systemic reactions were probably due to accidental injection into the adnexal veins. Although the dose in the Austrian study was considerably higher than that in our studies (Lindblom et al. 1990), the low therapeutic index of $PGF_{2\alpha}$ is a problem and there is a need for an agent with similar or better local effects and less systemic toxicity.

Compounds for local injection therapy of tubal pregnancy could exert their action on different target tissues (Table 20.2). There is limited knowledge of the effects on these targets and the mode of action is insufficiently explored. The effect on trophoblast cells is probably the key factor.

Lang et al. (1989) conducted a randomise controlled study between $PGF_{2\alpha}$ and hyperosmolar glucose injection in the treatment of ectopic pregnancy. The success rate was similar, indicating that $PGF_{2\alpha}$ may be replaced by the less harmful glucose. Since hyperosmolar glucose is a more powerful inhibitor of trophoblast growth in vitro than $PGF_{2\alpha}$ (Lindblom et al. 1991), it

**Table 20.2.** Target tissues for a pharmacological attack on a tubal pregnancy

| Target tissue | Effect | Desired result |
|---|---|---|
| blood vessels | vasoconstriction | ischaemia |
| tubal muscle | contraction | tubal abortion |
| trophoblast | growth inhibition | resolution |
| corpus luteum | antigonadotropic | luteolysis |

**Table 20.3.** Results of laparoscopically guided local injection therapy in unruptured tubal pregnancy

| Author | Agent | Success rate |
|---|---|---|
| Lindblom et al. 1987, 1990 | $PGF_{2\alpha}$ | 24/27 |
| Egarter and Husslein* 1988 | $PGF_{2\alpha}$ ($+PGE_2$) | 6/6 |
| Vejtorp et al. 1989 | $PGF_{2\alpha}$ | 10/11 |
| Lang et al.** 1989 | $PGF_{2\alpha}$ | 13/15 |
| Lang et al.** 1989 | glucose | 16/16 |
| Pansky et al. 1989 | MTX | 24/27 |
| Kooi and Kock* 1990 | MTX | 24/25 |
| Total | | 117/127 (92.9%) |

* Local and systemic therapy.
** Randomised trial.

seems reasonable that a combination of glucose, acting mainly on trophoblast, and a low dose of $PGF_{2\alpha}$, acting mainly on tubal muscle and local blood flow, could be an attractive combination for local injection therapy in tubal pregnancy. However, further studies should be controlled, randomised trials with adequate inclusion criteria including serum hCG profiles e.g. the "hCG- score" (Lindblom et al. 1989). The classification of cases according to the hCG-score and/or the pre-operative serum progesterone level may identify patients with increased risk of persistent trophoblast (Hagström et al. 1992).

Local injection of MTX by the laparoscopic route has been tried. A dose of 12.5–25 mg MTX was effective in 24 out of 27 cases (Pansky et al. 1989). Similar results were obtained with a dose of 100 mg MTX (Kooi and Kock 1990). Combinations of local and systemic treatment have been tested, but only in a small uncontrolled series (Zakut et al. 1989). The results of laparoscope-guided local injection are summarised in Table 20.3.

## Transvaginal Approach

The precision of ultrasound in localising the conceptus is still unsatisfactory and the results of ultrasonographic-guided injection therapy are therefore variable (Robertson et al. 1987; Feichtinger and Kemeter 1989; Timor-Tritsch et al. 1989; Ménard et al. 1990; Tulandi et al. 1991). But hopefully ultrasonographic methods can be improved and may replace laparoscopy in the diagnosis and treatment of ectopic pregnancy.

A randomised trial of ultrasound-guided injection therapy combined local

**Table 20.4.** Results of ultrasound-guided local injection therapy in unruptured tubal pregnancy

| Author | Agent | Success rate |
|---|---|---|
| Feichtinger and Kemeter 1989 | MTX | 8/9 |
| Robertson et al. 1987 | MTX | 4/9 |
| Ménard et al. 1990 | MTX | 13/17 |
| Tulandi et al. 1991 | MTX | 10/12 |
| Fernandez et al.* 1991 | MTX | 8/12 |
| Fernandez et al.* 1991 | $PGE_2$ | 6/9 |
| Total | | 49/68 (72.1%) |

* Local and systemic treatment.

**Table 20.5.** Reproductive performance

| Author | Approach | Agent | IUP rate/year |
|---|---|---|---|
| Lindblom et al. 1990 | Local injection | $PGF_{2\alpha}$ | 10/19 |
| Stovall et al. 1990 | Systemic | MTX | 10/14 |

and systemic therapy (by PG or MTX) and obtained success in 14 out of 21 treated cases (Fernandez et al. 1991). All ten cases with pre-injection hCG-levels of <1000 IU/l were successful, emphasising the significance of pre-operative hCG levels in predicting the risk of retained trophoblast after conservative surgery (Lundorff et al. 1991). Although it may not be valid to pool data from various studies and make comparisons between different investigations, it appears that laparoscopically guided injections give a higher success rate than do ultrasound techniques (Tables 20.3 and 20.4).

A recent and very promising development is the application of transuterine tubal cannulation for local injection therapy (see Chapter 21).

Few studies have addressed the important question of reproductive performance after application of the new modalities of treatment. In several studies, the fertility prospects were "evaluated by a post-operative hysterosalpingogram." However, the value of such an investigation to predict future fertility outcome is doubtful. However, the prospects for future fertility seem good when compared to conventional treatment (Table 20.5).

# Conclusion

A variety of non-surgical treatments for ectopic pregnancy have been proposed during recent years. So far, only cytotoxic agents such as methotrexate have been found effective for systemic medical treatment. With this therapy, a success rate of more than 95% can be anticipated if ectopic pregnancies with embryonic cardiac activity are excluded. The main disadvantage of MTX therapy is the 5%–10% risk of cytotoxic side effects and uncertainty about long-term teratogenic effects (Egarter 1991). Local injection of MTX would reduce the total dose, but the effectiveness of this has not yet been documented.

Laparoscopically guided injection of less harmful agents like prostaglandin $F_{2\alpha}$ and hyperosmolar glucose show similar effectiveness to MTX although few controlled trials have been conducted. Ultrasound-guided injection is a promising alternative but as yet effectiveness appears to be inferior to that of laparoscopically guided local treatment. Efforts to improve the sonographic localisation of active trophoblast (for example, by the use of colour doppler) could increase the efficacy of local treatment. Furthermore, new agents may substitute for the currently used cytotoxic drugs.

It is possible that, in the future, transcervical infusion therapy with non-cytotoxic agents will become the first-line treatment for most ectopic pregnancies, while systemic treatment (with MTX or other agents) may serve as a back-up if the local therapy fails. Surgery would then only be necessary as a third-line treatment in a very small proportion of cases.

*Acknowledgement.* Investigations by the author were supported by The Swedish Medical Research Council (grant 8683).

## References

Bengtsson G et al. (1990) Treatment of persistent ectopic pregnancy with methotrexate. Abstract, ESHRE Workshop on Retrotubal Catheterization, Paris, 1990

Bengtsson G, Bryman I, Thorburn J, Lindblom B (1993) Low dose oral methotrexate as a second line therapy for persistent trophoblast after conservative treatment of ectopic pregnancy. Obstet Gynecol – in press

Borten M, Friedman EA (1985) Ectopic pregnancy among early abortion patients: does prostaglandin reduce the incidence? Prostaglandins 30:891–905

Di Marchi JM, Kososa TS, Kobana TY, Hale RW (1987) Persistent ectopic pregnancy. Obstet Gynecol 70:555–558

Dumesic DA, Hafez GR (1991) Delayed haemorrhage of a persistent ectopic pregnancy following laparoscopic salpingostomy and methotrexate therapy. Obstet Gynecol 78:960–962

Ergarter CH (1991) Methotrexate treatment of ectopic gestation and reproductive outcome (letter). Am J Obstet Gynecol 164:698–700

Egarter CH, Husslein P (1988) Treatment of tubal pregnancy by prostaglandins. Lancet 1:1104–1105

Feichtinger W, Kemeter P (1987) Conservative treatment of ectopic pregnancy by transvaginal aspiration under sonographic control and injection of methotrexate. Lancet 1:381–382

Feichtinger W, Kemeter P (1989) Treatment of unruptured ectopic pregnancy by needling of sac and injection of methotrexate or $PGE_2$ under transvaginal sonography control. Arch Gynecol Obstet 246:85–89

Fernandez H, Baton C, Lelaidier C, Frydman R (1991) Conservative management of ectopic pregnancy: prospective randomized clinical trial of methotrexate versus prostaglandin sulprostone by combined transvaginal and systemic administration. Fertil Steril 55:746–750

Hagström H-G et al. (1992) Prediction of persistent trophoblast after laparoscopic surgery in ectopic pregnancy. XXVIII Nordic Congress of Obstetrics and Gynecology, Reykjavik, Iceland, Abstract

Hahlin M, Lindblom B (1986) Farmakologisk behandling av ektopisk graviditet – en framkomlig väg? Acta Soc Med Suec 95:OB 17

Hahlin M, Bokström H, Lindblom B (1987) Ectopic pregnancy: in vitro effects of prostaglandins on the oviduct and corpus luteum. Fertil Steril 47:935–940

Ichinoe K et al. (1986) Nonsurgical therapy to preserve oviduct function in patients with tubal pregnancies. Am J Obstet Gynecol 156:484–487

Keningsberg D, Porte J, Hull M, Spiz IM (1987) Medical treatment of residual ectopic pregnancy: RU486 and methotrexate. Fertil Steril 47:702–703

Kooi S, Kock HCLV (1990) Treatment of tubal pregnancy by local injection of methotrexate after adrenaline injection into the mesosalpinx: a report of 25 patients. Fertil Steril 54:580–584

Lang P, Weiss PAM, Mayer HO (1989) Local application of hyperosmolar glucose solution in tubal pregnancy. Lancet 2:922–923

Lindblom B, Hahlin M, Källfelt B, Hamberger L (1987) Local prostaglandin $PGF_{2\alpha}$ injection for termination of ectopic pregnancy. Lancet 1:776–777

Lindblom B, Hahlin M, Sjöblom P (1989) Serial hCG determination by fluoroimmunoassay for differentiation between intrauterine and ectopic gestation. Am J Obstet Gynecol 161:397–400

Lindblom B, Hahlin M, Lundorff P, Thorburn J (1990) Treatment of tubal pregnancy by laparoscope-guided injection of prostaglandin PGF2-alpha. Fertil Steril 54:404–408

Lindblom B, Bengtsson G, Wallin A, Sjöblom P (1991) Influence of methotrexate and hyperosmolar glucose on cultured human trophoblast cells. XIII World Congress of Gynecology and Obstetrics, Singapore (abstract 1917)

Lobel SM, Meyerovitz MF, Benson CC, Goff B, Bengtsson MJ (1990) Preoperative angiographic uterine artery embolization in the management of cervical pregnancy. Obstet Gynecol 76:937–941

Lundorff P, Hahlin M, Sjöblom P, Lindblom B (1991) Persistent trophoblast after conservative treatment of tubal pregnancy: prediction and detection. Obstet Gynecol 77:129–133

Ménard A, Créquat J, Mandelbrot L, Hauuy JP, Mandelenat P (1990) Treatment of unruptured tubal pregnancy by local injection of methotrexate under transvaginal sonographic control. Fertil Steril 54:47–50

Ory SJ, Villaneuva AL, Sand PK, Tamura RK (1986) Conservative treatment of ectopic pregnancy with methotrexate. Am J Obstet Gynecol 154:1299–1306

Pansky M et al. (1989a) Local methotrexate injection: a non-surgical treatment of ectopic pregnancy. Am J Obstet Gynecol 161:393–396

Pansky M et al. (1989b) Tubal patency after local methotrexate injection for tubal pregnancy. Lancet 2:967–968

Robertson DE, Moye MAH, Hansen JN (1987) Reduction of ectopic pregnancy by injection under ultrasonic control. Lancet 2:974–975

Sauer MV et al. (1987) Nonsurgical management of unruptured etopic pregnancy: an extended clinical trial. Fertil Steril 48:752–755

Segna RA, Mitchel DR, Misas JE (1990) Successful treatment of cervical pregnancy with oral etoposide. Obstet Gynecol 76:945–947

Stovall TG, Ling FW, Buster JE (1990) Reproductive performance after methotrexate treatment of ectopic pregnancy. Am J Obstet Gynecol 162:1620–1623

Stovall TG, Ling FW, Gray LA, Carson SA, Buster JE (1991) Methotrexate treatment of unruptured ectopic pregnancy: a report of 100 cases. Obstet Gynecol 77:749–753

Tanaka K, Hayshi H, Kuksuzaka WT (1982) Treatment of interstitial ectopic pregnancy with methotrexate: report of a success case. Fertil Steril 37:851–853

Timor-Tritsch I, Baxi L, Paeisner DB (1989) Transvaginal salpingo-centesis: a new technique for treating ectopic pregnancy. Am J Obstet Gynecol 160:459–461

Tulandi T, Bret PM, Atri M, Senterman M (1991) Treatment of ectopic pregnancy by transvaginal intratubal methotrexate administration. Obstet Gynecol 77:627–630

Vejtorp M, Vejerslev LO, Ruge S (1989) Local prostaglandin treatment of ectopic pregnancy. Hum Reprod 4:464–467

Ylöstalo P et al. (1990) Conservative treatment of ectopic pregnancy. Ann NY Acad Sci 626:516–523

Zakut H, Sadam O, Katz A, Dreval D, Berstein D (1989) Management of tubal pregnancy with methotrexate. Br J Obstet Gynaecol 96:725–728

Chapter 21

# Transcervical Tubal Cannulation and Ectopic Pregnancy

F. Risquez, R. Forman and J.-R. Zorn

## Introduction

The incidence of ectopic pregnancy continues to increase. In the USA, with a fourfold increase since 1970, it is the second commonest cause of maternal mortality, responsible for 10% of all maternal deaths (Center for Disease Control 1990). This figure reflects a decline in mortality since Parry reported a 69% rate in 1876. Nevertheless, this condition is an important contributor to maternal mortality, especially in third world countries. It is generally agreed that a large percentage of the maternal mortality due to ectopic pregnancy is preventable.

Some of the increase in incidence reflects the rise in the incidence of sexually transmitted disease, pelvic inflammatory disease, treatment of tubal obstruction, in utero exposure to diethylstilboestrol, intrauterine device use and treatment with clomiphene, gonadotrophins or GnRH analogues. The role of chronic luminal lesions in recurrent ectopic pregnancy was recently emphasised by Stock: in a series of 15 recurrent ipsilateral ectopic pregnancies, pathological analysis of the tubes revealed no lesion related to the previous implantation site or to previous conservative surgical incisions or manipulation, but all tubes displayed anatomical abnormalities (Stock 1990).

Progress in early diagnosis of ectopic pregnancy is an important factor for the increase in incidence and the parallel reduction in the death-to-case ratio. Transvaginal ultrasound and rapid hCG assays have significantly improved diagnosis of early asymptomatic tubal pregnancies.

Indeed these improved diagnostic techniques have led to the introduction of less aggressive surgical procedures (laparoscopic surgery, salpingectomy or salpingotomy when the tube can be conserved), and to medical treatment, either systemic or local. Furthermore, fertility after these new modalities of treatment appears to be improved.

The development of successful therapy, both surgical and pharmacological, for ectopic pregnancy has stimulated research into the normal physiology and pathophysiology of implantation of the human embryo.

The aim of the present chapter is to propose a new approach for ectopic pregnancies by transcervical tubal cannulation, and to describe the effects of methotrexate injected intraluminally into tubal ectopic implantation.

## Diagnosis of Ectopic Pregnancy

The traditional diagnosis of ectopic pregnancy was based on association of abdominal pain, irregular vaginal bleeding, amenorrhea and abdominal tenderness. The early stages simulate many other conditions. Nearly half of all cases of ectopic pregnancy are still missed on the first visit to a general emergency unit. The major problem is actually to recognise the pregnancy. It has been proposed that all female patients presenting to the emergency room should have a rapid immunoassay for urine hCG. Thereafter, investigations should be initiated to rule out ectopic pregnancy. The situation is different in patients who have conceived by assisted conception procedures. These women are at high risk: ultrasound and biochemical markers should be used routinely at the end of each successful treatment cycle.

Modern tests for hCG can distinguish pregnant from non-pregnant women, but do not readily differentiate normal from pathological pregnancies. Plasma hCG levels are lower in pathological than in normal pregnancies, but there is a large overlap between ectopic pregnancy and miscarriages. If the time of conception is unknown, hCG is of limited value.

Serial hCG assays and calculation of rates of increase can enhance the accuracy, but the diagnosis is delayed by at least two or three days. Pregnancy-specific beta-1-glycoprotein and pregnancy-associated plasma protein-A provide little additional information.

Progesterone (P4) levels are lower in ectopic pregnancy than in normal pregnancy. The association of low P4 and hCG predicts a pathological pregnancy, but not the site of implantation. Renin production by the corpus luteum is impaired in ectopic pregnancy: between 4 and 10 weeks of amenorrhea, immunoreactive active renin levels are lower in ectopic pregnancy than in normal or abnormal intrauterine pregnancy.

The indications for laparoscopy have changed with the development of biochemical markers and ultrasound. In very early ectopic pregnancy, laparoscopic inspection may be negative. Equally, the diagnosis can be made without laparoscopy and medical treatments are now available. However, laparoscopy is mandatory whenever the diagnosis is unclear.

Decreasing values of hCG during the course of therapy of ectopic pregnancy are the most useful markers of resolution. Nevertheless, the disappearance of hCG is still not well defined. Moreover, recent studies have suggested that declining values of hCG should not give the clinician a false sense of security (Gretz and Quagliarello 1987).

Transvaginal sonography is more accurate than abdominal sonography to examine early gestation. Evidence of a live embryo outside the uterine cavity is the definitive sign of ectopic pregnancy. This finding has been observed in only 10% of cases with abdominal sonography, compared with 17%–21% with transvaginal sonography. Other sonographic findings are nonspecific. Useful information might be obtained by adding Doppler to the transvaginal sonography probe, which could distinguish ectopic pregnancy from other adnexal masses, and true intrauterine nidation from pseudogestational sacs. Transvaginal ultrasound is more sensitive than transabdominal in detecting early ectopic pregnancy. Combined with hCG, transvaginal ultrasound has become a valuable diagnostic procedure. The association of a transvaginal sonography adnexal mass and an hCG level of less than 1000 mIU/ml has a sensitivity of 97%, and a specificity of 99%. We consider that a pathological pregnancy should be suspected when an intrauterine gestational sac is not visible after day 21; if hCG is over 1000 mIU/ml, ectopic pregnancy is likely.

The exact level of hCG at which an intrauterine gestational sac may be imaged is related to the reference standard used by the laboratory, to the ultrasound equipment, and to the skill of the person performing and interpreting the ultrasound.

Other diagnostic aids have been utilised, including combinations of sonography and hormonal determinations, hysterosalpingography, culdocentesis, curettage, colpotomy, laparoscopy and laparotomy.

The first two steps in diagnosis of ectopic pregnancy are i) hCG determination to ascertain pregnancy; and ii) transvaginal sonography to look for an intrauterine pregnancy. If a patient presents with symptoms and signs of an ectopic pregnancy, a high hCG level and no gestational sac seen on transvaginal sonography, the possibility of ectopic pregnancy is increased. The choice of subsequent procedures appears to depend upon technical facilities available to the clinician.

# Treatment of Ectopic Pregnancy

## Surgical Management

Until recently, laparotomy and salpingectomy have been the treatment of choice for ectopic pregnancy. Despite its efficacy, surgical treatment for ectopic pregnancy is associated with post-operative morbidity and risk of subsequent infertility. Early diagnosis has permitted conservative laparoscopic treatment of ectopic pregnancy without removing the tube.

Conservative management may lead to the so-called "persistent" ectopic pregnancy. Stock (1991) recently demonstrated that persistence was due to surgery directed at the most dilated portion of the tube, whereas histopathological examination revealed that the implantation site was located medially, towards the uterus.

## Non-surgical Management

Ectopic pregnancy is amenable to non-surgical treatment and medical treatment has become an accepted method for many patients (Pansky et al. 1991).

Expectant management has been proposed in selected patients with resolution rates of 57%–92% (Lund 1955). These reports suggest that, in asymptomatic patients with low and falling hCG levels, simple observation is enough (Garcia et al. 1987). However, low and declining hCG levels are not always associated with spontaneous resolution: tubal rupture can still occur (Tulandi et al. 1991). Despite the progress in biochemical markers and ultrasound, the course of ectopic pregnancy is often unpredictable.

Drugs such as methotrexate can arrest trophoblastic cell growth and thus stop the development of ectopic pregnancy. Pansky et al. (1991) have reviewed the outcome of conservative management. Systemic methotrexate was successful in 94% of 188 cases. Tubal patency was retained in 71%. There is a high incidence of side effects, and it has been suggested that the treatment should not be used if hCG values exceed 1500 mIU/ml or if the tubal ectopic mass is more than 3.5 cm in diameter. Other treatments include potassium chloride, prostaglandin, hyperosmolar glucose or only aspiration. However, methotrexate is still the most widely used product (Cannon and Jesionowska 1991). There is little difference between various forms of conservative treatments.

Methotrexate can be administered locally at laparoscopy (Cannon and Jesionowska 1991) or alternatively, by using transvaginal ultrasound, if the gestation sac can be accurately identified. However, in a series of 191 patients reported by Pansky et al. (1991), the ectopic pregnancy was only identified by ultrasound in 7%. Others have reported visualising a sac in more than 70% of ectopic pregnancies (Ménard et al. 1991). Although ultrasound is an excellent diagnostic aid, it is difficult to differentiate the trophoblastic ring from an adnexal myoma, hyperstimulated ovaries and/or other pelvic structures.

For these reasons Risquez et al. (1990c) proposed a new approach, using transcervical tubal cannulation under fluoroscopy or ultrasound for both diagnosis and treatment. With this technique, the diagnosis can be ascertained by direct visualisation of the ectopic sac and, at the same time, the disease is cured by luminal administration of a low dose of methotrexate. This offers an elegant one-step management of very early ectopic pregnancy. As there is no needling of the gravid tube, there is less risk of traumatic injury to vessels. Preliminary results are encouraging and the method is now under evaluation in a multicentre international trial.

Medical treatments do not appear to impair subsequent reproductive performance. Follow-up indicates 53%–100% success rate of tubal patency after subsequent hysterosalpingography (Pansky et al. 1991). The recurrent ectopic pregnancy and intrauterine pregnancy rates are comparable to laparoscopic salpingostomy.

Chemotherapy has also been used successfully for treatment of cervical, interstitial and abdominal pregnancies. Recently, Dumestic and Reza (1991) reported delayed haemorrhage from a persistent ectopic pregnancy following salpingostomy and methotrexate therapy. This case emphasises that close follow-up after conservative surgical or medical treatments of ectopic pregnancy should continue until the level of serum hCG is undetectable.

## Methodology of Transcervical Tubal Cannulation for the Diagnosis and Treatment of Ectopic Pregnancy

Selective tubal cannulation allows non-operative access to the fallopian tube. In order to avoid the difficulties encountered during previous tubal cannulation methods, we designed a new technique: the Risquez–Zorn catheter system (Nycomed-Ingénor, Paris, France), which facilitates retrograde tubal cannulation. Cannulation of the tubes from the vagina guided by tactile impression can be easily performed.

The equipment includes:

1) the introducer: an outer Teflon guiding cannula (length 26.6 cm, outer diameter 6 french = 2 mm) with a lateral curved tip, which is straightened by means of a metallic mandril.
2) two coaxial inner catheters: a first transparent inner catheter (0.6 mm) and a second outer radiopaque Teflon catheter (1 mm).
3) guide wire with a soft terminal tip pre-loaded into the two coaxial inner catheters.

All elements of the system can advance together or separately (usually together). A schematic representation of the Risquez–Zorn catheter system for tubal cannulation is shown in Figs 21.1 and 21.2.

In early studies, we demonstrated the use of this system for

(a) Human reproduction techniques, transcervical GIFT and tubal embryo transfer (Risquez et al. 1990).
(b) Contraception (tubal sterilisation by obstructing the tubal lumen).
(c) Tubal surgery (resection and implants).
(d) Diagnosis and treatment of tubal obstruction by selective cannulation, re-canalisation and dilatation of the fallopian tubes (performed under hysteroscopy, laparoscopy and fluoroscopy (salpingography).
(e) Investigation of silent tubal infection by chlamydia. Tubal samples were obtained during re-canalisation (direct and culture tests for chlamydia were negative) in 5 cases with bilateral blocked tubes.

In a preliminary series of transcervical tubal cannulations for the transfer of gametes and embryos, we obtained three ectopic pregnancies. It was, therefore, logical to manage such pregnancies using the same route. In 1989, we diagnosed and treated the first patient with a tubal pregnancy by direct injection of small amounts of medications using the transcervical route.

Transcervical cannulation of the tubal ostia can be achieved by curved catheters. Transcervical cannulation of the isthmic portion of the fallopian tube and advance of the catheter into the ampullary portion requires specialised catheters with small diameters and flexible yet firm properties.

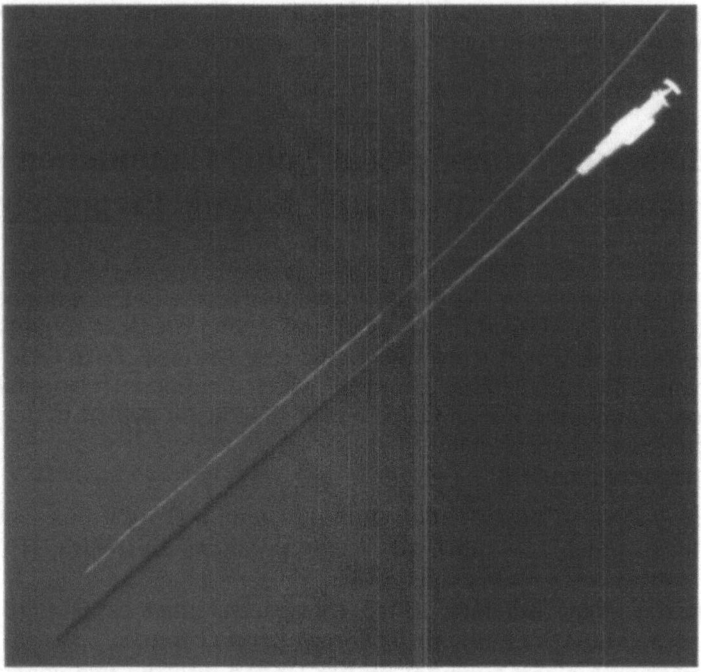

Fig. 21.1. The Risquez–Zorn catheter system (Nycomed-Ingénor, Paris, France).

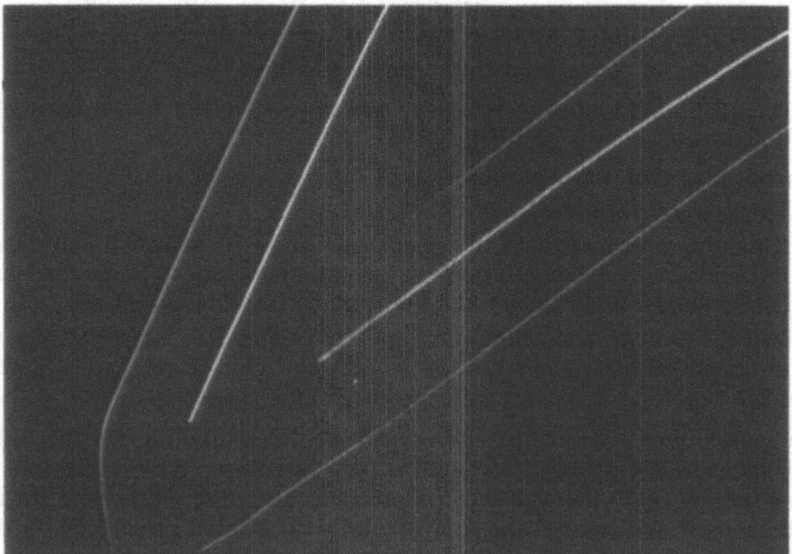

Fig. 21.2. Components of the Risquez–Zorn catheter system:
(1) The introducer: an outer Teflon guiding cannula with a lateral curved tip, which is straightened by means of a metallic mandril. (2) Two coaxial inner catheters: transparent inner catheter and outer radiopaque teflon catheter. (3) Guide wire with a soft terminal tip.

The first attempts at transcervical tubal cannulation are difficult, and experience is necessary. Performing tubal catheterisation under laparoscopy, sonography or fluoroscopy enables the operator to use only tactile impression in later procedures. Cannulation of the tubes during fluoroscopic and sonographic procedures and even by tactile impression is much easier than with the use of a rigid hysteroscope. If fluoroscopy is used, time should be limited to 10 min; thus the amount of radiation imposes very minor risk to future reproductive performance of the patient. Fluoroscopy may be replaced with either sonographic guidance or tubal catheterisation under tactile impression.

Gentle operation of tubal catheters is unfamiliar to many gynaecologists. Cannulas will easily slip into the endotubal lumen and advance along the tube but it is sometimes difficult to differentiate between an advancing catheter and one which bends and retracts back into the uterine cavity.

Tubal catheterisation has a low morbidity, comparable to that with hysterosalpingograms (Confino et al. 1990). Tubal cannulation can be performed under paracervical block, intravenous sedation, oral premedication and on most occasions without premedication.

## Technique

A diagrammatic representation of a transcervical tubal cannulation procedure is shown in Figs 21.3 to 21.6.

Retrograde cannulation serves to confirm the diagnosis and to allow therapeutic intraluminal injection of methotrexate. The introducer is placed in the uterine fundus. After withdrawal of the metallic mandril, the tip of the introducer is directed to the cornua. Moving the catheter from side to side will allow alternative cannulation of either the right or the left tubal ostium. The inner coaxial catheter is advanced into the proximal portion of the fallopian tube guided by tactile impression, without meeting any resistance. Gentle traction on the cervix may help to straighten the tube and allows easier negotiation of the acute curve by the intratubal catheter.

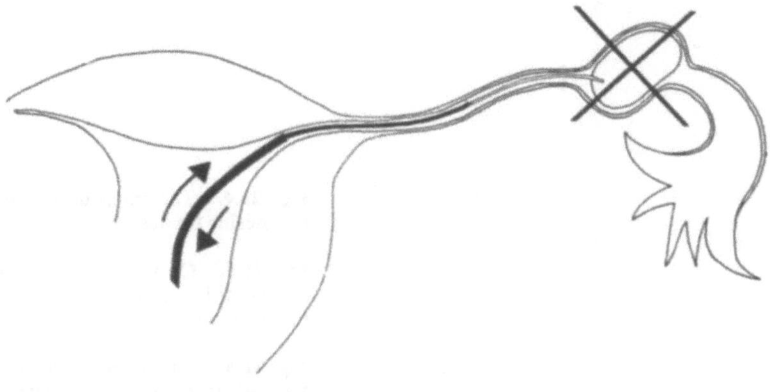

**Fig 21.3.** Transcervical tubal cannulation for the management of tubal pregnancy.

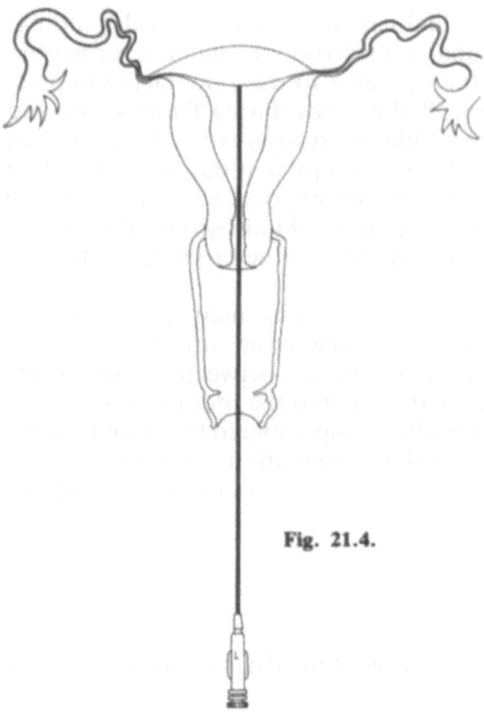

Fig. 21.4.

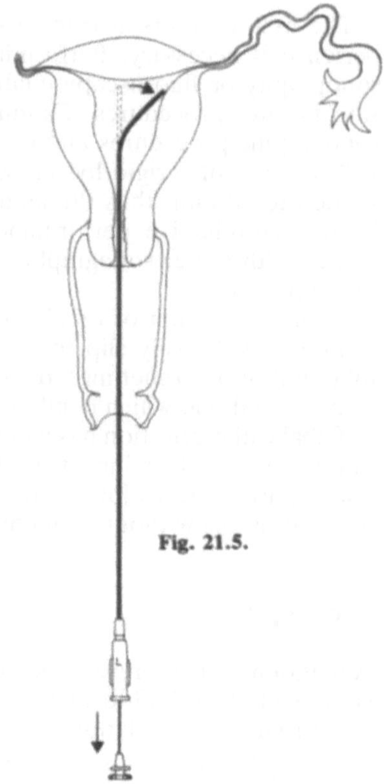

Fig. 21.5.

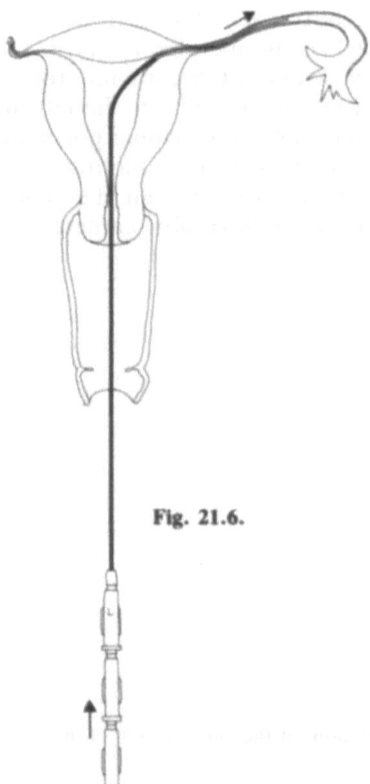

Fig. 21.6.

**Fig. 21.4.** The introducer is placed in the uterine fundus.

**Fig. 21.5.** On withdrawal of the metallic mandril, the tip of the introducer is directed to the cornua.

**Fig. 21.6.** The inner coaxial catheter is then advanced into the proximal portion of the fallopian tube guided by tactile impression, without meeting any resistance.

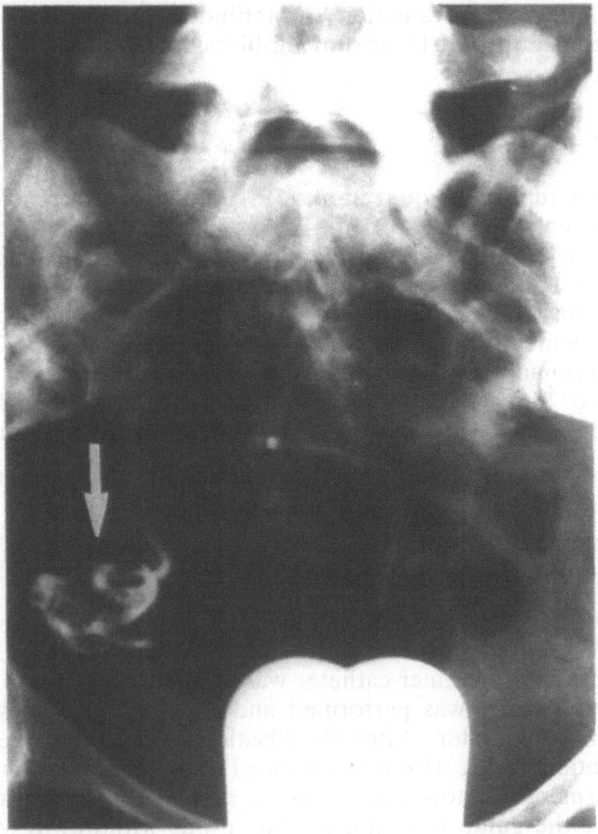

**Fig. 21.7.** The fallopian tube which is distended and distally occluded by a haloed mass (arrow, ectopic pregnancy).

A small flow of blood is sometimes observed at the proximal orifice of the catheter when its distal tip is advanced into the tube. Contrast medium is injected; visualising a distended tube which, in some cases, is distally occluded by a haloed mass, strongly suggesting an ectopic pregnancy (Fig 21.7). Contrast medium can reflux into the uterine cavity. In some cases, the correct placement of the catheter is verified using ultrasound. The coaxial catheter is thereafter withdrawn and replaced by a soft-tipped metallic leader which is pushed forward to the distal portion of the tube, and its position is confirmed by fluoroscopy or ultrasound. Advancement of catheters within the isthmic portion of the tube requires very gentle manipulation; the most difficult area is the isthmic cornual junction, where the fallopian tube acutely curves down and away from the uterine corpus. The coaxial catheter is advanced along the metallic leader. After removal of the latter, up to 50 mg of methotrexate is injected into the fallopian tube. Tubal catheterisation and drug injection can be visualised by ultrasound when the adnexal mass is clearly identifiable by this method.

Transcervical tubal cannulation does not require extensive pre-operative preparation, laboratory evaluation or antibiotic prophylaxis. In selected cases, we administer prophylactic oral antibiotics for 7 days.

## Study Design and Results

In a preliminary report, Risquez et al. (1990) described the use of this technique in 4 patients (Risquez et al. 1991). The study was expanded to 4 university-based gynaecology and radiology departments in three countries (France, England and Germany) (Risquez et al. 1992a).

The series consisted of 33 patients who presented with a clinical diagnosis of ectopic pregnancy. Pregnancy was confirmed by elevated hCG levels and intrauterine pregnancy was excluded by transvaginal ultrasound using a 5 or 7.5 MHz probe. Some patients were symptomatic. In others, the diagnosis was made after 6 weeks' amenorrhoea. The inclusion criteria were:

1. Desire for future fertility, personal preference for medical treatment
2. Unruptured tubal pregnancy with no active bleeding
3. Haemodynamic stability
4. Absence of intrauterine pregnancy.

Informed written consent was obtained. Transcervical tubal catheterisation was performed using the Risquez–Zorn catheter system. In 18 cases, correct placement of the inner catheter was verified using ultrasound. In the remainder, fluoroscopy was performed and contrast medium was injected through the inner catheter. After visualisation of the tubal pregnancy, the soft-tipped metallic guide wire was advanced to the implantation site and the position confirmed by fluoroscopy or echography. The coaxial catheter was advanced over the guide wire and the latter was withdrawn. Methotrexate was then injected through the coaxial catheter to the implantation site.

All patients were followed up using serial hCG measurements until baseline levels of hCG were reached or a further intervention became necessary.

The salpingographic appearance included either complete occlusion, semicircular filling defect or a clear circumferential margin. The tubal lumen might be trumpet-shaped, dilated or cloudy. If tubal patency was still present minimal spilling of dye into the abdominal cavity occurred.

The most frequent symptom during retrograde catheterisation is a unilateral continuous slight pain. In some cases, there was colicky pain on advancing the catheter, especially on motion of the affected tube or during injection.

We have often observed resistance to injection, reflux of contrast medium, and in a few cases, blood loss from the proximal orifice of the catheter. Blood and tubal fluids continued to have very high hCG levels when compared to blood hCG levels.

### *Results*

Thirty three patients were treated by methotrexate. Their ages ranged from 25 to 41 years (mean ± standard deviation, 32 ± 4.5). The mean (±SD) gestational age at presentation was 6.6 weeks (±1.7) (range 5–12 weeks). Eight patients were asymptomatic, 18 presented with abdominal pain and 16 had vaginal bleeding. Transvaginal ultrasound was performed in all patients and no intrauterine pregnancies were recorded. In 21 patients, a mass was documented lateral to the uterus. A fetal sac was observed in five of these but fetal heart activity was only present in one case. Free peritoneal fluid was documented in 17 patients.

On the day of transcervical tubal catheterisation (TCTC), the mean hCG level was 2250 (±2361) mIU/ml (range 217 to 10600). There was no significant correlation between gestational age and level of hCG ($r = 0.0374$, $p = 0.856$). The dose of methotrexate varied; 21 patients received 50 mg, 10 patients received 20–50 mg and 1 patient received 5 mg.

Two of the 33 patients elected to withdraw from the protocol following TCTC and methotrexate administration to have operative treatment. In the remaining 31 patients, there was complete resolution of the ectopic pregnancy (as shown by reduction of hCG to baseline levels) in 27 (87%). Surgery was performed in the remaining 4 patients. The first patient had methotrexate when the hCG was 10 600 mIU/ml. Despite reduction in the hCG level over the next 13 days to 2225 mIU/ml the ectopic pregnancy ruptured and an emergency laparotomy was required. A second patient had methotrexate when the hCG was 7250 mIU/ml. The level of hCG continued to rise over the 7 days following treatment to 10 200 and surgery was performed. The third patient required a laparoscopy for pain associated with intra-abdominal bleeding 23 days following methotrexate. The level of hCG had fallen from 1935 mIU/ml to 24 mIU/ml at the time of surgery. The fourth patient developed clinical symptoms of acute salpingitis 4 days after TCTC and methotrexate administration with severe lower abdominal pain associated with a fever of 40 °C. She underwent salpingectomy. At surgery, there was no evidence of pelvic infection. Examination of the removed fallopian tubes of those patients who underwent salpingectomy revealed chronic salpingitis in 2 patients, tubal bleeding in 1 patient, and evidence of tubal rupture in 1 patient. The mucosa was replaced by fragments of decidual tissue and fibrous placental villi. There was no pathological evidence of acute necrosis within the fallopian tubes.

In the 27 patients successfully treated, the time taken to achieve baseline levels of hCG was related to the initial hCG level on the day of methotrexate. The mean (±SD) number of days to achieve resolution was 18.0 (9.8), 25.8 (8.6) and 37.0 (12.7) when initial hCG level was <1000, 1000 to 5000 and >5000 mIU/ml respectively. None of these patients experienced any side effects.

Seventeen patients were available for follow-up to examine the return of reproductive potential after the procedure. Of these 17 patients, 14 desired pregnancies as soon as possible. All 7 patients who subsequently underwent hysterosalpingography had a normal uterus and patency of the affected tube, and 5 later had an intrauterine pregnancy. Two pregnancies arose spontaneously including one through the treated tube (the patient had previous salpingectomy for tubal pregnancy); another patient became pregnant after intrauterine insemination and two others after IVF (due to male factor infertility). Of these five pregnancies, one patient later had an early miscarriage, two had given birth to three normal babies (one twin pregnancy, one singleton) and two singleton pregnancies are still ongoing. The other patients remain symptom-free.

In a later series, Confino et al. (1992) reported five patients managed using the same approach. All patients with tubal ectopic pregnancies resolved and there were no complications (Confino 1992, personal communication).

The advantage of TCTC is that it is possible to attempt the technique in all patients with an unruptured ectopic pregnancy. As there is no needling of the gravid tube, there is less risk of traumatic injury to vessels (Hönigl et al. 1991). The results of our study agree with previous observations that conservative therapy with methotrexate as the antitrophoblastic agent has a higher failure rate when the hCG at the time of treatment exceeds 5000 mIU/ml. There was no apparent relation between treatment failure and increased gestation age. Indeed, gestation age was not correlated with hCG levels. In 65% of patients (20/31) hCG levels increased in the first 4 days following administration of methotrexate but, in those cases associated with resolution of the ectopic pregnancy, the hCG level had reached a plateau after 6 days. In-vitro studies using choriocarcinoma cells show that there is a tenfold increase in hCG synthesis in these cells following exposure to methotrexate (Speeg et al. 1976). A transient rise in hCG should, therefore, not be taken as a sign of treatment failure. Two other important practical points emerged from this work. First, tubal rupture can occur even when hCG levels are declining; second, surgical intervention may be necessary in the presence of nearly baseline hCG levels. The latter is a rare occurrence probably associated with continued bleeding from a necrotic area around the implantation site. However, all conservative surgical or medical therapeutic strategies need careful follow-up by hCG levels and possibly by repeated transvaginal ultrasound and clinical examination until the ectopic pregnancy has resolved both clinically and biochemically (Dumestic and Reza 1991).

In previous studies in which the methotrexate was injected into the gestational sac following aspiration of sac contents, it is possible that the aspiration itself was implicated in the success of therapy. This study demonstrates that intraluminal methotrexate per se is capable of causing regression of the ectopic pregnancy.

Transcervical tubal catheterisation in patients with tubal pregnancies is feasible and may be performed without anaesthesia or analgesia in most cases. The ease of the procedure, the non-surgical nature of this approach, the absence of drug toxicity and the efficacy of the treatment is promising. It is surprising that failure to catheterise the fallopian tube did not occur as in a previous report (Risquez et al. 1990). It is possible that hormonal changes induced by the ectopic pregnancies resulted in enlargement of the tubal ostium compared to the non-pregnant state allowing easy cannulation of the fallopian tubes. Other explanations may include increased tubal pressure, secretion of materials which cause smooth muscle relaxation or reflux of blood through the fallopian tube. While the procedure is easy to perform, it requires experience with catheterisation of fallopian tubes (Risquez et al. 1990).

Improvements in endoscopic technology permit transcervical introduction of small-diameter fibre optics and direct visualisation of the tubal lumen. In a recent study, we demonstrated that it is feasible to identify ectopic

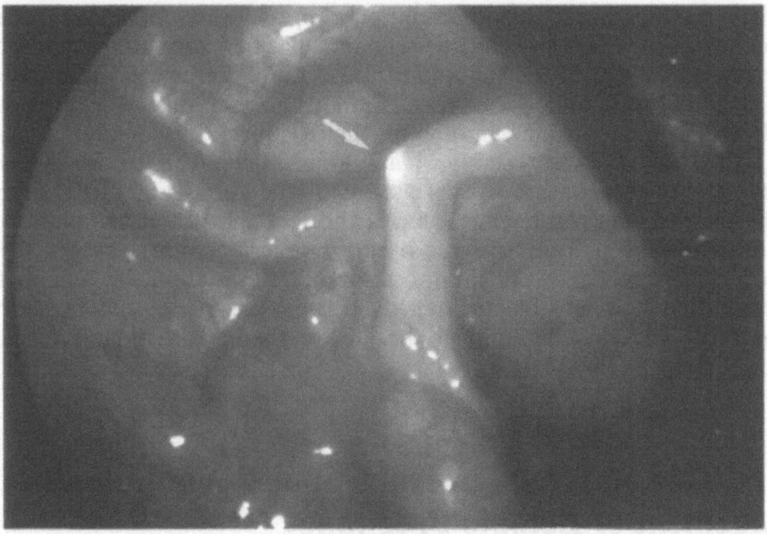

**Fig. 21.8.** The arrow shows the tip of the falloposcope in the medial part of the tube under laparoscopic vision.

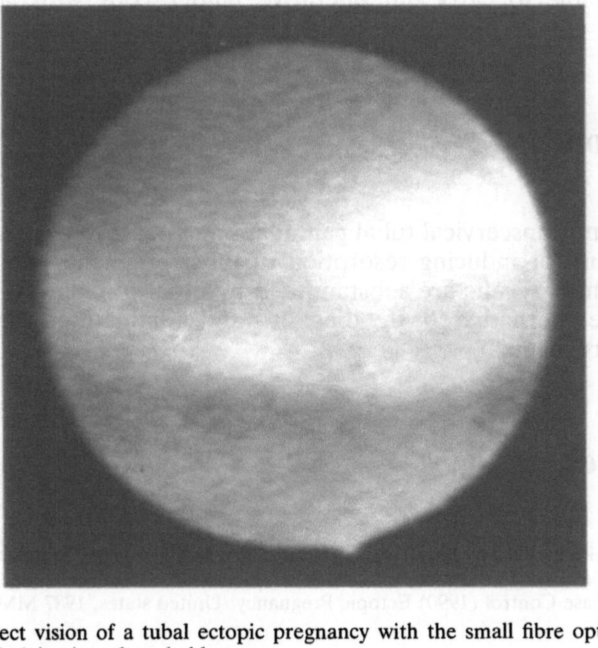

**Fig. 21.9.** Direct vision of a tubal ectopic pregnancy with the small fibre optic. The ectopic mass is visible, bulging into the tubal lumen.

pregnancy by the direct introduction of a small fibre optic. We recently described cases in which an ectopic pregnancy has been directly visualised via the uterotubal ostium of the fallopian tube. The procedure is relatively simple. A 0.5 falloposcope (Transcott, Geneva, Switzerland) is introduced through the 1-mm coaxial cannula of the Risquez–Zorn catheter system without the use of hysteroscopy, leaving insufficient space for adequate mobility of the fibre optics and irrigation of the tube (Fig 21.8). General anaesthesia was required because it was thought that tubal insufflation and irrigation would be painful. As micro-endoscopic techniques evolve, it may become possible to carry out falloposcopy under sedation. This report demonstrates that it is feasible to identify ectopic pregnancy by transcervical falloposcopy. The images confirm that the catheter can indeed reach the ectopic pregnancy (Fig 21.9).

## Future Role of Transcervical Tubal Cannulation in the Management of Ectopic Pregnancy

Transcervical tubal cannulation reduces the risk, cost and morbidity of surgical procedures. Future progress in optic technology will probably improve the diagnostic and therapeutic results. The technique could become a new diagnostic aid for suspected ectopic pregnancies. Catheterisation may allow collection of samples for assessment of tubal pathology and for local drug administration other than methotrexate. As techniques evolve, it may become possible to carry out operative falloposcopy with laser or other instruments.

## Conclusion

In conclusion, transcervical tubal cannulation appears to be a safe and effective treatment for inducing resorption of tubal pregnancy while preserving fertility. If these results are substantiated by other groups, TCTC may offer a new simple alternative for the diagnosis and treatment of selected patients with tubal pregnancy.

## References

Cannon L, Jesionowska H (1991) Methotrexate treatment of tubal pregnancy. Fertil Steril 55:1033–1038

Center for Disease Control (1990) Ectopic Pregnancy: United states, 1987 MMWR 39:24, 401–404

Confino E et al. (1990) Transcervical balloon tuboplasty: a multicenter study. JAMA 264:2079–2082

Dumestic D, Reza G (1991) Delayed haemorrhage of a persistent ectopic pregnancy following salpingostomy and methotrexate therapy. Obstet Gynaecol 78:960–962

Garcia A et al. (1987) Expectant management of presumed ectopic pregnancies. Fertil Steril 48:395–400

Gretz E, Quagliarello J (1987) Declining serum concentrations of the beta-subunit of human chorionic gonadotrophin and ruptured ectopic pregnancy. Am J Obstet Gynecol 164:940–941

Hönigl W, Lang P, Urdl W, Weiss PAM (1991) Rupture of tubal pregnancy after transvaginal puncture. Lancet 336:885–886

Lund JJ (1955) Early ectopic pregnancy treated non-surgically. J Obstet Br Empire 62:70–76

Ménard A, Créquat J, Maldelbrot L, Hanuy JP, Madelenat P (1991) Treatment of unruptured tubal pregnancy by local injection of methotrexate under transvaginal sonographic control. Fertil Steril 54:47–50

Pansky M, Golan SA, Bukovsky I, Caspi E (1991) Non-surgical management of tubal pregnancy: necessity in view of the changing clinical appearance. Am J Obstet Gynecol 164: 888–895

Risquez F et al. (1990a) Diagnosis and treatment of ectopic pregnancy by retrograde selective salpingography and intraluminal methotrexate injection: work in progress. Hum Reprod 5:759–762

Risquez F et al. (1990b) Retrograde tubal transfer of human embryos. Hum Reprod 5:185–188

Risquez F, Mathieson J, Zorn JR (1990c) Tubal cannulation via the cervix: a passing fancy or here to stay? (editorial). J In Vitro Fert Embryo Transfer 7:301–370

Risquez F, Mathieson J, Zorn JR (1991) Twin pregnancy after diagnosis and treatment of ectopic implantation by retrograde selective salpingography and intraluminal methotrexate injection. Fertil Steril 54:1168–1170

Risquez F et al. (1992a) Transcervical catheterization of the fallopian tube for the management of ectopic pregnancy: prospective multicenter study. Fertil Steril – in press

Risquez F et al. (1992b) Transcervical tubal cannulation and falloposcopy for the management of tubal pregnancy. Hum Reprod 7:274–275

Speeg KV, Clifford Azizkhan J, Stromberg K (1976) The stimulation by methotrexate of human chorionic gonadotrophin and placental alkaline phosphatase in cultured choriocarcinoma cells. Cancer Res 36:4570–4576

Stock RJ (1990) Histopathology of fallopian tubes with recurrent tubal pregnancy. Obstet Gynaecol 75:9–14

Stock R (1991) Persistent tubal pregnancy. Obstet Gynaecol 77:267–270

Tulandi T, Hemmings R, Khalifa F (1991) Rupture of ectopic pregnancy in women with low and declining serum β-human chorionic gonadotrophin concentrations. Fertil Steril 56:786–787

# Subject Index

MIX
Papier aus verantwortungsvollen Quellen
Paper from responsible sources
FSC® C105338

If you have any concerns about our products,
you can contact us on
**ProductSafety@springernature.com**

In case Publisher is established outside the EU,
the EU authorized representative is:
**Springer Nature Customer Service Center GmbH**
**Europaplatz 3, 69115 Heidelberg, Germany**

Printed by Libri Plureos GmbH
in Hamburg, Germany